T0394673

Practicing Biomedicine at the Albert Schweitzer Hospital 1913–1965

Clio Medica

STUDIES IN THE HISTORY OF MEDICINE AND HEALTH

VOLUME 103

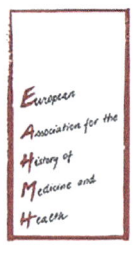

The titles published in this series are listed at *brill.com/clio*

Practicing Biomedicine at the Albert Schweitzer Hospital 1913–1965

Ideas and Improvisations

By

Tizian Zumthurm

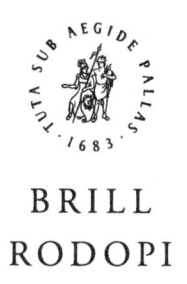

BRILL
RODOPI

LEIDEN | BOSTON

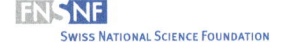 Published with the support of the Swiss National Science Foundation.

Cover illustration: The Swiss nurse Trudi Bochsler overseeing the dressing of wounds, 1950s. © Archives Centrales Albert Schweitzer Gunsbach.

The Library of Congress Cataloging-in-Publication Data is available online at http://catalog.loc.gov LC record available at http://lccn.loc.gov/2020024571

Typeface for the Latin, Greek, and Cyrillic scripts: "Brill". See and download: brill.com/brill-typeface.

ISSN 0045-7183
ISBN 978-90-04-40267-6 (hardback)
ISBN 978-90-04-43697-8 (e-book)

Contents

Acknowledgements

Many people have contributed in many ways to this book. I heartily thank all of them. Some deserve particular mentioning. Hubert Steinke provided the best setting one could wish for and invaluable inputs in regards of content and strategy. Walter Bruchhausen shared his endless expertise. Without Hines Mabika, this book would not exist and his advice was very welcome. Our advisory board (Wolfgang Eckart, Nancy Rose Hunt, Gesine Krüger, Elísio Macamo, Laurence Monnais, William Schneider, Joseph Tonda) travelled all the way to Bern and gave encouraging and treasured feedback. Neil Kodesh enabled my fruitful stay at UW-Madison and took time for stimulating discussions on my drafts. Florence Bernault also gave extremely useful comments. My colleagues from the IMG, especially Beat Bächi, Urs Germann, and Pascal German, provided valuable exchanges and inputs. Numerous peers, too many to name, at academic events commented various stages of my work and enabled good times. My favorite librarians Pia Burkhalter and Bruno Müller made life a lot easier. Romain Collot and the team at the Maison Schweitzer were a great help. Frank Huisman and an anonymous reviewer helped me to sharpen important things in this book, especially reformulating the Introduction. Rosanna Woensdregt from Brill was always very helpful. I want to specifically thank all the interviewees for sharing their experiences and thoughts. Jacques-Adrien Rolagho provided precious contacts and guide services. Benoit Moussavou-Wora and his family offered their very kind hospitality. I am very grateful to my parents who have always supported me in all my endeavors. My friends, and also my sister, are the best. I am happy, lucky, and thankful that I spent the time surrounding this book with Rahel.

Patrick Grogan has edited this book, which greatly improved the quality of the arguments and the writing. John Boonstra has corrected parts of the Introduction and the whole Conclusion. I have translated all the quotes from primary sources and secondary literature in German or French into English. Vincent Hischier has created Maps 1–3 for me. The 'Association Internationale Albert Schweitzer' and the 'Schweizer Hilfsverein für das Albert-Schweitzer-Spital in Lambarene' supported this project, also financially. The doctoral research, out of which this book has developed, has been funded by the Swiss National Science Foundation (SNSF) as part of the project 100011_149880 (2014–2017).

Illustrations

Tables

Introduction

News on medical issues from Africa and other parts of the Global South often come with triumphant images of biomedical personnel fighting scary diseases using sophisticated technologies that are met with local incomprehension or rejection. Ebola workers are depicted in their white body suits; coverage on AIDS interventions emphasizes the seemingly strange reactions that those therapeutic and preventive measures provoke. To the historian, the colonial heritage of such global health interventions is rather obvious.

Historical research on medicine in Africa and other colonial contexts frequently analyzes what might be called the domineering side of biomedicine. Studies that examine health policies, public health campaigns, or public-private cooperation often focus on the spectacular aspects of colonial medicine, on what today are represented by the white suits or antiretroviral drugs.[1] Such scholarship illustrates how racist and forcible biomedicine can be. It stresses biomedicine's top-down nature and explains how it suppresses vernacular practices and knowledge. Emphasizing global or inter-colonial transfers, research of this kind frequently neglects to assess how biomedicine is transformed locally.

Historical research that focuses on how biomedicine is instantiated in the colonies, on local incomprehension, or on the agency of the colonized often analyzes what can be called biomedicine's interactive side.[2] Such studies, frequently drawn from missionary contexts, investigate biomedicine's contact with other forms of healing and with local conceptions of health and disease. They illustrate that biomedicine was highly adaptive: it incorporated local ideas and practices, and it was incorporated by them. Concerned with issues of translation and hybridity and often working with memories and material evidence, this strand of scholarship frequently disregards how biomedicine aims for dominance and suppression. Many historical studies, of course, examine both the domineering and the interactive aspects of biomedicine.[3]

---

1 Recent examples of studies with such a focus include: Lachenal, *Le médicament qui devait sauver l'Afrique*; Ngalamulume, *Colonial Pathologies, Environment, and Western Medicine in Saint-Louis-Du-Senegal, 1867–1920*; Pearson, *The Colonial Politics of Global Health*. For a chronological overview of the historiography, see: Hunt, 'Health and Healing'.

2 Recent examples include: Hardiman, *Missionaries and Their Medicine*; Kalusa, 'Medical Training, African Auxiliaries, and Social Healing'; Langwick, *Bodies, Politics, and African Healing*.

3 Greenwood, *Beyond the State*; Hokkanen, *Medicine, Mobility, and the Empire*; Tappan, *The Riddle of Malnutrition*.

What is poorly understood about colonial medicine, and about global health today, despite this rich literature, is how it operated on a daily basis. Routines and practices have rarely been the focus of historical or anthropological studies on colonial medicine. Medical historians working on Europe or North America, on the other hand, have recently started to acknowledge the importance of practical work in medicine. They have, however, rarely been interested in Africa. My study, while not necessarily limited to an African context, aims to be locally grounded.

My monograph shows how an examination of practices and routines increases our understanding both of everyday medical work and of biomedicine itself. The domineering and interactive sides of biomedicine are equally important in this respect. My focus demonstrates, however, the centrality of uncertain theories and unproven experimentations, therapeutic half-successes and half-failures – in short, *improvisations* – to the practice of biomedicine. Equally importantly, this approach takes a step toward better comprehending local experiences and understandings of medicine, illness, misfortune, and health, as patients and their kin, auxiliaries and nurses, come to the fore as individuals and subjects.

A microhistorical lens is the most useful tool for an in-depth study of daily routines.[4] Considering the hospital as a microcosm for biomedical practices allows us to study not only processes, connections, and blind spots within the institution, but also interactions with individuals and structures outside the institution. An extensive and deep archive and a careful scrutiny of the material therein are central for recreating such a microcosm. While analyzing the various wards and treatments of a hospital reveals patterns, it uncovers even more incoherences. Practices that were instantiated differently within the same institution can be considered examples of the 'normal exception'.[5] Such an analysis thus avoids quick conclusions and illuminates the complex links between the micro- and macro-levels. It allows for multiperspectivity, prevents the formation of reductionist arguments, and reveals the improvised nature of biomedicine.

Biomedicine, in theory, functions with respect to various key concepts. Among them, I have chosen to analyze order, control, knowledge, standardized experimentation, and 'civilization', because these are also helpful for studying colonial relations. In practice, these ideas and ideals are very brittle in their application. The pursuit of control in surgery and trial-and-error testing in the

---

4   For informative discussions on microhistory see chapters 8–11 of: Renders, *Theoretical Discussions of Biography*.

5   For a discussion of the value of this concept, first developed by Italian historian Edoardo Grendi and also translated as 'exceptional normal' or 'exceptional typical', see: Peltonen, 'Clues, Margins, and Monads'.

treatment of infectious diseases may seem contradictory, but they are both readily employed in the same hospital. The same is true for staff who, on the one hand, seek to understand patients' psyches, while at the same time ignoring their obstetric practices. Such contradictions, as they unfold in practice, demonstrate one of the ways in which I understand improvisations: as pragmatic approaches and solutions to local challenges. My focus on improvisations as such undermines the self-image of a biomedicine that understands itself as universally applicable and unrelated to context. Improvisations of this kind result from the fact that actors do not simply follow an ideological plan or idea. Medical-scientific principles, health-policy strategies, and even institutional rules often prove to be futile in practice.

The Albert Schweitzer Hospital in Lambaréné, established in 1913, is particularly well suited for conducting a microhistory of biomedical practices, given the extraordinary amount of source material that it left behind. It provides an alternative vantage point that looks beyond the dominant governmental or missionary institutional frameworks of colonial medicine. In discussions on the spread and adaptation of biomedicine, Nobel Peace laureate Albert Schweitzer from Alsace and his hospital in the French territory of Gabon quickly come to the fore. Yet, no historian has considered the institution in detail, and thus far no scholarly book has examined its medicine within its spatial and temporal context (Maps 1–3). An analysis of the hospital's medical practices thus also contributes to revising the myth surrounding the institution.

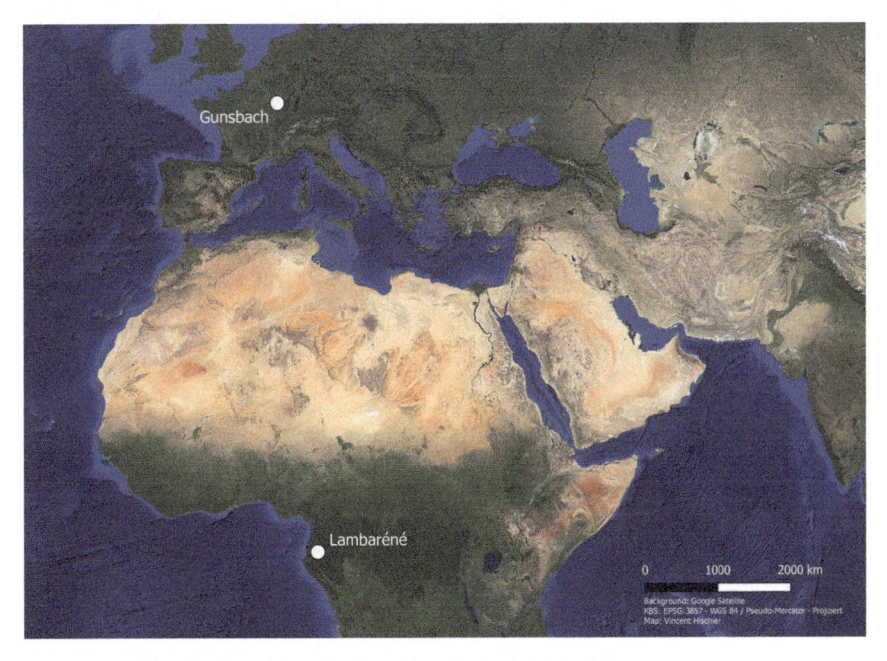

MAP 1   The location of Gunsbach and Lambaréné on the globe

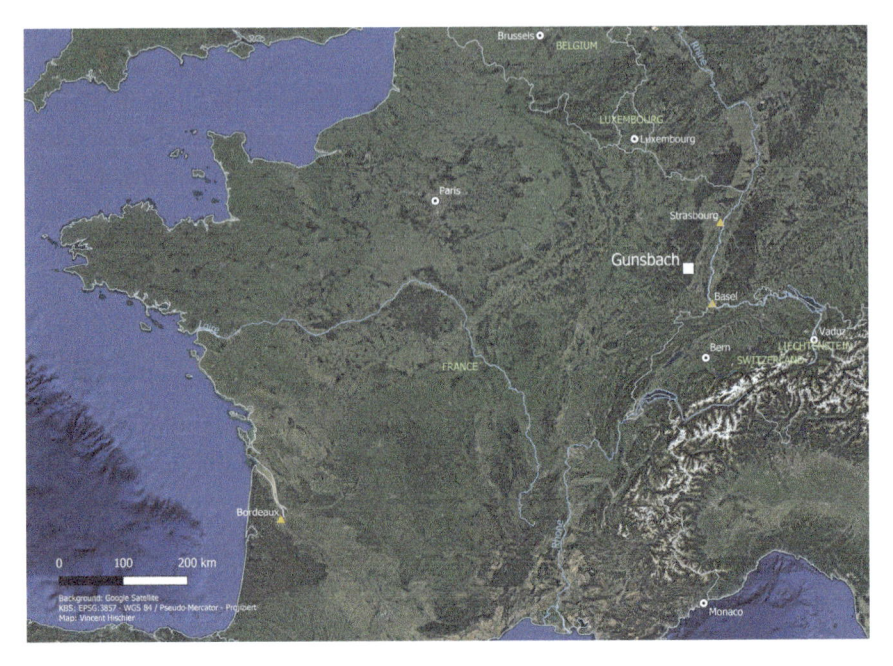

MAP 2   Location of Gunsbach in France

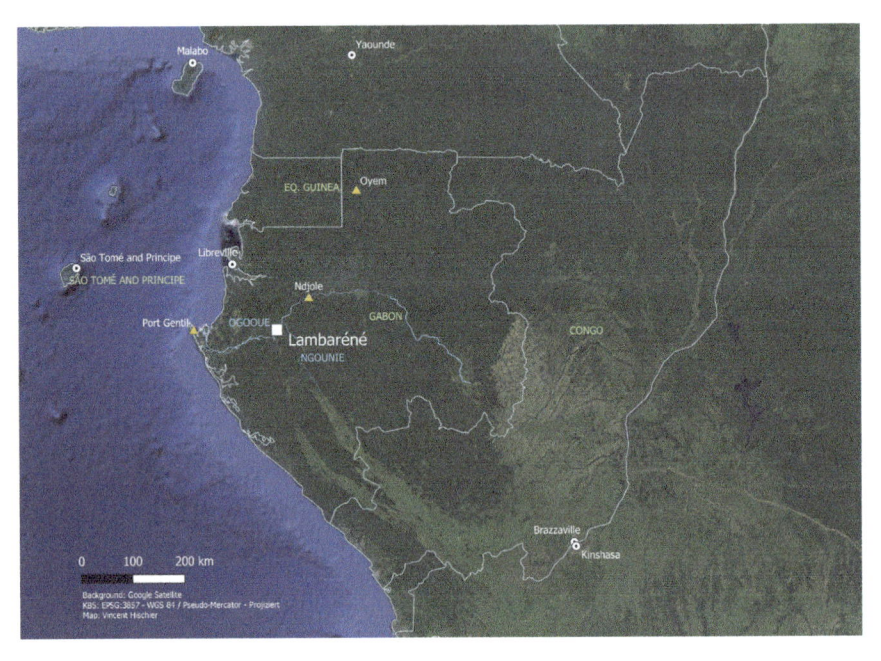

MAP 3   Location of Lambaréné in Gabon

1 Utilizing a Colonial Archive in Gunsbach, Alsace

In 1967, two years after Albert Schweitzer died, the Dutchwoman Ali Silver, who had served at the Albert Schweitzer Hospital as a nurse and secretary since 1947, began transferring Schweitzer's papers to what had been the hospital's organizational base in Europe until his death. This was a house that had been constructed in 1928 in Gunsbach, the small Munster Valley village where Schweitzer had grown up. Sonja Poteau, who had worked in Lambaréné as a nurse for four years during the late 1950s, soon came to Silver's assistance in the immense task of cataloguing the documents, before taking over full responsibility for this work herself in 1990. Assisted by their friends, family, and volunteers, Silver and Poteau classified correspondence, manuscripts, and photographs, while seeking to acquire as many additional letters as possible that Schweitzer had sent to his countless correspondents all over the globe. In 2010, a new team assumed the running of the Maison Albert Schweitzer Gunsbach, which became the headquarters of the Association Internationale de l'Oeuvre du Dr. Albert Schweitzer de Lambaréné in 1966, the year the organization was founded. Its goal is 'the diffusion of the ethical values proposed by Albert Schweitzer'; to this end, 'the conservation and maintenance of the archives in Gunsbach are a major contribution', they claim on their website.[6]

Today the Maison Albert Schweitzer Gunsbach houses a comprehensive library of books by and on Schweitzer, as well as a museum containing, among many other things, the piano on which he used to play after dinner in Lambaréné and the bed in which he slept when in Europe for his extensive fundraising tours. In addition to a number of his philosophical and theological manuscripts, drafts of sermons he gave, and a collection of photographs taken by various visitors and numbering in the thousands, the archive holds at least 70,000 letters addressed to Schweitzer as well as 10,000 letters that he composed. These are arranged by topic rather than in a strictly alphabetical or chronological order, but an alphabetical card index of correspondents aids research. The archive is currently being reorganized and partly digitized; nevertheless, many uncategorized documents that are held in the cellar still await filing, including the medical records used for this study, such as operation protocols and patient lists. For this book, I have consulted all catalogued letters

---

6 http://www.schweitzer.org/aisl/qui-sommes-nous (2 June 2020).

written by Schweitzer on relevant topics,[7] as well as all the letters from staff in Lambaréné that were addressed to Schweitzer during his trips to Europe.[8]

Letters to Schweitzer proved to be the most useful sources, with staff frequently writing about medical practices. The letters composed by Schweitzer concern themselves overwhelmingly with organizational and financial affairs, especially with issues of how to recruit personnel or acquire, pay for, and ship medication and other material. A large number of published memoirs by hospital employees and travel accounts by visitors also describe aspects of life at the hospital, including some that offer valuable insights into the daily practices of biomedicine. To supplement my research, I conducted interviews with Swiss medical personnel who were employed at the hospital as well as with Gabonese who lived on the hospital grounds during Schweitzer's lifetime, usually the children of hospital personnel. I have also consulted the archives of the colonial administration, maintaining a particular focus on records relating to its health services.[9]

The archival documents relating to the Albert Schweitzer Hospital are extraordinary in their narrative quality. They are exceptionally detailed and varied, not only for an African hospital, but in a global context. It is important, however, to recognize that these records are colonial sources. Scholars have long cautioned about the validity of colonial historical material, outlining how their authors drew from a long tradition of fiction and travel writing that had combined to produce a prejudiced image of Africa and the colonial world. In these works, whole territories and their inhabitants were feminized, infantilized, and/or romanticized, while at the same time rendered as dangerous and unhealthy.[10] The images invoked in the process could then serve to justify colonial penetration and exploitation, as well as the imposition of radical changes in colonized societies.[11] In Gabon itself, colonial officials and

---

7   Namely 'Médecine', 'Hôpital', 'Lambaréné', 'Gabon', 'Lambaréné Personnel', 'Lambaréné Malades', and 'Lambaréné Hôpital'; a total of roughly 900 letters, which have all been digitized.

8   These letters amount to 900–1000 pages.

9   The records of the French colonial Service de Santé are now archived at the Service Historique de la Défense (SHD) in Toulon. This proved to be the most useful state archive for the purposes of this study. I have also consulted documents in the Archives Nationales d'Outre-Mer in Aix-en-Provence (ANOM), in the Archives Nationales du Gabon in Libreville (ANG), as well as in the archives of the Wisconsin Historical Society in Madison (AWHS).

10   Bhabha, 'Signs Taken for Wonders'; Comaroff and Comaroff, *Christianity, Colonialism and Consciousness in South Africa*, 109–17.

11   See Mudimbe, *The Invention of Africa*, 69. Valentin Mudimbe identifies 'three complementary genres of "speeches" contributing to the invention of a primitive Africa: the

missionaries alike produced knowledge designed to nourish and uphold colonial stereotypes. The former often spoke of the 'laziness' of the local population,[12] while the latter were more concerned with customs that they considered barbaric, such as 'fetishism'.[13] Not only did medical knowledge and texts play a crucial role in the construction of such ideas, but they also drew from these very stereotypes.[14]

Sources by and on Schweitzer borrowed from and contributed to all of these genres, as identified by Osaak Olumwullah, who starts his study on colonial medicine in Kenya by quoting from the first page of Schweitzer's memoir *On the Edge of the Primeval Forest*, in which he wrote: 'out there in the colonies ... sits wretched Lazarus'. In this book, Schweitzer compared himself and his fellow Europeans to the rich man of the biblical parable: despite possessing superior medical knowledge and means, they had long ignored the health of Africans. Olumwullah highlights how such narratives fed into 'the idea of Africa as both patient and nature'.[15] Identifying these limitations in the archival record is the first and perhaps most important step for the historian to take when engaging with such sources.

Thereafter, a range of strategies presents themselves for analytical purposes, of which reading against the grain is one of the most promising. I understand this approach as the distilling of information from a source that its author did not intend to provide, a method especially useful for microhistories such as this study.[16] While this technique is crucial for uncovering patients' perceptions and their attitudes towards biomedicine, the reconstruction of medical practices often follows the grain; it was usually medical practitioners' intention to inform their superiors about treatments and challenges. Ann Laura Stoler shows how a critical reading along the grain corrects the 'familiar plots' of colonial knowledge production. She demonstrates that colonial power was intent on a 'selective winnowing and reduction' rather than an accumulation of

---

    exotic text on savages, represented by travelers' reports; the philosophical interpretations about a hierarchy of civilizations; and the anthropological search for primitiveness'.

12   Pourtier, *Le Gabon: espace, histoire, société*, 1:220–22.

13   For an insightful discussion of colonial writings on Gabon, see: Cinnamon, 'Of Fetishism and Totemism'.

14   Vaughan, *Curing Their Ills*, 5.

15   Olumwullah, *Dis-Ease in the Colonial State*, 4. See also: Schweitzer, *Zwischen Wasser und Urwald*, 1.

16   For a discussion of this concept, see: Myscofski, 'Against the Grain'; Ratschiller and Weichlein, 'Der schwarze Körper als Missionsgebiet 1880–1960. Begriffe, Konzepte, Fragestellungen', 23. Classic works that apply the approach include: Ginzburg, *The Cheese and the Worms*; Spivak, 'Can the Subaltern Speak?'.

knowledge.[17] Tracking the medical concerns of hospital staff retraces how specific kinds of knowledge were favored and how particular sets of behaviors and attitudes were cultivated in biomedical settings. Another major strength of this approach is the space it gives to individuals, colonizing and colonized alike; this renders characters, motivations, and experiences of humans in a palpable manner. Walter Bruchhausen warns how individuals often disappear behind Foucauldian discourse analyses. These tend to foreground universal generalizations that ignore the role of local developments, which may be equally important for understanding the bigger picture.[18]

2   Theorizing Hospitals in Africa and the Practice of Biomedicine

Biomedicine is an imprecise yet useful term; despite its shortcomings, the expression is worth retaining, as its alternatives are even more misleading.[19] Commonly, it refers to the body of medical practices that rely on the biological sciences to explain life processes. The term is notoriously ambiguous, as it describes research as well as practice. The close interaction between theory and praxis results in varieties of biomedicine that take on diverse local forms.[20] This perspective is particularly valuable for historical empirical studies of biomedicine in general and its practices in particular. Both Claire Wendland and Julie Livingston have highlighted the improvised aspects of biomedicine. These become especially obvious when analyzing how biomedicine is practiced in twenty-first century Africa. Their studies reveal that it is an adaptable field that manifests itself in different configurations depending on its specific context.[21]

In this book, I concentrate on an understanding of practice in its plural form, namely as 'a sequence of activities' rather than the 'generic [...] work of

---

17   Stoler, *Along the Archival Grain*, 50.
18   Historians of colonial medicine have typically concluded that colonial medical practitioners, missionary and governmental alike, neglected preventive and rural medicine while dismissing traditional local forms of healthcare. In his microstudy, Bruchhausen shows that while missionaries in particular were engaged in rural areas and attempted to implement some forms of preventive medicine, they failed for a variety of complex reasons relating to the nature of both biomedicine and African societies. See: Bruchhausen, *Medizin zwischen den Welten*, 23–24.
19   For a discussion of the term and its scholarly history, see: Bruchhausen, '"Biomedizin" in sozial-und kulturwissenschaftlichen Beiträgen'; Löwy, 'Historiography of Biomedicine'.
20   For the value of conceptualizing biomedicine as localized, see: Anderson, 'Making Global Health History'.
21   Livingston, *Improvising Medicine*; Wendland, *A Heart for the Work*.

cultural extension and transformation in time', a useful distinction drawn by Andrew Pickering.[22] However, these definitions are sometimes difficult to distinguish; the latter is then considered for this study. I follow Joseph Rouse's observation that knowledge is mediated as much by 'models, skills, instruments, standardized materials and phenomena and situated interactions among knowers, in short, by *practices*' as by language.[23] A close-up and localized empirical analysis of practices thus allows me to describe biomedicine not only in 'relation to its own theory of itself (as found, for instance, in textbooks)' but in its 'local instantiations'.[24]

Historians of medicine are increasingly following the 'practice turn' in science studies, an approach that has been the subject of much recent scholarly discussion,[25] but they still lament the lack of understanding of physicians' daily routines.[26] Publications that aim to fill this gap usually rely on practice records or casebooks, both of which are particularly well suited to answering questions on medical practices.[27] Other potentially relevant sources include a great variety of records, from doctors' diaries to invoices and medical instructions for patients. These documents draw attention to the recording process and the fact that writing has always formed an essential part of clinical practice. They are also particularly useful for reconstructing everyday clinical practices.[28]

The operation and delivery protocols, monthly patient lists, patient casebooks, and annual statistics for the Albert Schweitzer Hospital – and even Schweitzer's notebooks[29] – are notably less discursive than those used for

---

22   Pickering, *The Mangle of Practice*, 4–5.

23   Rouse, 'Two Concepts of Practices', 204. Italics in the original.

24   Wendland, *A Heart for the Work*, 23.

25   Dinges, 'Arztpraxen 1500–1900. Zum Stand der Forschung'; Schatzki, 'Introduction: Practice Theory'.

26   Dinges and Stolberg, 'Medical Practice, 1600–1900, Introduction', 1–2; Löwy, 'Historiography of Biomedicine', 122.

27   See the many contributions in this edited volume: Dinges et al., *Medical Practice, 1600–1900: Physicians and Their Patients*. The pioneering study in this regard was: Duffin, *Langstaff*.

28   Hess and Schlegelmilch, 'Cornucopia Officinae Medicae: Medical Practice Records and Their Origin'; Hess, 'Krankenakten als Gegenstand der Krankenhausgeschichtsschreibung'; Warner, 'The Uses of Patient Records by Historians'.

29   Schweitzer's original 123 notebooks are held at Syracuse University. The AMS has copies, which were scanned for the purposes of this study. In these notebooks, Schweitzer recorded his observations on what he read in books, newspapers, and letters. They include his thoughts on philosophy and theology, notes on contemporary political events and scientific findings, and quotations from famous persons. Addresses of individuals with whom Schweitzer wanted to remain in contact or names of drugs that he considered

similar historical studies. These records proved more useful for compiling statistics or verifying claims made in other types of sources. Letters written by hospital personnel that update Schweitzer on medical issues take the place of casebooks in my study, for example when they describe treatment methods in great detail.

Most practice-oriented studies by medical historians focus on individual doctors. Although the hospital, alongside the laboratory, is considered the quintessential setting in which biomedicine takes place,[30] scholarship that explores the medical practices of individual hospitals is more rare, possibly due to the limitations of the archival record. Hospitals are by their very nature local institutions. They have been defined by and reflect the political, social, and economic power structures that manifest themselves in architectonic and organizational preferences as well as medical principles.[31] Because of these interactions, historians of colonialism often view individual hospitals as offering 'important case (studies) in tensions between tradition and modernity'.[32] Historical studies on medicine in Africa that rely heavily on hospital sources exemplify this point. Often using mission records they frequently explore these tensions.[33] Contributions on hospitals in South Africa have concentrated on how political and social contestations unfolded around biomedicine.[34]

This book regards biomedicine as a lens through which to study the colonial encounter and the tensions to which it gave rise. It pays particular attention to daily hospital routines and where they collapse. It is precisely here where we can discern agency and learn more about African patients as they went about negotiating their hospital stays. Despite every hospital's unique local form, it is important to emphasize that hospital treatment represents an exceptional experience for each patient. As patients leave their familiar social setting, they

---

useful are also recorded. I have closely examined those nine notebooks with a title suggesting medical content.

30   Cunningham and Andrews, *Western Medicine as Contested Knowledge*, 5.

31   Borck, 'Quo vadis, Krankenhausgeschichte?', 20; Howell, 'Hospitals', 503; Risse, *Mending Bodies, Saving Souls*, 5; Van Der Geest and Finkler, 'Hospital Ethnography'.

32   Harrison, Jones, and Sweet, *From Western Medicine to Global Medicine*, 23.

33   Linda B. Kumwenda examines how missionaries saw the training of biomedical personnel as a means to 'Westernize' Africans, an endeavor that was understood quite differently and used to dissimilar ends by the latter. See: Kumwenda, 'African Medical Personnel of the Universities' Mission to Central Africa in Northern Rhodesia'. Markku Hokkanen investigates biomedicine's relationship to local forms of medicine and religion. See: Hokkanen, 'Quests for Health and Contests for Meaning'. Walima Kalusa discusses how Africans incorporated biomedicine and its practitioners into their own medical world. See: Kalusa, 'Missionaries, African Patients, and Negotiating Missionary Medicine'.

34   Digby and Phillips, *At the Heart of Healing*; Horwitz, *Baragwanath Hospital*; Parle and Noble, *The People's Hospital*.

encounter new or more apparent power structures to which they have to submit or against which they resist.[35] Focusing closely on medical practices is particularly insightful in this respect.

An important exercise throughout this book is to place my findings in their local and global contexts, and to compare them to contemporary medical trends and broader colonial socio-political patterns. Early colonial governments established medical services in their respective colonies for the primary benefit of European officials and settlers. From the second half of the nineteenth century, missions were the main providers of biomedical services in rural parts of Africa.[36] A number of historians have observed that Africans often preferred attending mission hospitals due to these institutions' propensity to adapt to local demands, their more compassionate staff, and their less rigid rules.[37] Initial attempts to secularize missionary medicine occurred in the interwar period.[38] After World War Two, governments in much of the colonial world, including Gabon, started to expand their medical services, becoming more interventionist in the process.[39]

Recent research highlights that medical missions likewise implemented preventive medicine programs. They trained Africans, provided healthcare education, offered pre- and postnatal care, and participated in or planned vaccination campaigns; their focus on curative services, meanwhile, was often a response to the demands of the local population.[40] Missions were thus pivotal for the 'popularization of biomedicine, or at least certain aspects of biomedicine', as David Hardiman argues.[41] The hospital under study in this book also played a role in popularizing biomedicine, but in many of its other features represented an alternative model to the prevailing missionary- or government-led approaches to healthcare in Africa.

---

35   Howell, 'Hospitals', 511; Lammel, 'Das Hospital als Raum dazwischen', 125; Risse, *Mending Bodies, Saving Souls*, 9–10.

36   Wall, *Into Africa*, 4; Hardiman, *Healing Bodies, Saving Souls*, 1; Harrison, Jones, and Sweet, *From Western Medicine to Global Medicine*, 15; Giles-Vernick and Webb Jr, *Global Health in Africa*, 4.

37   Debusmann, 'Médicalisation et pluralisme au Cameroun allemand', 234; Good, *The Steamer Parish*, 261; Kalusa, 'Christian Medical Discourse and Praxis on the Imperial Frontier', 249.

38   Bruchhausen, 'Medicine between Religious Worlds', 188; Wall, *Into Africa*, 8–9.

39   Hardiman, *Healing Bodies, Saving Souls*, 20; Mabika Ognandzi, *Médicaliser l'Afrique*, 220.

40   Bruchhausen, *Medizin zwischen den Welten*, 110–11; Jennings, 'Healing of Bodies, Salvation of Souls', 43–47.

41   Hardiman, *Healing Bodies, Saving Souls*, 48.

3   The Context: Trade, Politics, and Health in Colonial Lambaréné

The settlements on the confluence of the Ngounié and Ogooué rivers were important nodes in far-reaching African trading networks of the nineteenth century. The Galoa king Nkombe founded Adolinanongo in about 1860 on the
same land to which Schweitzer would move his hospital in 1927.[42] The two
decades following Adolinanongo's establishment marked the first economic
boom of the region around the town, which is today known as Lambaréné.
Nkombe encouraged trading companies and factories to establish their headquarters in the vicinity, possibly to decrease his reliance on middlemen to facilitate trade. Missions as well as the French army soon established their own
bases in the area, but many were moved further up the Ogooué River to the
town of Ndjolé in the late 1880s and early 1890s.[43] In 1910, Gabon became one
of the four territories that made up the new French colony of Afrique Equatoriale Française (AEF); it retained this status until it gained its political independence in 1960.

The Galoa and the Fang formed the two largest groups of patients who attended the Albert Schweitzer Hospital. Each group had their own separate accommodation there, while the hospital employed resident interpreters for
both languages.[44] The Galoa people, who speak a language belonging to the
Myene cluster of Bantu languages, had been present in the Lambaréné region
since at least the early nineteenth century.[45] They were known for embracing
Catholic and Protestant missionary education, both of which were represented in local schools.[46] The Galoa were sandwiched between Gabon's two biggest

---

42   For more on the move of the hospital, see Chapter 1. The location of Nkombe's house,
      where Schweitzer would build his own, was slightly above that of the landing site on the
      river, where the main hospital buildings would emerge. Pounah translates 'Adôlinanôngô'
      as 'Looking over the nations'. Pounah, *Notre passé*, 37.

43   On the history of Lambaréné and Adolinanongo, see: Ambouroue-Avaro, *Un peuple gabo-
      nais à l'aube de la colonisation*, 222–32; Gardinier, *Historical Dictionary of Gabon*, 179; Mer-
      let, *Légendes et histoire des Myéné de l'Ogooué*, 63–66; Pounah, *Notre passé*, 32–37;
      Raponda-Walker and Soret, *Notes d'histoire du Gabon*, 67.

44   Joy, Arnold, and Schweitzer, *The Africa of Albert Schweitzer*, 144; Munz and Munz, *Mit dem
      Herzen einer Gazelle und der Haut eines Nilpferds*, 116; Nessmann, *Avec Albert Schweitzer de
      1924 à 1926*, 198.

45   On the history of the Galoa, or the Galwa as they are also known, see: Ambouroue-Avaro,
      Un peuple gabonais à l'aube de la colonisation, 219–21; Gaulme, *Le pays de Cama*, 65; Des-
      champs, *Traditions orales et archives au Gabon*, 21. 107; Pounah, *Notre passé*, 11–13, 22–28;
      Weinstein, *Gabon : Nation-Building on the Ogooué*, 22, 81.

46   Gardinier, *Historical Dictionary of Gabon*, 180; Mebiame Zomo, 'Le travail des missions
      chrétiennes au Gabon pendant la colonisation', 55; Weinstein, *Gabon : Nation-Building on
      the Ogooué*, 40–44.

ethnic groups, the Eshira people to the south and the Fang to the north. The political scientist Brian Weinstein argued in 1966 that the French regarded the Fang, who had migrated to the area in the late 1870s as superior, not because they 'submitted to French material superiority but because (they) did not'.[47] A feeling of Fang exceptionalism was widespread not only among the Fang themselves, but also among Europeans and other ethnic groups of Gabon, as has been highlighted by historians working on present-day Gabon.[48] To this day, the majority of ethnographic work on Gabon has focused on the Fang. While the Fang would later become the preferred employees of the army, the government, and the Catholic missions, the Galoa were regarded as elitist and separatist by the colonial apparatus during the interwar period.[49]

Movement and migration was routine for people of the Lambaréné region throughout the first half of the twentieth century. Local residents usually relocated their settlements after a maximum of ten years.[50] The pressures of World War One as well as the colonial administration's resort to forced labor for the construction of roads and the Congo-Ocean Railway in the 1920s compelled men to leave their families, which then drove women to seek work, such as the gathering of rubber, beyond their settlements.[51] The colonial government unsuccessfully tried to control these movements of men and women by enacting a series of 'village regroupement' schemes,[52] which aimed to facilitate tax collection and to satisfy the exigencies of capitalism and the monetary system.[53] Scholars emphasize the dramatic impact of global trade on the region, which transformed disparate structures ranging from modes of agricultural

---

47   Weinstein, *Gabon : Nation-Building on the Ogooué*, 37.

48   Bernault, 'Dévoreurs de la nation'; Cinnamon, 'Colonial Anthropologies and the Primordial Imagination in Equatorial Africa'.

49   Gray, *Colonial Rule and Crisis in Equatorial Africa*, 209; Weinstein, *Gabon : Nation-Building on the Ogooué*, 38–43, 68.

50   Grébert, *Au Gabon*, 64–65. In the ethnographic section of his book, the missionary Grébert explained that villages had to be relocated due to soil exhaustion. Sixty years later, the geographer Roland Pourtier argued that this relocation process also served to resolve social tensions, but was less certain of the exact reasons that motivated its participants. In his view, residents may have moved simply because the surrounding land was empty enough to allow them to do so. See: Pourtier, *Le Gabon: espace, histoire, société*, 1:233–35.

51   Gardinier, *Historical Dictionary of Gabon*, 140, 145–46; Gray, *Colonial Rule and Crisis in Equatorial Africa*, 154–57; Gray and Ngolet, 'Lambaréné, Okoume and the Transformation of Labor', 87; Weinstein, *Gabon : Nation-Building on the Ogooué*, 49–51.

52   The first was enacted in 1911, the final one after World War Two. Gray, *Colonial Rule and Crisis in Equatorial Africa*, 111, 179–81; Sautter, *De l'Atlantique au fleuve Congo*, 772–73; Weinstein, *Gabon : Nation-Building on the Ogooué*, 67.

53   Nzenguet Iguemba, *Colonisation, fiscalité et mutations au Gabon*, 393.

production to gender relations.[54] In a 1952 study commissioned by the colonial administration, the sociologists Georges Balandier and Jean-Claude Pauvert concluded that 'the current situation can be explained by the demographic crisis affecting the totality of Gabon, by social disorganization and moral disarray, by the persistence of a only rudimentary economy; it is the inevitable result of a certain type of colonization'.[55]

Throughout the study period, Gabon's most important export was Okoumé, a relatively soft wood. Timber extraction was a seasonal activity as it depended on the water level of the rivers for transportation. Its production intensified after 1900, attracting a large number of migrant laborers. Despite various economic crises, such as during the world wars or the Great Depression, the local timber industry usually recovered quickly. In time, the dominant lumber companies strengthened their influential position in the relevant political and economic circles of the colony.[56] Sanitary conditions in the lumber camps were often substandard and accidents occurred frequently.[57] A considerable percentage of the patients who sought care at government healthcare facilities or at Schweitzer's hospital came from lumber camps, as will be discussed in Chapter 2. Many of those patients came to repair hernias, which was a very common intervention in various hospitals of the region.

In the late 1920s, up to 25,000 workers were employed in the industry in Lower Ogooué and Middle Ogooué, the two administrative districts that stretched from Ndjolé westwards to the mouth of the river.[58] The colonial administration counted 6,000 laborers under contract plus an unknown number of workers 'in an irregular situation' in the Lambaréné Subdivision alone.[59] During the 1930s, the town itself was estimated to have approximately 1,000 inhabitants,[60] while the wider subdivision had an estimated population of about 15,000 people.[61] The period after World War Two until Gabonese independence is less

54   Metegue N'Nah, *Histoire du Gabon*, 80–81; Pourtier, *Le Gabon: espace, histoire, société*, 1:217–19; Jean-Baptiste, 'A Black Girl Should Not Be With a White Man', 66.
55   Balandier and Pauvert, *Les villages gabonais*, 9.
56   Gray and Ngolet, 'Lambaréné, Okoume and the Transformation of Labor', 99, 103–4; Metegue N'Nah, *Histoire du Gabon*, 138; Ombigath, 'La Crise économique de 1930', 150–53, 165; Sautter, *De l'Atlantique au fleuve Congo*, 757, 768.
57   Gray and Ngolet, 'Lambaréné, Okoume and the Transformation of Labor', 102–3.
58   Ibid., 100.
59   Sautter, *De l'Atlantique au fleuve Congo*, 769.
60   Metegue N'Nah, *Histoire du Gabon*, 118.
61   The 1932 politcal annual report for Gabon mentions 14,815 inhabitants. The one for the second semester of 1936 mentions 15,734. 4(1)D 36–38 (1930–32) and 4(1)D 44 (1936), ANOM.

well researched. It is assumed that the overall population of Gabon remained relatively stable during this period,[62] but the population of the Lambaréné Subdivision appears to have risen slightly.[63] The timber industry still remained central to the colony's economy.[64]

Many Gabonese historians underline the complicit attitude adopted by missions towards these overtly colonial and capitalist processes, as missionaries were concerned with assimilating Gabonese into a European value system. To this end, they fought against what they perceived as local 'superstitions', seeking to eradicate 'fetishism' and reconfigure the relationship between individuals and their communities, for example by aiming to alter family structures. Schooling was envisaged to play a pivotal role in this process.[65] Chapter 5 describes how Schweitzer positioned himself in this 'civilizing mission'.

European and North American scholars, on the other hand, have often focused on the aspects of central African life that missionaries meant to eliminate. They show how Gabonese resorted to the 'supernatural' and how this was intertwined with what is commonly labeled as the separate spheres of religion and politics, a distinction that most present-day scholars of central Africa consider misleading or useless.[66] The Gabonese sociologist Joseph Tonda insists that commodity capitalism was and still is entangled in this complex too, a nexus that also included healing and medicine.[67]

---

62   According to Mabika, an estimated 430,000 to 450,000 people lived in Gabon in the mid-1930s, while approximately 440,000 people were resident in the country at the time of its first census after independence in 1960/61. His population estimates for the early 1950s are slightly lower, ranging from 388,000 to 405,000. Headrick has also commented on Gabon's remarkably stable population in the period from 1920 to 1960. Her estimates range from 370,000 in 1921 to 404,000 in 1935. She estimates that Gabon had a population of 384,000 in 1950. See: Mabika, 'Médicalisation de l'Afrique centrale', 352–57; Headrick, Colonialism, Health and Illness in French Equatorial Africa, 106–7.

63   The 1953 annual report of the Service de Santé of Gabon mentions 17,249, ZK 005-005, SHD.

64   Metegue N'Nah, Histoire du Gabon, 138; Pourtier, Le Gabon: état et developpement, 2:158–60.

65   Mebiame Zomo, 'Le travail des missions chrétiennes au Gabon pendant la colonisation'; Mekodiomba, 'Rôle et influence des églises missionnaires dans la mission civilisatrice au Gabon'; Nguema Minko, 'L'évangélisation comme forme religieuse de la conquête politique du Gabon'.

66   Bernault, 'De la modernité comme impuissance', 764–66; MacGaffey, 'Changing Representations in Central African History', 205–7; Schatzberg, Political Legitimacy in Middle Africa, 107.

67   Tonda, 'Capital sorcier et travail de Dieu'.

The exertion of power in all these domains relied on forces that could simultaneously strengthen and weaken, heal and harm.[68] In precolonial Gabon, the indigenous term for 'medicine' or 'remedy' went well beyond the biomedical conception attached to pharmaceutical products. Medical objects were not only used to combat disease, but also to attract good fortune, attain greater success in trade, or repel bad luck, among other objectives. Colonial observers termed such objects 'fetishes'.[69] Jan Vansina, the eminent historian of Central Africa, refers to them as 'charms'. He notes that they were regarded as being able to function on a collective level, often targeting 'crucial problems: control of the rains, defense of the village, help in war and hunting, and, not least, detection and eradication of witchcraft'.[70] Tonda confirms that this broad conception of the term 'médicament' is still maintained in the region today.[71] This is not to say that local inhabitants did not exploit plants with the aim of inducing effects that more closely corresponded to the biomedical concept of a drug; a wide range of herbal medications have long been employed to treat a large variety of afflictions in Gabon.[72] Chapter 1 will provide more details on local vocabulary and actors of healing.

The interrelatedness of what Western scholars would label religion, politics, economics, and healing is often exemplified in the (diseased) body, which can be presented as a fertile site to demonstrate where the views of colonizers and the colonized differed and where they overlapped, as Florence Bernault convincingly does. As she writes, the 'fetish value of the human body, far from being confined to African societies during colonialism, haunted the minds, the laboratories and the markets of French rulers'; one of their main shortcomings

---

68   Cinnamon, 'Spirits, Power and the Political Imagination in Late-Colonial Gabon', 192. The close association between healing and harming has been widely observed across the African continent. See: Hunt, 'Health and Healing'.

69   Bernault, 'Witchcraft and the Colonial Life of the Fetish'; Cinnamon, 'Of Fetishism and Totemism'.

70   Vansina, *Paths in the Rainforests*, 96. In Fang, 'charms' were called 'Biang'. According to the anthropologist James Fernandez, they served 'to increase or decrease the capacities of whatever they were applied to, whether inanimate objects or living beings'. Fernandez, *Bwiti*, 221.

71   Tonda writes that: 'the "natives" do not use the word "fetish", they speak of medicines ("medicaments"), an ambivalent and polysemous term: medicine is also what would correspond to the biomedical meaning of this word, but it is also a poison, real and not only symbolic – in the fictional sense – it is also an object supposed to act at a distance against a person or against forces in nature and that can be inscribed in the magical, in the technical meaning of this term' Tonda, 'Capital sorcier et travail de Dieu', 56.

72   Morel, 'Au Gabon avant l'arrivée du Docteur Schweitzer', 186; Grébert, *Au Gabon*, 142; Fernandez, *Bwiti*, 625; Vansina, *Paths in the Rainforests*, 96.

was that 'they refused to envision the coexistence of material and ritual power as compatible with moral norms and social good'.[73] In the same way, biomedicine separated the figure of the priest from that of the doctor, as Tonda argues, before they would later be reconciled again in the form of prophet figures.[74] Syncretic cults like *Bwiti* or anti-witchcraft movements such as *Mademoiselle*, which integrated the realms of politics, religion, and healing, had possibly been present in Gabon since precolonial times, but appear to have grown in support during the 1950s. The rise of these organizations has usually been interpreted as a reaction to the above-mentioned rapid social changes that occurred under colonialism and the capitalist economic system,[75] but has also occasionally been seen as primarily linked to the emerging political contestations that marked the period leading up to Gabonese independence.[76] For the historian of Africa studying Schweitzer's hospital, it is at first striking, then intriguing, and ultimately frustrating that the hospital sources rarely discuss local religion, politics, economics, or healing practices.

Since the various healthcare services offered by the colonial government will be discussed in detail in each of the main chapters, I will now provide only a very short overview of government medical services in Gabon, doing so by drawing from the comprehensive histories written by Hines Mabika Ognandzi and Rita Headrick respectively. Headrick underlines that while there were more doctors per inhabitant in AEF during the 1920s than in other French colonies, much less money was spent on healthcare than in other colonies.[77] Gabon itself, meanwhile, received 24 percent of the medical supplies allocated to AEF, but made up only 12 percent of its population.[78] The first biomedical services in Gabon were offered in the 1860s on an army ship off the coast of Libreville. A hospital was established there in 1896, and three years later 'medical posts' had been founded in Port-Gentil and Ndjolé.[79] The colonial government made some efforts to expand healthcare provision during the interwar years,[80] but only after World War Two did medical funding, personnel, and facilities increase significantly. For example, the total number of hospital

---

73   Bernault, 'Carnal Technologies', 185.

74   Tonda, *La guérison divine en Afrique centrale*, 107, 227.

75   On Bwiti, see: Fernandez, 'Symbolic Consensus', 904–5; Mary, 'L'alternative de la vision et de la possession', 283–84. On Mademoisselle, see: Tonda, 'Capital sorcier et travail de Dieu', 61–63; Weinstein, *Gabon : Nation-Building on the Ogooué*, 53–55.

76   Cinnamon, 'Spirits, Power and the Political Imagination in Late-Colonial Gabon', 201.

77   Headrick, *Colonialism, Health and Illness in French Equatorial Africa*, 405–7.

78   Ibid., 216.

79   Mabika Ognandzi, *Médicaliser l'Afrique*, 126.

80   Ibid., 203.

beds in government institutions rose from 400 in 1946 to 3,000 in 1956.[81] From the late 1920s to the early 1950s, Schweitzer's hospital provided approximately one-third of all hospital beds in Gabon. Mabika illustrates that missionaries played a relatively minor role in introducing biomedicine to Gabon.[82] In the Lambaréné area, however, they had already provided basic medical services from before Schweitzer's arrival, as had itinerant army surgeons.[83]

The Gabonese colonial government first opened a healthcare facility in Lambaréné in 1921. This was closed when Schweitzer returned to Gabon in 1924, but was reopened in 1926.[84] There is evidence to suggest that Schweitzer urged the authorities to do so to offer his hospital a respite from the increasing numbers of patients arriving with beriberi and sleeping sickness.[85] Subsequent government reports occasionally express a relatively hostile attitude towards Schweitzer and his hospital, a perspective usually infused with anti-German and anti-Protestant sentiments.[86] However, this did not prevent the two clinics in Lambaréné from cooperating in certain areas, including their agreement that all sleeping sickness patients would be treated at the government facility.[87] Comparisons between the two institutions are made throughout this book. Towards the end of the 1950s, Balandier visited the government facility, whose status had been upgraded from 'infirmerie' to 'hospital'. The resident physician there, a former student of philosophy, was rather disillusioned by the state of the hospital's equipment and its general condition, comparing it unfavorably to the Albert Schweitzer Hospital:

---

81   Ibid., 220.

82   Mabika, 'Médicalisation de l'Afrique centrale', 288.

83   Emane, *Docteur Schweitzer: une icône africaine*, 56–57; Morel, 'Au Gabon avant l'arrivée du Docteur Schweitzer'; Schweitzer, *Zwischen Wasser und Urwald*, 65.

84   This information is taken from a historical overview of the Assistance Médicale Indigène in: 'Rapport Annuel du Service de Santé de la Colonie du Gabon 1932', ZK 005-127, SHD.

85   Mai, *Albert Schweitzer und seine Kranken*, 115. Mai does not provide any references for this statement.

86   As he suggested in the Service de la Santé's 1932 annual report, the Médecin Général spoke of Schweitzer's 'German or pro-German ties' that weren't broken by his recent French nationalization, 'whose degree of sincerity should be questioned and clarified'. 'Rapport Annuel du Service de Santé de la Colonie du Gabon 1932', ZK 005-127, SHD. Jacques Bessuges, the colonial government physician in Lambaréné during the early 1950s, claimed that Schweitzer was not always on best terms with government representatives. See: Bessuges, *Lambaréné à l'ombre de Schweitzer*, 92.

87   Schweitzer claimed that this arrangement had been in place since 1928. See: Schweitzer, *Das Spital im Urwald: Aufnahmen von Anna Wildikann*, 11–12. It was not strictly implemented or would be lifted, as sleeping sickness patients are listed in the monthly patient records, the *appels mensuels*, that commence in 1932. More details on this arrangement, which was definitively in place by 1936, will be given in Chapter 4, on the *appels mensuels* in Chapter 2.

Look, I was called to a hospital without any equipment. What you see here is fictional, out of order. The autoclave is from the founding days, we could make it a pantry. Do you take your meals at the hotel? Then you risk appendicitis. I'll operate on you and you'll have every chance of staying for lack of asepsis. Dies irae, dies illa ... No, I'll send you to Schweitzer. That's what I'm reduced to! I become a supplier, while I should be a competitor.[88]

4   Albert Schweitzer and His Hospital in Lambaréné: a Short Historiography

Books on Schweitzer often indulge in colonial genre-writing, as outlined above, thereby focusing on particular stories. Like Schweitzer's own account of his life in Lambaréné, many memoirs of visitors or employees start with a description of their author's outward voyage by ship or, later, airplane. Most biographers repeat what Schweitzer had written himself, such as when recounting the reasons behind his initial decision to move to Lambaréné or how he put together the final pieces of his ethical philosophy.[89] Bertrand Taithe and Katherine Davis remind us that Schweitzer played an active role in molding his own legacy. They argue that he lived long enough to 'be able to shape his own reputation', labeling scholarship on him as 'something of a cottage industry'.[90] Ruth Harris observes that biographies do not situate Schweitzer, his thought, or his hospital into the broader context of colonial medicine, humanitarianism, or missionary endeavors, with their authors ignoring relevant historiographical trends, such as transnationalism.[91]

Most publications on Schweitzer rely heavily on already published secondary sources or on material published by Schweitzer himself. One explanation for this is that much of this writing is concerned with his theology or philosophy.[92] Schweitzer held a doctorate in the latter discipline and a habilitation in the former. While current research agrees that his prospects for an academic

---

88   Balandier, *Afrique ambiguë*, 218.

89   Oermann, *Albert Schweitzer 1875–1965*.

90   Taithe and Davis, 'Heroes of Charity?', 915. On how Schweitzer shaped his own reputation, see: Moll, *Albert Schweitzer: Meister der Selbstinszenierung*.

91   Harris, 'Schweitzer and Africa', 1110.

92   For a recent example of this kind of writing, see: Spangenberg and Landman, *The Legacies of Albert Schweitzer Reconsidered*. See also the contributions to the series *Études Schweitzeriennes: revue annuelle de l'Association française des Amis d'Albert Schweitzer*, sometimes with the alternative subtitle: *revue d'étique, de théologie et de philosophie* (*Strassbourg 1990–2003*). This series was then renamed as the *Cahiers Albert Schweitzer*.

career were more than reasonable, it does not place him at the forefront of either field or consider his contributions to them as his main legacy, an assertion that Schweitzer readily acknowledged himself.[93]

According to his own narrative, Schweitzer quit both disciplines in 1905 at the age of thirty and began to study medicine with the goal of traveling to Africa to salvage the African 'Lazarus' already referred to and redeem the sins of colonialism.[94] Balandier, writing during Schweitzer's lifetime, and James Carleton Paget, writing more recently, have both underlined how uninterested he was in the fate of the continent and its people, and how marginal a role the local context that he encountered in Lambaréné played in his writing and thinking.[95] His estimations of the local people to whom he administered medical care did not improve during his long stay in Gabon; rather they lowered over time even though he refrained from saying so publicly. In private letters and in conversations with visitors, Schweitzer voiced a particular distaste towards the new African elite.[96] He was disillusioned about their embrace of Western political and economic values in particular. In his view – an opinion that he shared with many contemporaries, notably Protestant Swiss[97] – 'European civilization' was on the decline due to the rise of materialism and nationalism as well as technology's ever-increasing permeation of society. Schweitzer specifically lamented that those trends were not accompanied by a corresponding shift in ethical thinking. For him, the two world wars were proof of this development.[98] Nevertheless, he still believed in the superiority of 'European civilization', an argument that he justified by invoking a cultural rather than a racial discourse.[99]

---

93   Carleton Paget and Thate, 'Introduction: Questioning the Relevance of Albert Schweitzer', 2; Körtner, '"Ehrfurcht vor dem Leben" – Zur Stellung der Ethik Albert Schweitzers in der ethischen Diskussion der Gegenwart', 100.

94   Schweitzer, *Zwischen Wasser und Urwald*, 161–62. Schweitzer wrote there: 'We and our civilization are burdened, really, with a great debt. We are not free to confer benefits on these men or not, as we please; it is our duty. Anything we give them is not benevolence but atonement'.

95   Balandier, *Afrique ambiguë*, 225; Carleton Paget, 'Albert Schweitzer and Africa'; See also: Harris, 'The Allure of Albert Schweitzer', 804.

96   Schweitzer to Thiébaud, 24 July 1953, AMS; Barthélemy, *Wie ich Lambarene erlebte*, 57–58; Günther and Götting, *Was heisst Ehrfurcht vor dem Leben?*, 153–54; Jilek-Aall, *Working with Dr. Schweitzer*, 114–15; McKnight, *Verdict on Schweitzer*, 242. See also Chapter 5.

97   Harries, 'From the Alps to Africa', 215.

98   Oermann, *Albert Schweitzer 1875–1965*, 151–59; Rehm-Grätzel, 'Albert Schweitzers Philosophie der "Ehrfurcht vor dem Leben" und der Friedensgedanke', 95–96; Scholl, *Von der Ehrfurcht vor dem Leben zur transkulturellen Solidarität*, 93.

99   Arnold, 'Vous les noirs, nous les blancs', 438; Harris, 'Schweitzer and Africa', 1110.

Given his sentiments described above, it would appear surprising that Schweitzer showed any interest in going to Gabon at all. Indeed, Carleton Paget concludes that his 'decision to go to Africa arose almost by chance'.[100] Prior to this, Schweitzer had attempted to participate in a number of charitable endeavors, such as looking after orphans. In such activities, however, he was forced to adhere to the narrow prescripts of charities or governments, a circumstance that conflicted with his strong desire for personal independence.[101] 'In seeking to distance himself from the restraints of European civilization, he was not unlike other adventurers and explorers of a more openly imperialistic cast of mind', Harris argues.[102] Schweitzer's reasons for joining the Paris Evangelical Missionary Society, an organization that was highly suspicious of his liberal theological views as well as his German origins, are similarly obscure. With this decision, he might have sought to nurture a peculiar form of Alsatian transnationalism; alternatively, he may have recognized in the society's call for missionaries to salvage Africa a personal vocation from Christ.[103]

Schweitzer's move to Lambaréné – and, indeed, his whole life thereafter – is probably best understood as an enactment of his own ethics, the moral system that he termed 'Ehrfurcht vor dem Leben' and which is commonly translated as 'Reverence for Life'. Its basic tenet is that all living beings, including animals, share the same will to live, and thus possess an identical inherent value and right to life. That Schweitzer's life and hospital represented an embodiment, a practice so to speak, of this theory had already been argued during his lifetime.[104] The British reporter Gerald McKnight suggested in 1964 that Schweitzer 'went to Lambaréné to serve his own purpose, not *primarily* to heal sick primitives'.[105] There is evidence that Schweitzer himself saw his life in a similar light.

---

100 Carleton Paget, 'Albert Schweitzer and Africa', 301.
101 Ibid., 281.
102 Harris, 'The Allure of Albert Schweitzer', 813.
103 Carleton Paget, 'Albert Schweitzer and Africa', 283; Harris, 'Schweitzer and Africa', 1112–13.
104 For an overview of the various thinkers, from W.E.B. Du Bois in the 1940s to Ludwig Watzal in the 1980s, who suggested such an interpretation, see: Thate, 'An Anachronism in the African Jungle?'.
105 Italics in the original. McKnight went even further by arguing that Schweitzer wanted to prove that any person with sufficient willpower can become a new Jesus Christ. McKnight, *Verdict on Schweitzer*, 241. Shortly after its publication, *The New York Review of Books* commented on McKnight's book as follows: 'having shattered the Legend of Lambaréné—no difficult task, since the camera does most of it—he pursues the Man (*i.e.* *Schweitzer*) with a dull, pertinacious hostility, an obsessive anxiety to find discreditable interpretations of the most innocuous biographical data, which can only make one reflect how much greatness must still smoulder, even in the wreck of Schweitzer, to arouse so much envious malice'. Italics mine. http://www.nybooks.com/articles/archives/1964/aug/20/the-schweitzer-legend (2 June 2020).

To the American journalist Norman Cousins, who visited Lambaréné in 1957, Schweitzer explained his reasons for moving to Gabon: 'instead of trying to get acceptance for my ideas, involving painful controversy, I decided I would make my life my argument'.[106] He answered other interviewers in a similar manner: 'when you portray me it shall not be as the doctor who ministers to the sick. It is my contribution of reverence for life that I consider my primary contribution to the world'.[107]

In order to contextualize these interpretations and gain initial insights into the Albert Schweitzer Hospital, I now provide a brief overview of how the institution has been evaluated. A more detailed analysis on three of the hospital's most remarkable features is conducted in another book.[108] It sketches out how Schweitzer's international networks were created and maintained. These were also important for sustaining what we call the 'Lambaréné Spirit', which was the ideal atmosphere under which living and working at the institution occurred. This concept included, among many other things, to consider the hospital's offers as simple medical services, which people were free to use or not.

Negative assessments of the hospital increased in the late 1950s, a time during which Schweitzer's global reputation was growing.[109] Replies that defended the hospital suggest that there was indeed something more to the endeavor than the desire to care for sick Africans. Furthermore, many reports reveal that improvisation was important at the hospital not only in medical matters. It was also a central feature of its general organization, as will be examined in Chapter 2; and indeed, Schweitzer's hospital as such is sometimes regarded as an improvised enactment of the 'Reverence for Life'.[110]

---

106   Cousins, *Dr. Schweitzer of Lambaréné*, 191. In general, Cousins interprets Schweitzer's work in a very positive, almost allegoric, light: 'the point about Schweitzer is that he brought the kind of spirit to Africa that the dark man hardly knew existed in the white man' (ibid., 215); and: 'if Albert Schweitzer is a myth, the myth is more important than the reality' (ibid., 219).

107   Melamed and Melamed, 'Albert Schweitzer in Gabon', 191. Melamed and Melamed took this quotation from a poster advertising the 'Albert Schweitzer International Symposium on Health', which was held at the United Nations in New York in 1994.

108   Mabika Ognandzi, Steinke, and Zumthurm, *Schweitzer's Lambaréné: A Hospital in Colonial Africa*.

109   For an overview of Schweitzer's global reception, see: Mbondobari, *Archäologie eines modernen Mythos*.

110   An argument put forward by: Ohls, *Improvisationen der Ehrfurcht vor allem Lebendigen*. Walter Munz claims that Schweitzer himself also suggested such a reading, see: Munz, *Albert Schweitzer im Gedächtnis der Afrikaner und in meiner Erinnerung*, 28.

André Audoynaud, the government physician in Lambaréné in the early 1960s and perhaps Schweitzer's harshest critic, compared the hospital to a 'bidonville', a slum.[111] The well-known anthropologist James Fernandez, who traveled to Gabon with his wife in 1958 to conduct fieldwork for a period of two years, spent some time at the hospital towards the end of his stay. In a stimulating article about this visit, Fernandez recounted that he was not overly mystified by what he observed at the hospital. 'Unlike those many visitors who were yesterday in Paris or New York we were not especially struck with the hurly-burly of hospital life', he wrote.[112] 'The ragged inmates in barracks' and a 'Teutonic desire for order' reminded him of a concentration camp, but he recognized that 'a humanitarian ethic is the organizing rationale at work at Lambaréné, and that is the crucial difference'.[113] Jacques Bessuges, the government physician in Lambaréné in the early 1950s, maintained good relations with Schweitzer. During his first visit, he also associated Schweitzer's hospital with a concentration camp, mainly due to its architectural style and overcrowded conditions. The large number of domestic animals roaming freely all over the hospital grounds caused him added disconcertion. When Bessuges left, however, he sensed that the patients at the hospital were happy; he now bemoaned the contrasting conditions in more conventional hospitals that saw patients left to give birth or die without the support of their families, who were encouraged to stay at the Albert Schweitzer Hospital.[114]

A reevaluation of first impressions is a typical feature of accounts of the Albert Schweitzer Hospital, as exhibited in a letter by Dr. Victor Nessmann, the first physician to practice alongside Schweitzer in Lambaréné. In October 1924, Nessmann wrote to his parents about how he had been initially struck by the disorder that he found at the hospital. However, this feeling soon dissipated, and two weeks after his arrival he had already come to appreciate Schweitzer's 'wise and powerful spirit and methods and his guiding ideas'.[115] The South African surgeon Jack Penn, who visited Lambaréné in 1956, subsequently wrote an article about his stay in a medical journal. He noted how 'the wards at first glance look overcrowded and shocking'; the practice of permitting family members to stay alongside patients and cook in front of their wards particularly

---

111 Audoynaud, *Le docteur Schweitzer et son hôpital à Lambaréné*, 14. Audoynaud's poorly structured book reads like a personal attack on Schweitzer, his legacy and the medicine that was practiced at the hospital.

112 Fernandez, 'The Sound of Bells in a Christian Country', 540.

113 Ibid., 557.

114 Bessuges, *Lambaréné à l'ombre de Schweitzer*, 65–72.

115 Nessmann, *Avec Albert Schweitzer de 1924 à 1926*, 62.

disturbed him, but he was quick to add that 'everything Schweitzer does has a reason for it'.[116]

Former nurses whom I interviewed were appalled by the unhygienic conditions that they discovered on arrival.[117] The numerous animals and cooking fires on the hospital grounds also generated further dismay among newly arriving nurses.[118] Dr. Walter Munz, who would become the hospital's medical director after Schweitzer's death, was similarly perturbed by the conditions that he encountered on arrival, but soon recognized that Schweitzer had created order in this apparent chaos that could be understood by patients and staff only.[119] Cousins held a similar view:

> much of what you saw for the first time at the Hospital seemed so primitive and inadequate as to startle. But when Dr. Schweitzer walked through the grounds, everything seemed as it should be. More than that: the profound meaning of Lambaréné suddenly came to life.[120]

Dr. Greet van der Kreek, who completed a total of almost six years of service at the hospital in the late 1950s, recalled her stay in much the same manner. Like Penn and others, she compared the hospital to a village. 'In my memories, Lambaréné is first and foremost this fascinating village, living and alive, whose rhythm the Great Doctor regulated like a poet', she recounted in an interview.[121] In 1931, the nurse Emma Haussknecht, who would become one of the hospital's most dedicated staff members and serve as a secretary and nurse until her death in 1956, wrote that Africans spoke of the 'village of the doctor'.[122] When Schweitzer described the design and construction of the hospital's second site, he wrote that 'the new hospital will become a real village'.[123] One of the first additional physicians to arrive at the hospital, the Alsatian surgeon Frédéric Trensz, later claimed that this had been planned to make the patients feel at home.[124] Van der Kreek repeated this argument, explaining to Cousins that the hospital was

---

116   Penn, 'A Visit to Albert Schweitzer', 165.

117   Schnee et al., Group Interview Speicherschwendi; Interview Munz and Munz.

118   Stocker, 'Diary 1961–63', 2.

119   Interview Munz and Munz.

120   Cousins, *Dr. Schweitzer of Lambaréné*, 11.

121   Becht, 'Témoignage d'une chirurgien, Mme Le Docteur Greet Barthélémy', 170.

122   Schweitzer, 'Briefe aus dem Lambarene Spital Pfingsten 1931', 12.

123   Schweitzer, *Mitteilungen aus Lambarene. Drittes Heft, 1925–1927*, 26.

124   Trensz, 'Le médecin', 209.

a jungle village with a clinic. If Dr. Schweitzer had put up a fully equipped modern hospital of the kind you see in large cities, I am not sure the natives would come to it. They would probably be afraid of it. The hospital here they understand. It is very simple. If a person gets sick and the local remedies are of no use and the sickness stays on, the entire family gets into a pirogue and paddles – sometimes many, many miles – to the clinic here at Lambaréné. When they arrive, they find an African village very much like the one they left.[125]

Although the village metaphor still finds currency in current research on Schweitzer, it was already under challenge in the 1960s.[126] Fernandez highlighted that the 'crowded sick huts' were also found in mission hospitals. In his experience, African settlements were less crowded and offered 'more healthy space and orderly living arrangement', adding that 'the virtue of equatorial life lies in moving the village to a completely fresh site every eight or nine years'.[127] Two nurses noted independently, and not without surprise, that the settlements that they visited appeared to be much cleaner than the hospital.[128] The Gabonese jurist Augustin Emane conducted approximately sixty interviews with people who had stayed at the hospital as patients or attendants. In addition to the points already identified, they specified a range of further differences. A Gabonese village housed fewer people per room than the Albert Schweitzer Hospital and did not see women cooking outside, as the courtyard was a masculine space. Unlike the hospital, a village had toilets and no one imposed a night-time curfew from 8 p.m. A patient's stay at Schweitzer's hospital was transitory; a village, meanwhile, implied sedentariness.[129]

Fernandez observed that the living quarters for African staff were significantly inferior to those of their European colleagues, remarking that 'when one compares them to the quarters available to the *infirmier* working for the administration, one asks how Schweitzer can keep any competent Africans at all'.[130] This sentiment is supported by the fact that these facilities were among

---

125 Cousins, *Dr. Schweitzer of Lambaréné*, 71.

126 Carleton Paget, 'Albert Schweitzer and Africa', 293; Harris, 'The Allure of Albert Schweitzer', 813.

127 Fernandez, 'The Sound of Bells in a Christian Country', 543.

128 Balsiger, 'Ein helles Band und ein Sonntag', 148; Stocker, 'Diary 1961–63', 16.

129 Emane, *Docteur Schweitzer: une icône africaine*, 92–98. Although Emane provides an intriguing and useful study, his methodology lacks a degree of transparency. He frequently does not support his claims with references, he does not provide details of his informants, and repeatedly cites the same four to five interviewees.

130 Fernandez, 'The Sound of Bells in a Christian Country', 544. Italics in the original.

the first to be modernized after Schweitzer's death.[131] In a volume edited by Dr. Walter Munz, in which he and various Gabonese reflect on Schweitzer's deeds in Lambaréné and his legacy in Africa, the Gabonese pastor Anatole Wora, who claims to have been a close friend of Schweitzer's, rejects this criticism by explaining that the needs of Europeans could not be considered equivalent to those of Africans. According to Wora, Schweitzer understood this, respected every human being equally, and 'wanted everyone to live in his milieu'.[132] Various other Gabonese contributors defended Schweitzer in a similar manner in this volume, which contains exclusively positive views on Schweitzer and his hospital.

My interviews similarly suggest that the quality of their living quarters was not considered particularly important by African staff. Not unlike medical personnel from Europe, Africans who were involved in Schweitzer's work for a longer period of time assessed it in an overwhelmingly positive light. Children of Schweitzer's African staff members emphasized that he represented a sort of father or grandfather who cared well for them, for instance by providing clothing, food, and school utensils, as well as paying for their school fees.[133] They also insist that the salary offered to African employees was more than sufficient.[134] Emane summarizes his interviewees' points of view: 'what seemed most important to them was that this man who had left his country had come to settle among them and really behaved as someone from elsewhere should. He did not disrupt their lives or beliefs'.[135] This book will shed light on the specific ways and areas in which Schweitzer and the medical practices at his hospital disturbed, ignored, and/or reinforced African ways of life and beliefs.

More critical African voices are persistent, but usually mediated by visitors. Notable exceptions can be found in a recent collection of essays from Gabonese scholars.[136] More prominent is the Nobel Laureate in Literature V.S. Naipaul who contends that Schweitzer's reputation among Africans remains 'that of a man who was "harsh" to Africans and was not interested in their culture'.[137]

---

131 'Statistiques de l'Hôpital 1966', L – A – S3, AMS.

132 Munz, *Albert Schweitzer im Gedächtnis der Afrikaner und in meiner Erinnerung*, 117.

133 Interview Daudette Azizet Mburu; Interview Léontine Nsowe; Interview Anne-Marie Padje-Poabalou.

134 Group Interview Port-Gentil; Interview Marie-Joséphine Ndiaye-Boucah.

135 Emane, *Docteur Schweitzer: une icône africaine*, 272.

136 Boundzanga and Ndombet, *Le Malentendu Schweitzer*.

137 Naipaul, *The Masque of Africa,*, 204–5; See also: Achebe, *The Education of a British-Protected Child*, 80, 158; or the film by the Cameroonian director Bassek ba Kobhio, *Le grand blanc de Lambaréné* (1995).

Balandier wrote of the 'apparent ingratitude' displayed by Gabonese towards Schweitzer. Contrary to the above-cited opinions, he claims that Africans disliked 'his authoritarian behavior and resented that they had to pay by enforced labor for the healing of their wounds'. Balandier's informants did not approve of the way Schweitzer approached Africans, 'perceiving them as human machines to be restored with souls to be saved'.[138]

This introduction has revealed considerable ambiguities in Schweitzer's ideas and actions, as well as in the way that these have been assessed by colleagues, visitors, staff, and scholars alike. These contradictions cannot be fully explained by analyzing the medical practices at the Albert Schweitzer Hospital, nor is this my book's primary aim. It will show that practices, including improvised biomedical ones, often are contradictory. It is crucial to consider, however, the thought and motivations that enabled and framed these practices, as well as the social environment in which they occurred and by which they were shaped.

---

138   Balandier, *Afrique ambiguë*, 225.

Between Pragmatism and Order: Medical Organization and Daily Routine

The following introduction to hospital life and services outlines changes and continuities and presents the various actors involved. The mid-1930s, by which time the hospital had cast off its provisional character, and the mid-1960s, when it again expanded considerably after Gabonese independence, serve as the two major points of reference. The spatial organization, the structural hierarchy, and the development of infrastructure illustrate how the Albert Schweitzer Hospital reflects trends and concerns of other health institutions on the continent. A precise comparison is often difficult as these matters varied greatly in different African hospitals, which, moreover, have usually left behind much less detailed documentation.

The hospital authorities attempted to maintain an underlying order, but staff and patients alike approached their stay with a pragmatic attitude. The former had very broad responsibilities, while the latter embedded treatment at the hospital within their conceptions of health and therapeutic practices. This balancing act between order and pragmatism is also a striking feature of the specific medical practices to be analyzed in the chapters that follow. It will thus be insightful to begin by considering the extent to which these principles underlay the hospital's organization and routine.

1   The Hospital Prior to 1927: Establishment and Adaptation

The hospital's development can be divided into four phases, with the first occurring from 1913–1917.[1] One and a half years before the outbreak of World War One, Schweitzer and his wife Helene, who served as a nurse, arrived on the grounds of the Paris Evangelical Missionary Society on the Ogooué River. The story goes that they started to practice in what had been a chicken coop (see Illustration 1). After four months, they had a building constructed with a concrete foundation and a ribbed roof. It had two rooms and served as a consultation space and pharmacy, as well as a sterilization and storage unit. In addition,

---

1   Mabika, 'L'hôpital Albert Schweitzer de Lambaréné', 202.

© TIZIAN ZUMTHURM, 2020 | DOI:10.1163/9789004436978_003

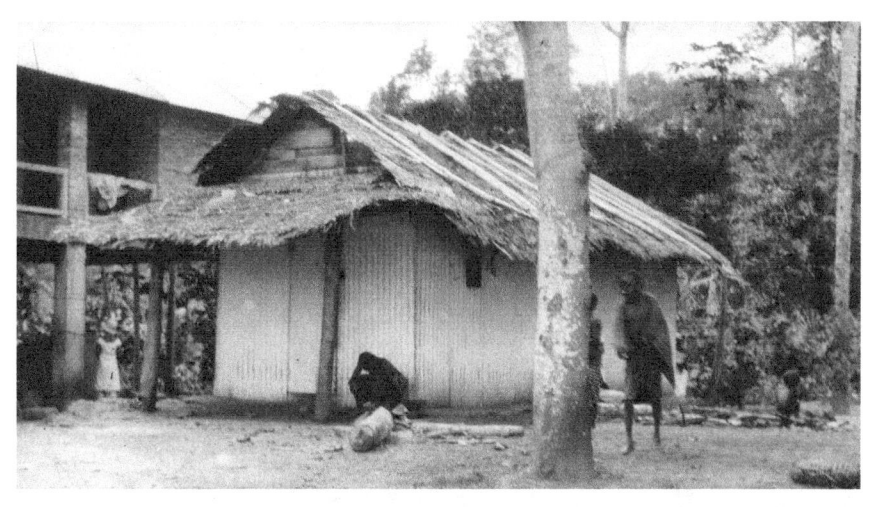

ILLUSTRATION 1   The former chicken coop at the mission station in Andendé, undated
© ARCHIVES CENTRALES ALBERT SCHWEITZER GUNSBACH

there was a waiting area, a dormitory for patients, and dwellings for the first African auxiliaries, Joseph Azoawanié and N'zeng.[2] Schweitzer claimed to have treated thirty to forty patients per day in this period.[3] The vast majority required ambulant treatment; he recorded an average of only four inpatients per day between June 1913 and October 1917.[4] When World War One started, the Schweitzers, as German citizens, were put under detention on the on the mission grounds. In 1917, they were forced to leave the French colony and were interned in France until the war was over, when they became French citizens. It took Schweitzer some time to recover from his internment and to collect the necessary funds for a recuperation of the hospital. Arriving back in Gabon in April 1924, Schweitzer had to undertake extensive renovations of the hospital buildings, which marked the beginning of the second phase (see Illustration 2). Due to tuberculosis, Helene was compelled to remain in Europe temporarily. He was accompanied by Noel Gillespie, a student at Oxford, whose mother, Emily Rieder, maintained close contact with Schweitzer. When in late 1924, a famine and a dysentery epidemic, which

---

2   Schweitzer, 'Notes et Nouvelles de la part du prof. Albert Schweitzer. Deuxième rapport', 32–35. African medical personnel was usually refered to as '(Heil-) Gehilfe', more rarely as 'Pfleger'. I will use auxiliary, assistant, and aide interchangeably. When I do not give their full names, it is because they are not mentioned in the sources.

3   Ibid., 14.

4   In total, 4,153 inpatients were accommodated at the hospital in this period. See the 'cahiers des patients', L – P – C1, L – P – C2, AMS.

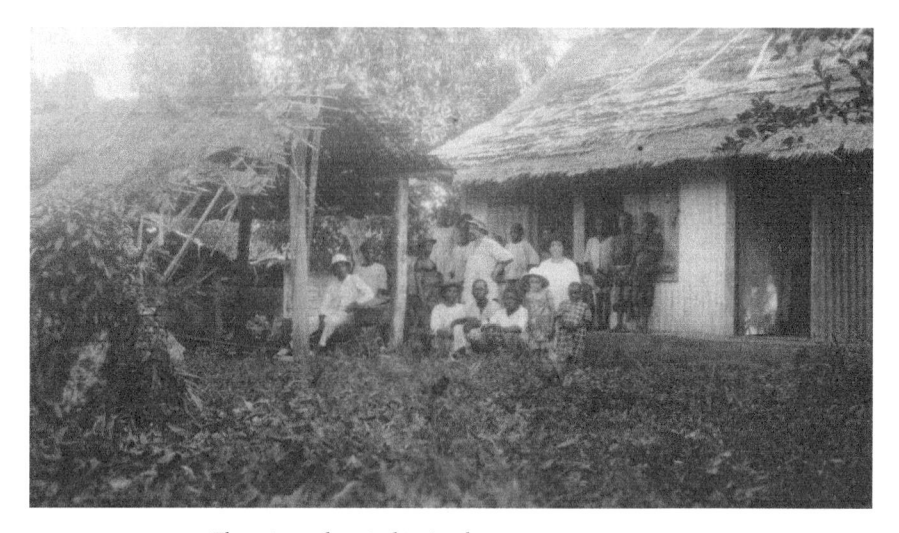

ILLUSTRATION 2   The ruinous hospital in April 1924
© ARCHIVES CENTRALES ALBERT SCHWEITZER GUNSBACH

would both last in varying intensity for two years, hit the region, Schweitzer concluded that the capacity of his hospital was insufficient.[5] Increasingly tense relations with the mission facilitated his decision.[6] Gillespie wrote to his mother in 1924 that Schweitzer was looking for a new site, because he was 'in very bad odour with the French official circles of the Paris Mission'.[7] By February 1926, with patient numbers steadily increasing, it seems that he was pushed to leave the mission grounds.[8]

Schweitzer thus acquired land three kilometers upriver to construct a new hospital, which he designed himself. He mentioned only in passing that King Nkombe, he referred to him as the 'Sun King', had lived there.[9] After 1924, Schweitzer was constantly supported by at least one doctor from Europe. Consequently, he was able to dedicate himself more frequently to working on the construction site. He was particularly proud of his architectural style: one-story wooden buildings on timber piles with ribbed roofs and excellent air

5   Schweitzer, 'Mitteilungen aus Lambarene. Zweites Heft, 1924–1925', 156–61. For more on the famine see: Mabika, 'La famine dans les Nouvelles de l'hôpital Albert Schweitzer'.
6   Scholl, *Von der Ehrfurcht vor dem Leben zur transkulturellen Solidarität*, 94–98. In 1923, Schweitzer had concretely considered to establish a hospital under the auspices of the Basel Mission in Cameroon in case the PEMS would obstruct his plans in Lambaréné.
7   Gillespie to Rieder, 26 April 1924, AWHS.
8   Schweitzer to Royden, 22 February 1926, AMS.
9   Schweitzer, 'Neues von Albert Schweitzer Pfingsten 1927', 5.

circulation.[10] Another priority was the establishment of plantations, especially for plantains, which were to guarantee the institution some degree of self-sufficiency.[11] Just like the rest of the hospital, these plantations would grow considerably in both extent and variety over the years.

2 Patient Numbers: Reflecting Global and Local Events in Orderly Records

At the beginning of 1927, the whole enterprise was moved to its new location. This marks the beginning of the third phase, which would last until 1981, when the new hospital, still in use today, was opened.[12] For the purposes of this study, it is helpful to subdivide this phase. Patient numbers serve as a useful guideline. They reflect how local realities, including the presence of a large timber industry, and global events, such as the Great Depression or World War Two, influenced hospital consultations.

Schweitzer had introduced a rigorous order in his files, which was maintained during his lifetime: the 'appels mensuels'. These were consistently recorded in a similar manner throughout the study period, thus equipping the historian with a continuous set of records. In 1935, Schweitzer described the recording procedure as follows: on the last day of each month, Dominique Bouka, an African assistant who was particularly trusted, summoned the patients by their place of origin, namely from which lumber station or region they came. They then had to enter the consultation room, where all the doctors, nurses, auxiliaries and interpreters would be seated at a table, before the patients' names, places of origin and diagnoses were recorded in the books (see Illustrations 3 and 4). Many relevant issues would also be discussed, including diagnosis and care, possible date of release, ability to work, and supply of food. The whole procedure lasted for only about four hours.[13]

Figure 1 shows the total number of inpatients treated each year. There is a high degree of uncertainty for many of these numbers, primarily because of the inconsistency and irregularity of the records.[14] Figure 2 is based on the

---

10 Schweitzer, *Mitteilungen aus Lambarene. Drittes Heft, 1925–1927*, 19–27.

11 Ibid., 9–13.

12 Mabika, 'L'hôpital Albert Schweitzer de Lambaréné', 207.

13 Schweitzer, 'Briefe aus dem Lambarene Spital November 1935', 13.

14 The numbers haven been compiled with information from the following documents: 'Statistiques de l'Hôpital', L – A – S1–3, AMS; *appels mensuels*, L – P – C1–16, L – P – AM3–11, AMS; Association française des Amis d'Albert Schweitzer, 'L'activité de l'Hôpital de Lambaréné 1965', AMS.

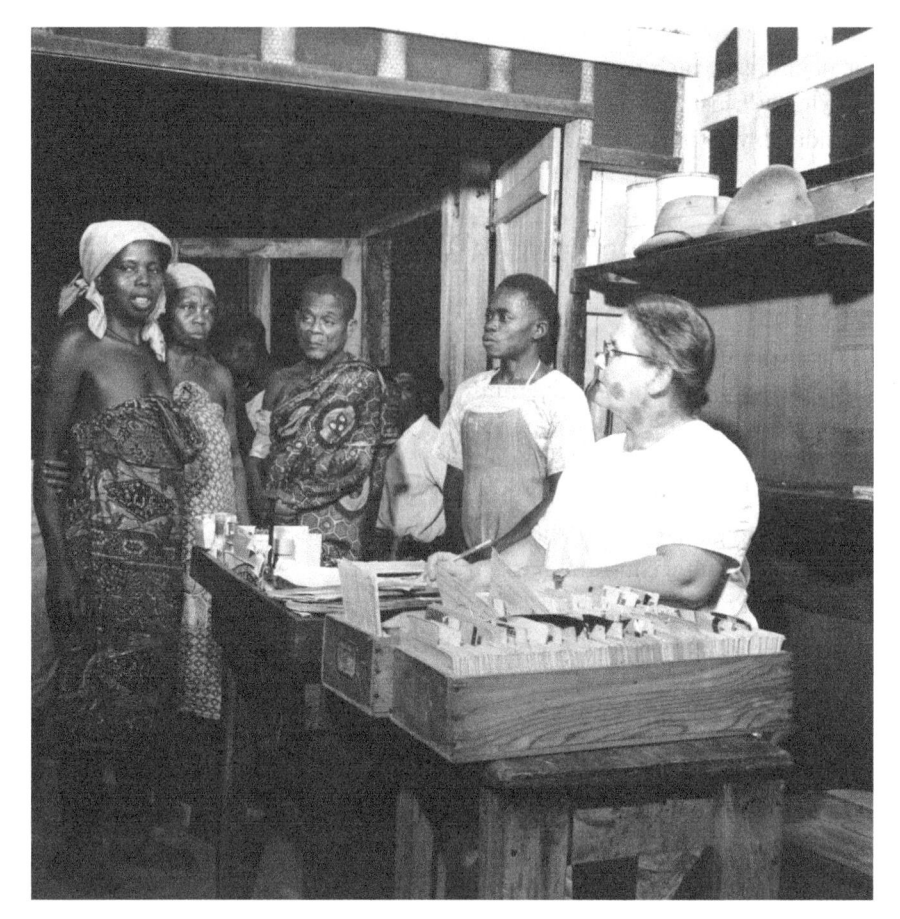

ILLUSTRATION 3   The nurse Gertrude Koch and the interpreter Auguste at the appels
                   mensuels, ca. 1950
                   © ARCHIVES CENTRALES ALBERT SCHWEITZER GUNSBACH

appels mensuels and illustrates the approximate average number of inpatients present at any moment within the year.[15] The graphs show three notable decreases in patient numbers. The first in 1930/31 has to do with the Great Depression, when numerous laborers left the region, while that from 1940 to 1943 is connected to World War Two, during which Schweitzer lost much of his funding and had to consequently turn away a considerable number of patients. The third drop, in the early 1950s, is due to a change in recordkeeping. From 1951 onwards, leprosy patients, of whom there had previously been as many as 160 on the list, were no longer recorded. The greatest influx of patients

---

15   The number for each year is the sum of the monthly figures divided by twelve.

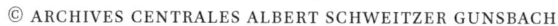

ILLUSTRATION 4   A page of the appels mensuels of 1 March 1936. Patients from maisons
were recorded separately (left side)

© ARCHIVES CENTRALES ALBERT SCHWEITZER GUNSBACH

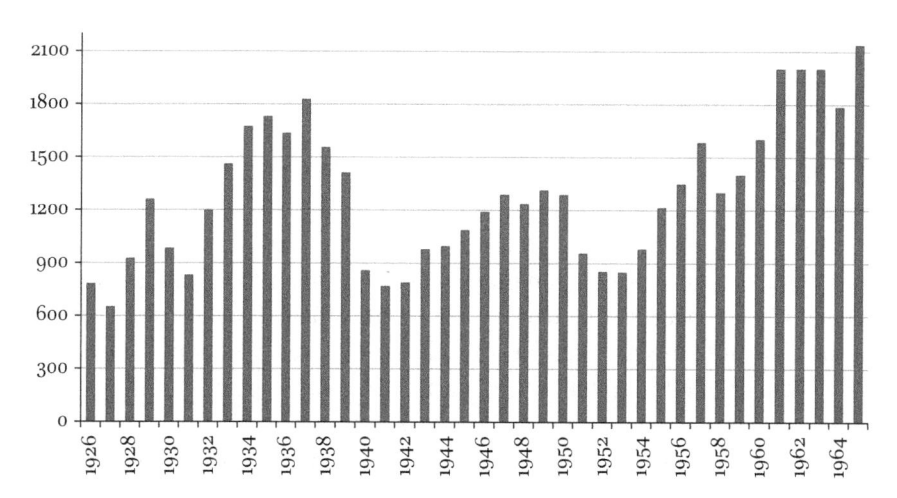

FIGURE 1   Total inpatients

only happened in the late 1950s and early 1960s, coinciding with Gabonese
Independence that started to take shape in 1958. Mabika argues that in its
wake government health services functioned less reliably.[16] Only at this point

---

16   Mabika Ognandzi, *Médicaliser l'Afrique*, 233–36.

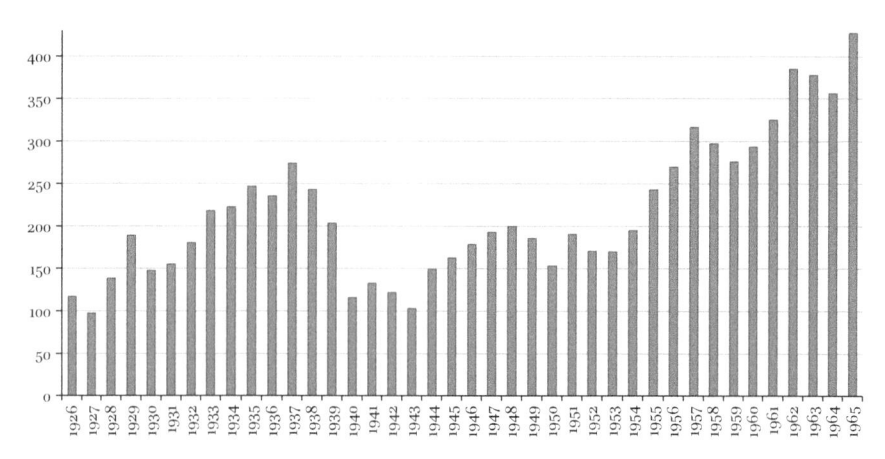

FIGURE 2   Average number of patients present

the Albert Schweitzer Hospital exceeded the initial importance that it had established for itself in the mid-1930s, at least if we judge its status solely by the numbers of patients treated.

Another major weakness of both of these graphs, and indeed of most sources, is that they do not include the outpatients. Dr. Rolf Müller claimed that in the late 1950s and early 1960s, two thirds of all patients were outpatients.[17] This suggests that they significantly increased in proportion: the statistics available for the 1930s and early 1940s indicate an outpatient percentage of between 50 and 60.[18]

Figure 3 shows the percentage of patients who came from 'maisons', sampled for every even year. *Maisons* were primarily lumber factories in the area, but also included smaller trading companies or missions.[19] These patients may have tended to stay longer than others due to the severity of their afflictions, which might constitute one reason for their disproportionate representation in the statistics. However, Rita Headrick has also observed that in the 1920s as many as half of all hospital patients in Gabon were loggers from the timber industry. This illustrates that health services were concentrated in areas of administrative or economic interest.[20] Schweitzer's hospital was no exception.

---

17   Müller, '50 Jahre Albert-Schweitzer-Spital', 4.

18   See the 'Statistiques de l'Hôpital', L – A – S1–3, AMS. The highest percentage of outpatients during this period was recorded in 1931 (1441 or 63 percent of the total). The lowest was in 1935 when 1510 outpatients made up 46 percent of all patients recorded.

19   Presumably for reasons to do with payment, the *appels* list patients from *maisons* separately.

20   Headrick, *Colonialism, Health and Illness in French Equatorial Africa*, 213.

Figure 3 reveals the profound influence of the timber industry in the surrounding region. Before the severe economic crisis of the early 1930s, between two-thirds and three-quarters of all inpatients at the hospital came from *maisons*. Thereafter, other patient groups predominated, with still an average of approximately a third of all inpatients listed as coming from *maisons*. An unsurprising drop in patient numbers occurred during World War Two, followed by a less explicable decrease in 1950. Finally, the graph shows that the rise in patients after independence was mainly due to the arrival of new categories of patients, particularly women as evidenced in Figure 4.[21] A more detailed discussion of female patients in their own right follows in Chapter 3.

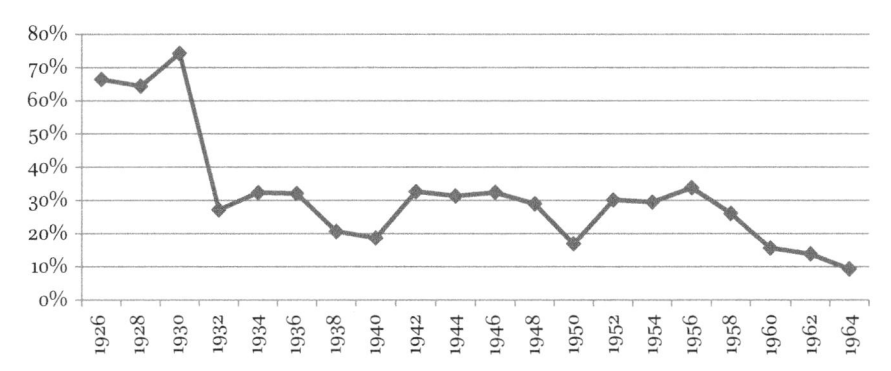

FIGURE 3   Percentage of inpatients from 'maisons'

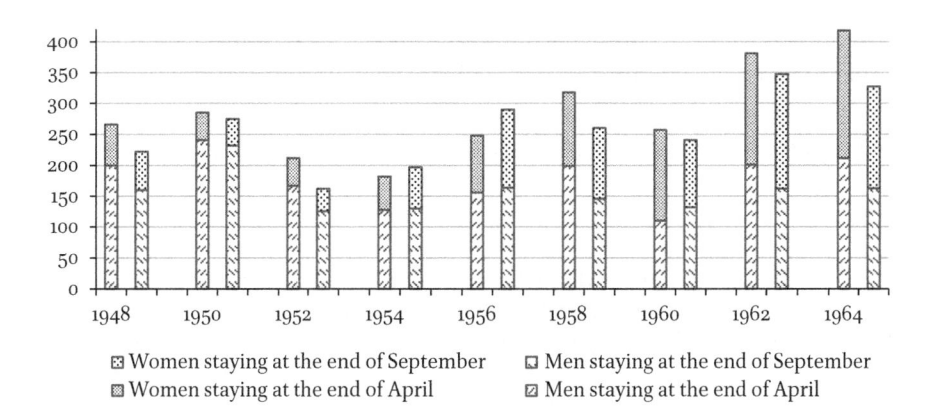

☒ Women staying at the end of September   ☐ Men staying at the end of September
▨ Women staying at the end of April   ▨ Men staying at the end of April

FIGURE 4   Gender ratio of inpatients

---

21   The data for Figure 4 is taken from the *appels mensuels* and is based on surnames; prior to 1948, these were not consistently and clearly recorded. I have sampled every even year.

3   Patients and Their Stay: Strict Conditions, Varied Degrees of Enforcement

Patients did not usually arrive at the hospital on their own, but were accompanied by family members, the 'therapy managing group'.[22] In fact, hospital rules dictated that each patient had to bring at least one 'gardien', as the staff referred to a patient's companion. These were to provide basic care, including cooking for and washing the patient. In practice, Schweitzer admitted that many patients came without their *gardiens*.[23] Indeed, the *appels mensuels* show that the number of *gardiens* present was normally between one-quarter and one-third of that of patients, while this ratio decreased slightly further towards the end of the study period. However, the appearance of *gardiens* in the sources is so consistent that it is likely that the presence of many were not recorded officially in the *appels mensuels*.

In the 1930s, patients regularly arrived by boat, some from as far afield as 500 kilometers away.[24] On arrival, they would wait with their relatives in the yard in front of the 'Grande Pharmacie', the hospital's central building (see Illustrations 5 and 6). This was a pile construction, which provided shade and shelter. After being summoned by a doctor, the patients proceeded to the consultation room.[25] At the first consultation, each patient received a ticket, a system that Schweitzer had introduced during his first stay. Patients rarely lost this small piece of cardboard and they often brought it around their neck along with a mark that the colonial government distributed to confirm the payment of the head tax.[26] Specified on this ticket were the patient's name, date of arrival, age and hometown as well as a diagnosis. The patient was assigned a number in order to be easily found in the records.[27] To facilitate patients' journey home, staff attempted to negotiate lifts with every passing boat. Moreover, departing patients were provided with food and those who had worked received a gift.[28]

Based on this data, April was most frequently the month with the highest number of patients present, September most often the one with the lowest.

22   Janzen, *The Quest for Therapy*, 4. Janzen defines the therapy managing group as 'kinsmen or their advocates' who oversee and organize the patient's illness and therapy.

23   Schweitzer, 'Briefe aus dem Lambarene Spital November 1935', 8.

24   Schweitzer, 'Briefe aus dem Lambarene Spital Juli 1933', 9.

25   Schweitzer, 'Briefe aus dem Lambarene Spital November 1935', 4.

26   Schweitzer, 'Notes et Nouvelles de la part du prof. Albert Schweitzer Lambaréné', 8.

27   Schweitzer, 'Briefe aus dem Lambarene Spital November 1935', 9.

28   Ibid., 11.

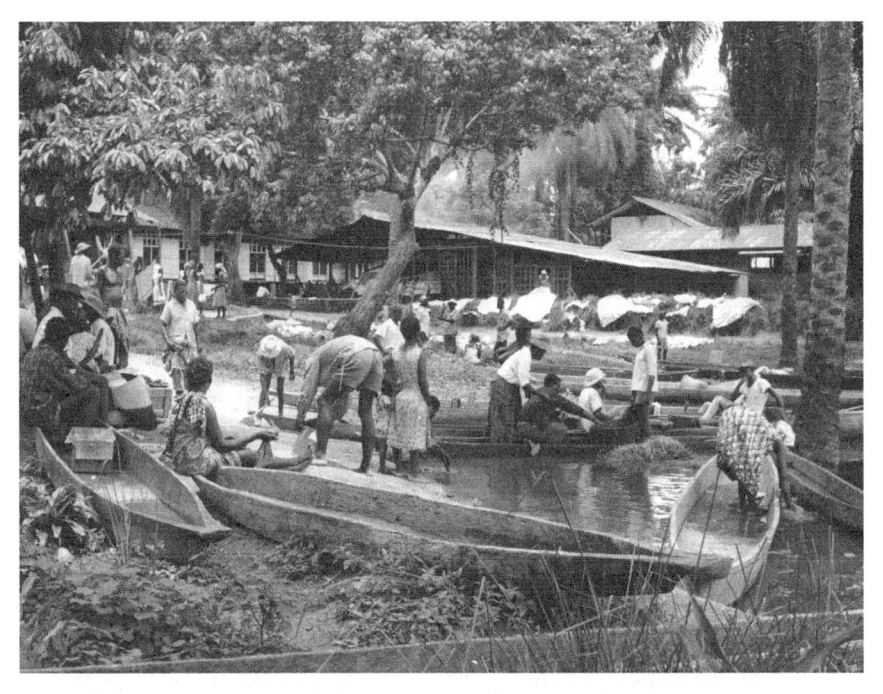

ILLUSTRATION 5   Patients and gardiens at the landing area during rainy season, late 1940s
© ARCHIVES CENTRALES ALBERT SCHWEITZER GUNSBACH

In 1925, this reportedly consisted of knifes, pots, cloth or similar items.[29] In later years, salt, linen bags and money were mentioned.[30]

Additional details about patient routines at the hospital from the early 1960s can be reconstructed through interviews.[31] On arrival, possible since 1939 by a road linking Libreville and Lambaréné, patients waited in the aforementioned yard next to a sign indicating 'new patients'. A nurse or auxiliary would then refer them to a doctor, assisted by an interpreter, in one of the three consultation rooms in the Grande Pharmacie (see Illustration 7).[32] These contained tables behind curtains. According to a long-standing schedule, operations were performed on Tuesdays, Thursdays and Saturdays. On these days, only one

---

29   Schweitzer, *Mitteilungen aus Lambarene. Drittes Heft, 1925–1927*, 7.
30   Zellweger, 'Grosskampftag im Spital', 97–98.
31   Interview Elisabeth Anderegg; Group Interview Speicherschwendi; Interview Munz and Munz; Interview Hedwig Schnee.
32   Interview Munz and Munz.

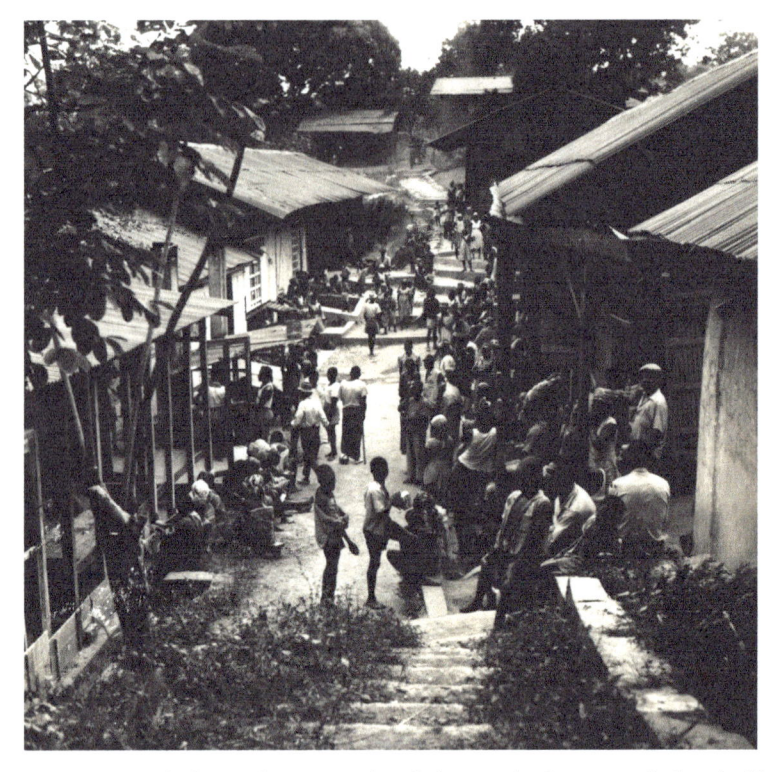

ILLUSTRATION 6   The hospital's 'main road' with the Grande Pharmacie, the long building
to the left, mid-1950s
© ARCHIVES CENTRALES ALBERT SCHWEITZER GUNSBACH

table and one doctor were available for consultations. This schedule, however, was not overly strict due to the regular demand for emergency treatments.

If it were not a patient's first consultation, he or she would present the ticket to allow the doctors to check the registers, which dated back to 1913. There was always an interpreter present, even though many patients spoke at least some French. According to Dr. Walter Munz the patient-doctor encounter of the early 1960s occurred in a typically biomedical fashion: the doctor would listen to the patient's history and eventually establish a diagnosis.[33] Recurring reports suggest that patients often expected the physician to know what was wrong with them before the consultation commenced.[34] According to the

---

33   Ibid.
34   Group Interview Speicherschwendi; Mai, *Albert Schweitzer und seine Kranken*, 11–13.

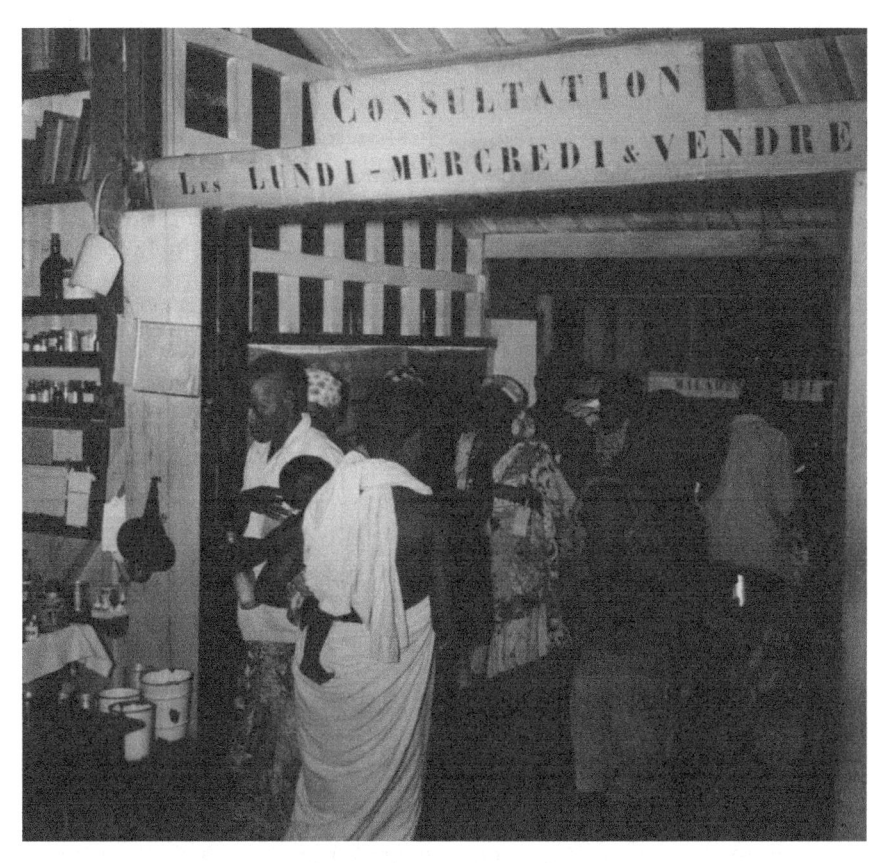

ILLUSTRATION 7   Patients at the consultation space, mid-1950s
© ARCHIVES CENTRALES ALBERT SCHWEITZER GUNSBACH

nurse Elisabeth Anderegg, in the frequent case of overtly visible conditions such as elephantiasis, ulcers and hernias, this was often easy to achieve.[35] From the doctors' perspective, patients tended to seek help when their afflictions were already too advanced, a frequently formulated complaint.[36] Eventually, the doctor would write the proposed treatment on a piece of paper. This was then handed to the patient, who was instructed to do as advised. Treatments could include, for example, taking an antibiotic for a specified number of days, visiting the injection room, or undergoing blood tests in the laboratory.[37]

---

35   Interview Elisabeth Anderegg,
36   Two examples from different periods: Cousins, *Dr. Schweitzer of Lambaréné*, 138; Schweitzer, *Mitteilungen aus Lambarene. Drittes Heft, 1925–1927*, 46.
37   Interview Munz and Munz.

The nurses from the ward to which the patient was assigned checked the ticket. Many wards maintained their own registers. After the prescribed therapy was completed, patients returned to the doctor for further consultations.[38] When patients had to take a certain medication they were ordered to go to the pharmacy with their ticket whenever the on-duty nurse or African assistant rang a bell. There they received a pill, which they had to swallow on the spot to ensure compliance with the treatment regime and because the hospital authorities wanted to make sure that the patient did not sell it.[39] The nurse Marianne Stocker recalled this to be a very impersonal process. 'It's like a factory', she noted in her diary.[40]

The hospital provided food to people coming from further than forty kilometers away (see Illustrations 8 and 9). For Schweitzer, the ideal diet for his patients consisted of manioc and plantains. In reality, often half of the food given to patients consisted of rice.[41] In the 1930s, approximately sixty kilograms of rice were distributed each day. In addition, patients received a daily portion of salt and palm oil, as well as imported dried fish on two or three occasions per week.[42] In the early 1960s, patients received alternating meals of rice and plantains and manioc or dried fish 'every now and then'.[43] Siegfried Neukirch, who worked as a mechanic at the hospital from 1959 to 1965, claimed that four to six tons of plantains were required per week, which he fetched from surrounding villages.[44] In addition, local women continued to bring agricultural produce and other goods to the hospital each Thursday.[45]

Patients were free to choose their own beds. With equipment in the quarters being sparse, they had to bring their own blankets and sheets.[46] Housing was segregated; the Galoa and the Fang had their own buildings.[47] To the proposal by Anderegg that these should be combined, Schweitzer replied: 'That doesn't work. They would kill each other'.[48] It is not clear if this segregation was

---

38 Ibid.; Group Interview Speicherschwendi.

39 Interview Elisabeth Anderegg; Interview Hedwig Schnee.

40 Stocker, 'Diary 1961–63', 20.

41 Zumthurm, 'Food at the Albert Schweitzer Hospital'.

42 Schweitzer, 'Briefe aus dem Lambarene Spital November 1935', 7–9.

43 Stocker, 'Diary 1961–63', 36.

44 Neukirch, 'Bananeneinkauf und Transporte', 41.

45 Stocker, 'Diary 1961–63', 5; Nüesch-Wohlfender, 'Hausfrauliches', 156.

46 Cousins, *Dr. Schweitzer of Lambaréné*, 92; Interview Hedwig Schnee.

47 Østergaard Christensen, *At Work with Albert Schweitzer*, 45; Siefert, *Meine Arbeitsjahre in Lambarene 1933–1935*, 178.

48 Interview Elisabeth Anderegg. This is one of the few points on which Audoynaud agrees with Schweitzer. Like Schweitzer, he argues that the different ethnic groups were very suspicious of each other. Ethnic segregation was thus not an innovation, he contends, but

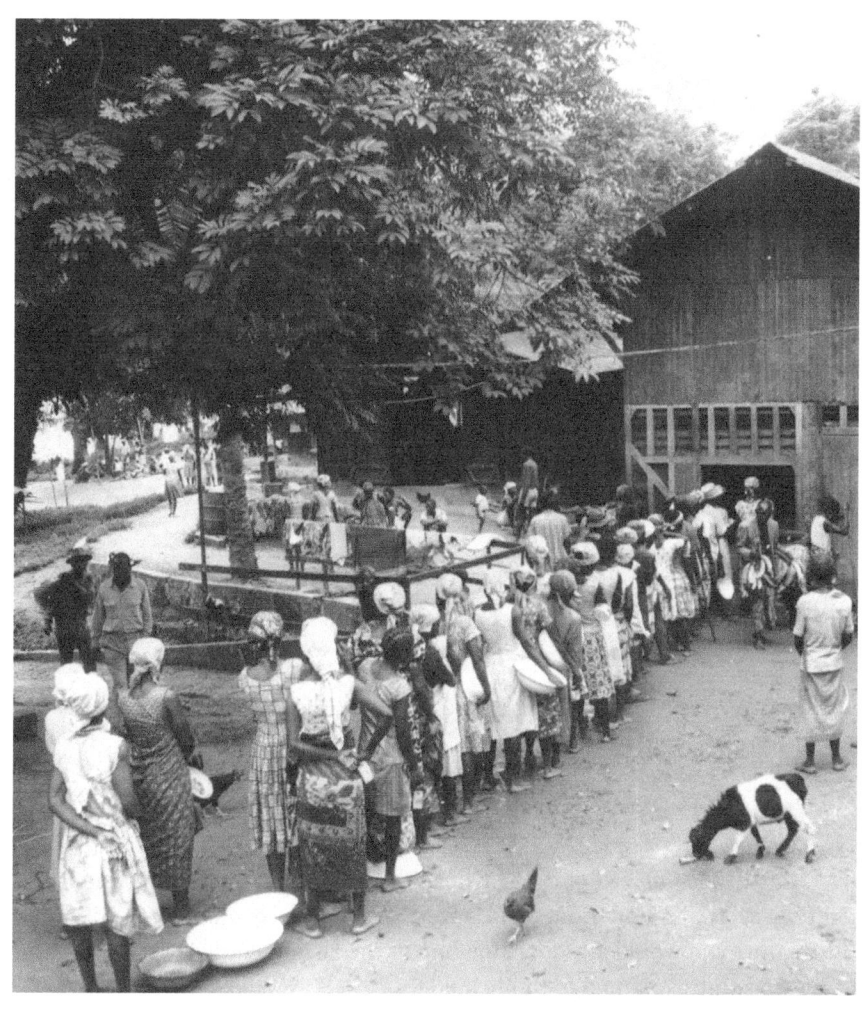

ILLUSTRATION 8   Patients or gardiens collecting their ration of food, mid-1950s
© ARCHIVES CENTRALES ALBERT SCHWEITZER GUNSBACH

intentionally ordered or if it was the outcome of patients' free choice of beds. The fact that Schweitzer had not mentioned maintaining different buildings for different groups in his otherwise very detailed description of the new hospital in 1927 hints towards the latter.[49] In any case, five years later, segregation

the inevitable result of the practical realities. See: Audoynaud, *Le docteur Schweitzer et son hôpital à Lambaréné*, 206.

49   Schweitzer, *Mitteilungen aus Lambarene. Drittes Heft, 1925–1927*, 51–53.

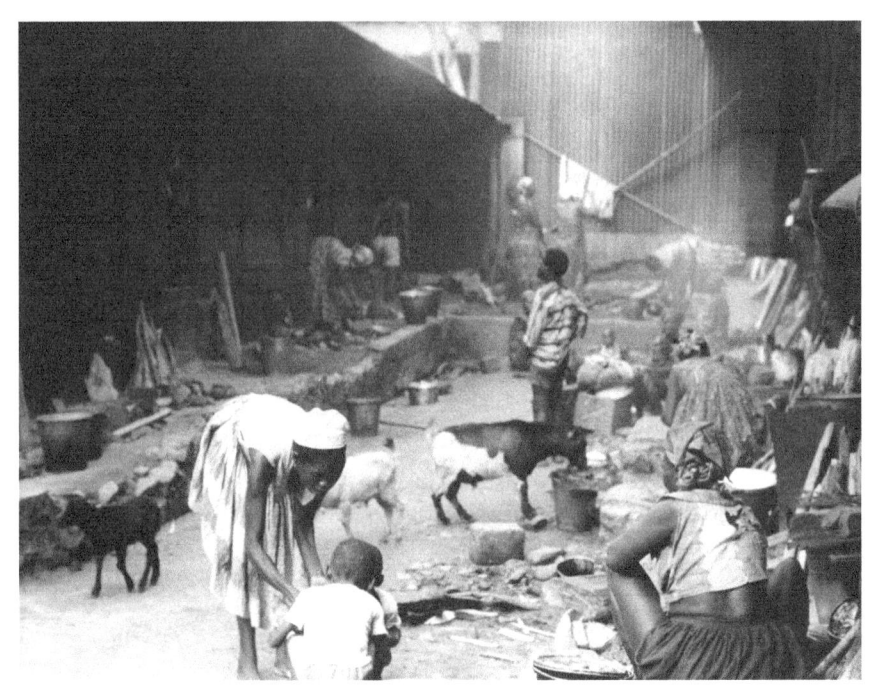

ILLUSTRATION 9   Patients or gardiens cooking their meals behind the sleeping quarters, mid-1950s
© ARCHIVES CENTRALES ALBERT SCHWEITZER GUNSBACH

had already become evident.[50] The hospital did adapt to patients' demands in relation to accommodation, as a letter dating from 1929 suggests. Mathilde Kottmann, who would later become one of the key individuals in the running of the hospital, explained to Emily Rieder:

> Two of the six hospital buildings house patients only, natives. Some of these buildings are even equipped a little more comfortably for the notables of the Galoas, who often refused to reside in the hospital because they could not be accommodated according to their status due to lack of space.[51]

---

50   I found this particular reference in a government report on Schweitzer's hospital: 'Rapport Annuel du Service de Santé de la Colonie du Gabon 1932', ZK 005–127, SHD. Schweitzer himself first mentioned this arrangement in the 1940s. See: Schweitzer, *Das Spital im Urwald: Aufnahmen von Anna Wildikann*, 15.

51   Kottmann to Rieder, 13 March 1929, AWHS.

Treatment had to be paid for according to each patient's means. In this manner, Schweitzer hoped to ensure their gratitude. In 1931, he stated that he was satisfied when one-quarter or one-fifth of the expenses was covered. While he asked for twenty *régimes* of plantains and the presence of two workers during a patient's stay to cover the costs of an operation, he often had to be satisfied with only five *régimes* and a single worker. A patient who could not pay was treated free of charge.[52] The Gabonese I interviewed reformulated this. They insisted that treatment at the hospital was 'gratis'. In their view, a patient did not have to pay, but gave a 'gift' or 'donation' in the form of fruit or chicken, for which Schweitzer showed his gratitude, saying 'thank you'.[53] Emane reports a similar attitude among his informants.[54]

Everyone staying at the hospital, who was sufficiently fit, was expected to work. This included *gardiens*, but also recovering patients or those with minor illnesses. Jobs were gendered and work was constantly supervised by European doctors or nurses. Each Saturday at 2 p.m., every woman who was able to work was ordered to clean the hospital grounds. This procedure often continued until dusk. Waste was dumped into the river.[55] Daily tasks were assigned before breakfast. At least six people were sent to gather wood from the forest, which was being rapidly denuded and had already been pushed back to a half hour's walk away by the mid-1930s. One man was responsible for cutting this wood for the entire day. Others were assigned to the task of constructing new buildings. A dozen women were instructed to do the hospital's laundry. They had to wash bandages and hospital clothing as well as the clothes and bedding of European staff. Four women prepared palm oil from nuts gathered by two men, separating the oily mass from the kernels, which were later exchanged for rice.[56] The compulsory gathering of palm nuts evoked painful memories in the area. During some of the interwar period, local residents who were unable to pay taxes to the French authorities were forced to collect palm nuts under a forced labor regime.[57] Forced labor was also not uncommon at the hospital itself. For

---

52   Albert Schweitzer, 'Le secours médical aux colonies' in *Revue des Deux Mondes September 1931*. Cited in: Sorg, *Schweitzer, le médecin*, 39–40.

53   Group Interview Port-Gentil; Interview Daudette Azizet Mburu; Interview Jacques Boucah; Interview Anne-Marie Padje-Poabalou. More details and personal information on these interviewees follow in the subsequent chapters, when their individual stories contribute to the analysis of specific issues.

54   Emane, *Docteur Schweitzer: une icône africaine*, 117–18.

55   Schweitzer, 'Briefe aus dem Lambarene Spital November 1935', 12.

56   Ibid., 3.

57   Gray, *Colonial Rule and Crisis in Equatorial Africa*, 182.

example, the nurse Marie Woytt-Secretan described the process of producing palm oil in great detail:

> If the women had been left to themselves, they would have gone up and away in the first unguarded moment, taking the oil with them. To prevent this, Doctor Schweitzer had built a large wire cage into which they were let in the morning with everything they needed to prepare the oil: Palm nuts, wood, water, kettles, etc. Then the cage was locked, and the sister did not have to check the work again until noon and let the workers out.[58]

Such drastic forms of supervision are frequently described in the sources, affecting not only workers but also patients. For the latter, this usually occurred in conjunction with a specific medical treatment. In 1926, for example, patients with intestinal worms were given thymol, which interacts dangerously with any kind of oil. Patients were suspected of not adhering to this dietary restriction; they were summarily confined behind bars. This measure had little effect: friends secretly brought them oily palm nuts.[59] In 1935, Schweitzer reported that Dominique Bouka summoned patients to their injections with a cow bell. As their number was considerable and the waiting period often lengthy, to reduce patients' temptation to spend their time elsewhere, they were locked in a barred area in front of the consultation room, from where they were fetched one after another.[60] In 1939, Schweitzer proudly reported a new treatment for worms derived from chenopodium oil. To mitigate the risk that it could 'cause fatal bowel inflammation if the necessary precautions are not strictly adhered to', he ordered that the 'patients, large and small, are kept locked in a spacious wire mesh cage in front of the consultation room, so that they are under constant supervision'.[61] Thereafter, reports of detention decrease.[62] This might be due to the spread of more progressive attitudes, but may also be the result of the introduction of antibiotics. Further details on pharmaceutical treatment and confinement can be found in Chapter 4.

Such severe measures encouraged resistance. Instances of undesirable patient behavior frequently surface in the sources. Besides the theft of equipment,

---

58   Woytt-Secretan, *Albert Schweitzer baut Lambarene*, 71. She served as a nurse from 1929 to 1931.

59   Schweitzer, 'Neues von Albert Schweitzer Februar 1925', 5.

60   Albert Schweitzer, Schweitzer, 'Briefe aus dem Lambarene Spital November 1935', 4f.

61   Albert Schweitzer, Schweitzer, 'Briefe aus dem Lambarene Spital Februar 1939', 3f.

62   With the exception of 1948, when patients with amoebic dysentery were isolated in a house with a barred yard: Schweitzer, *Das Spital im Urwald: Aufnahmen von Anna Wildi-kann*, 13.

such as nets or bedding, a main concern throughout the study period was that patients did not rest enough.[63] For example, some would go bathing in the river on the same day on which they were due to undergo an operation.[64] Others left the hospital in the middle of a treatment that they viewed as hopeless, choosing instead to return to their villages.[65] When Stocker went on a Sunday stroll in 1961, she met tuberculosis patients who had been prescribed strict bed rest. Their excuse was straightforward: it was a Sunday.[66]

4   Patient Motivation: Conceptions of Health and Other Treatments

Patients too were rather pragmatic in their approach towards their health and their selection of therapy. When asked about why patients would choose to go to the Albert Schweitzer Hospital, the answer given by my Gabonese interviewees was usually straightforward: it simply was the best hospital in Gabon, providing care that was patently superior to that offered in any government clinic.[67] Included in this conception of superior care was the provision of food to patients and the opportunity for them to cook it themselves, as was the possibility of being accompanied by friends and family.[68] Emane's informants confirm the centrality of food and cooking.[69] Bringing companions relates to Emane's repeated claim that the hospital was valued locally because it did not simply treat the sick body; people there acknowledged that patients were human beings in their own right. Indeed, the 'humanity' exuded by the hospital and its staff is constantly underlined throughout his book.[70] Similarly, most of my interviewees recalled the warm 'reception' that they received at the hospital.[71] Ngouawiri Suzanne Rembendambja, one of the few former patients to whom I was able to talk, recounted that when she was sent to the hospital by her father in 1954, 'ah ... it was the loving reception, really that has cured me'.[72]

---

63   Haussknecht, *Emma Haussknecht, 1895–1956*, 111; Barthélemy, *Wie ich Lambarene erlebte*, 52.

64   In 1937, Schweitzer reported that this had been a regular occurrence throughout the hospital's history. See: Schweitzer, 'Briefe aus dem Lambarene Spital Mai 1937', 3.

65   Group Interview Speicherschwendi.

66   Stocker, 'Diary 1961–63', 16.

67   Interview Jacques Boucah; Interview Jacques-Adrien Rolagho.

68   Interview Albert Bouassa; Interview Jacques Boucah; Interview Jacques-Adrien Rolagho.

69   Emane, *Docteur Schweitzer: une icône africaine*, 44.

70   Ibid., 47, 177–80, 217.

71   Interview Daudette Azizet Mburu; Interview Marie-Joséphine Ndiaye-Boucah; Interview Léontine Nsowe; Interview Jacques-Adrien Rolagho.

72   Group Interview Port-Gentil.

Readers of historical studies on colonial hospitals will have found many familiar issues in this examination of patient routines. Two themes are worthy of further emphasis. Firstly, it has long been observed that hospitals in Africa were often more open than their Western counterparts in permitting patients relatives or friends to stay with them for a prolonged period of time.[73] This seems to be especially true for mission hospitals.[74] The reasoning behind this approach was twofold. On the one hand, such openness and permeability were demanded from the therapy managing group and thus represented a precondition for luring patients to the hospital in the first place. On the other hand, companions provided basic nursing services that were often necessary given the lack of personnel in colonial hospitals. In Kalene Hospital in early-twentieth-century Zambia, this went so far that companions constructed the huts in which patients were accommodated.[75] Schweitzer's insistence on manual labor and 'handicraft', as well as his demand that everyone at the hospital be put to work, are traces of the institution's missionary context. Chapter 5 explains the peculiar ideology that lay behind this approach.

Another issue that has been raised in this overview is the prevalence of medical pluralism in Gabon, an attitude that persists in both urban and rural settings today.[76] Mabika argues that it only emerged after the colonial introduction of biomedicine and hospitals.[77] Elsewhere on the continent, especially in regions where Islam was present, it remains unclear to what degree medical pluralism had already been a precolonial phenomenon.[78] Many colonial doctors were aware of the fact that their patients regularly used a variety of different treatments.[79] John Janzen has famously observed great pluralism in very few cases in postcolonial Congo.[80] Ever since, the issue has attracted the attention of historians. Julie Livingston, for instance, provided an insightful

---

73   Feierman and Janzen, 'The Social Basis of Health and Healing in Africa, Introduction', 18.

74   These have also been the more frequent subject of historical research than government hospitals; they might have better preserved records. Examples of studies that mention patients' relatives staying at the hospital: Debusmann, 'Médicalisation et pluralisme au Cameroun allemand', 237–38; Pringle, 'Neurasthenia at Mengo Hospital, Uganda', 243; Ranger, 'Godly Medicine', 271; and one for a government context: Havik, 'Reconsidering Indigenous Health', 246.

75   Kalusa, 'Missionaries, African Patients, and Negotiating Missionary Medicine', 289.

76   Ebang, 'De la diversité des itinéraires thérapeutiques au Gabon'.

77   Mabika, 'Médicalisation de l'Afrique centrale', 436.

78   Dirar, 'Curing Bodies to Rescue Souls'; Iliffe, *East African Doctors*, 12; Olumwullah, *Dis-Ease in the Colonial State*, 11.

79   Debusmann, 'Médicalisation et pluralisme au Cameroun allemand', 237; Bado, 'Histoire, maladies et médecines en Afrique Occidentale', 256.

80   Janzen, *The Quest for Therapy*, 150.

expansion of the notion by examining 'productive misunderstandings', thereby increasing our understanding of how different medical systems operated together.[81] The idea of medical pluralism, and indeed of medical systems themselves, has been widely criticized and refined.[82] A central critique is that definitions are often imprecise and/or too broad.[83] Walter Bruchhausen points out that this represents a genuine conceptual contradiction. Pluralism, he argues, 'refers to diversity as a necessity and claims to describe some unifying aspect. Thus at one and the same time it emphasises and denies the worth of a single concept'.[84]

Outside of the Western world, illness has usually not been considered accidental.[85] As Vansina, posits for Central Africa, 'illness was the quintessential manifestation of abnormality and abnormality always resulted from the neglect of spirits or attacks by witches'.[86] In the case of the Fang of Gabon for the period around 1960, James Fernandez insists that 'any illness could be attributed to the maleficence of unseen forces', but that it could also be seen to be caused by 'contagion, worms, or accident'.[87] Specialists thus had to be consulted to clarify the exact cause.[88]

The most prominent of these specialists was the 'Nganga'. According to sociologist Bernadin Mve Minko, a *Nganga* possessed a versatile set of tools. 'He

---

81   Livingston, 'Productive Misunderstandings'.

82   Stacey Langwick instead calls for a deeper analysis that 'looks at the times and ways that healers, clinical practitioners, government bureaucrats, medical scientists, and patients implicate the modern in the traditional, the clinic in the home of the healer, science in the nonbiomedical, and vice versa'. In: Langwick, *Bodies, Politics, and African Healing*, 236. On the questioning of systems, see most famously: Last, 'The Importance of Knowing about Not Knowing'.

83   Waltraud Ernst, for instance, provides two definitions of medical pluralism, with the second more or less foregoing Langwick's call (see above footnote): (1) 'a variety of medial approaches existing alongside each other, at times in competition and at times in collaboration with or complementary to each other'. (2): 'the plural or multi-dimensional qualities inherent in medical practices and experiences, as these draw on and are open to different approaches, are "bastardised" or hybridised, syncretic, and versatile'. Ernst, *Plural Medicine, Tradition and Modernity*, 8.

84   Bruchhausen, 'Medical Pluralism as a Historical Phenomenon', 100.

85   Last, 'Non-Western Concepts of Disease', 642.

86   Vansina, *Paths in the Rainforests*, 98.

87   Fernandez, *Bwiti*, 190–91.

88   Ibid., 194. Fernandez identifies the *Ngungan* and the *Nsônkngang*. In his glossary, he defines the former as a '"doctor", person powerful in the knowledge of hidden things, also a courageous one in dealing with the demon'. The entry for the latter is: 'he who searches out hidden things, "doctor" of powerful revelation'. Fernandez further states that the *Nsônkngang* is more powerful but, having been targeted by the colonial authorities as a 'diviner', is now rarely found. Ibid., 222.

knew magical practices: knowledge of plants, access to spirits, to ancestors and to prophylactic formulas', Minko writes. These corresponded to his broad responsibilities. A *Nganga* 'relieved human and physical misery and addressed the problems between the individual and his environment'. His expertise centered on his knowledge of the '*Tout Autre*' and his ability to interpret the 'diverse levels of reality'.[89] In his study on the Nkomi, a group that, like the Galoa, speaks the Myene language but lives further west, François Gaulme notes that 'any operation related to the supernatural can be within the domain of the oganga and also require his intervention'.[90] These accounts illustrate the difficulty to provide an accurate definition of what constitutes a *Nganga* without using European categories that are based on a separation of different levels of reality. As indicated in the Introduction, Gabonese did not necessarily make such a separation. For them, the invisible, for instance in the form of spirits, was an inherent part of Nature's reality.

Gaulme, who conducted his ethnological research in the 1970s, observes that descriptions of *Nganga* from late-sixteenth-century documents did not differ much from those found in studies written during his own lifetime. He further underlines that the *Nganga* did not necessarily remain in one village or treat only patients from his or her own ethnic group.[91] In their book from 1962, Sillans and Raponda-Walker emphasized that *Ngangas* could be found in any ethnic group. According to them, the term had two meanings. The first was simply 'the one who makes a profession of caring for people' and explicitly included European doctors. The second related to '*occult practices* – such as divination, magic'. According to the authors, most *Ngangas* combine these two roles in one person. As such, they are 'the intermediary between the visible world and the invisible world'.[92]

In some of these accounts, another actor, more loosely defined, is present as a counterpart to the *Nganga*: the 'sorcerer',[93] 'witch',[94] or 'spellcaster'.[95] As

---

89   Minko Mve, *Gabon entre tradition et post-modernité*, 136–37. Minko Mve's spelling is 'Nguegan'. Italics in the original.

90   Gaulme, *Le pays de Cama*, 209.

91   Ibid.

92   Sillans and Raponda-Walker provided the following spellings: *Ngang* or *Uganga* in Fang; *Oganga* in Myene; and *Nganga* in Eshira, Mitsogo and many other languages. They insisted that *Ngangas* did not practice witchcraft, but instead used their powers to find out if a particular affliction was provoked by witchcraft. See: Raponda-Walker and Sillans, *Rites et croyances des peuples du Gabon*, 32–33. Italics in the original.

93   Minko Mve, *Gabon entre tradition et post-modernité*, 139. His French term is 'sorcier'.

94   Fernandez, *Bwiti*, 222.

95   Raponda-Walker and Sillans, *Rites et croyances des peuples du Gabon*, 33. They use the term 'jeteurs de sorts'.

discussed in the Introduction, more recent research on the region generally insists on the impossibility of separating the spheres of religion, politics, and medicine. As a result, the two figures are usually grouped together. Hines Mabika suggests that there was a variety of *Ngangas*, with some specializing in different areas.[96] Their overall aim, however, was to 'prevent evil or disease, in the form of disrupted life-force balances, or in the form of a separation between the normal and the pathological'.[97] Florence Bernault highlights in the case of the French Congo that the dichotomy between 'banganga (fetisher)' and 'bandoki (sorcerer)' has seldom stood up to scrutiny. Instead, it was a colonial construction with its roots in the politics of the day.[98]

After this discussion of treatments options one is tempted to conclude that good health according to local conceptions depended on an 'equilibrium',[99] a 'wholeness',[100] a 'general integrity of feeling and thought in human affairs'.[101] Janzen suggests that the unwillingness of biomedical practitioners to explore the social and personal contexts of disease accordingly reinforced 'the popular image of Western medicine's limited competence'.[102] However, various scholars remind us of the 'harming' side of African healing.[103] It was not necessarily 'benign and benevolent' for everyone involved.[104] This view is supported by the indistinctiveness of what were considered the destructive 'sorcerer' and the constructive 'fetisher' from above. I will discuss these themes in more detail in Chapter 5.

To return to the issue of pluralism it is instructive to ask when patients would seek to consult the *Nganga*. Mabika, writing of the pre-colonial era, highlights that patients would try to treat themselves or consult family members before going to the *Nganga*.[105] During colonial times, Minko argues the *Nganga* remained the final option, being consulted only after the biomedical doctor.[106] In our sources, however, there are abundant reports of patients having undergone earlier treatments. In any case, it might be misleading to distinguish between an African *Nganga* and a European physician. For Emane, it is

---

96   Mabika Ognandzi, *Médicaliser l'Afrique*, 81–82.
97   Mabika, 'Médicalisation de l'Afrique centrale', 94.
98   Bernault, 'De la modernité comme impuissance'.
99   Mabika Ognandzi, *Médicaliser l'Afrique*, 85.
100 Vansina, *Paths in the Rainforests*, 328.
101 Fernandez, *Bwiti*, 192.
102 Janzen, *The Quest for Therapy*, 215.
103 Hunt, 'Health and Healing'.
104 Vaughan, 'Healing and Curing', 293. See also: Bernault and Tonda, 'Dynamiques de l'invisible en Afrique'.
105 Mabika, 'Médicalisation de l'Afrique centrale', 408.
106 Minko Mve, *Gabon entre tradition et post-modernité*, 138.

obvious that Schweitzer was considered to be an *Nganga*; there were many similarities. Just like a *Nganga*, Schweitzer trained successors, played music and was attached to a specific location.[107] Schweitzer asserted that locals called him *Nganga* during his first stay.[108] Munz also claims to have been addressed as *Nganga*,[109] which suggests that the term was applied broadly. Such congruities or 'productive misunderstandings' are important to understand why Gabonese would choose the Albert Schweitzer Hospital for treatment.

Another point concerning the acceptance of new medical treatments is worth bearing in mind when asking why people came to the hospital. 'Proof of efficacy is less important than efficacy itself. New ideas can be adopted not because they are logical or even consistent, but because they appear to work', as Murray Last argues.[110] For this reason, Gabonese continued to consult local *Ngangas*, but also took advantage of newly available hospital facilities.[111] Headrick argues that the case of Schweitzer's hospital proves how perceptively patients could evaluate the quality of care that they received and their chances of recovery.[112] Emane agrees, contending that no Gabonese expected Schweitzer and his staff to 'treat everything', but rather that they would be able to cure a specific set of diseases.[113] In this regard, it is important to note that when I enquired about 'traditional medicine', almost all of my informants, African or European, strongly denied the existence of any alternative practices within the hospital's premises. This absence is similarly apparent in the written sources. Occasional cases, however, illustrate that medical pluralism was practiced.

Furthermore, medical options shared similarities in how they dealt with the sick, as is evident in specific examples throughout this book: autopsies resemble surgeries; a pregnant woman's voyage away from her village may lead to either her mother's home or a hospital; herbal remedies are applied like biomedical drugs against infectious diseases, and community care for the mentally ill is found in hospitals and villages alike.

A brief comparison between hospital treatments and those offered by *Ombwiri* serves to further illustrate this point. For Myene speakers, *Imbwiri* were 'fairies', 'ghosts', or 'functional spirits' that resembled humans.[114] They were associated with a specific location and could cause physical diseases. They could

---

107   Emane, *Docteur Schweitzer: une icône africaine*, 65–69.
108   Schweitzer, *Zwischen Wasser und Urwald*, 36. Schweitzer's spelling of the term is 'Oganga'.
109   Munz, *Albert Schweitzer im Gedächtnis der Afrikaner und in meiner Erinnerung*, 216.
110   Last, 'Non-Western Concepts of Disease', 648.
111   Mabika, 'Médicalisation de l'Afrique centrale', 417.
112   Headrick, *Colonialism, Health and Illness in French Equatorial Africa*, 401.
113   Emane, *Docteur Schweitzer: une icône africaine*, 128.
114   Swiderski, 'L'Ombwiri', 128–29.

be pacified through the *Ombwiri* ceremony, which was widely practiced among most ethnic groups of the region by the 1960s. This ceremony, which has frequently been referred to as the 'hospital' by scholars and their informants, was clearly therapeutic in scope.[115] Its leaders, the majority of whom were women, were usually former patients. It was not unusual for nurses from a biomedical hospital to participate. The ritual had to be paid. Purification occurred in a very tangible manner in which cleanliness was paramount: the diseased was bathed; freshly laundered sheets were spread on the walls and pillars; and purgatives were administered, sometimes forcibly, including psychedelic substances from iboga and herbal medication. *Ombwiri* also targeted the health of the whole family; relatives were thus present during the ceremony.[116] Parallels to practices in biomedical hospitals in general and Schweitzer's hospital in particular are immediately identifiable: African biomedical personnel had often first stayed as patients, hygiene was important in most units, and family members were allowed to accompany patients. The degree of interaction between these two and other healing institutions would merit further research, but is beyond the scope of this study.

5 Staff from Europe: Clear Guidelines and Flexible Duties

In August 1935, Schweitzer described a typical day at his hospital in his *Letters from Lambaréné Hospital*, regular leaflets he compiled for his supporters in Europe.[117] This very detailed account offers a window into what he pictured as the ideal organizational structure for his institution. While clearly focused on the role of European staff, his discussion of their various duties provides a useful overview of the frequency of certain diseases and the workload in different wards.

Employees from Europe usually committed themselves to staying a term of two and a half years. At the time of Schweitzer's account, three doctors were practicing at the hospital; this had not always been the case, however, as for some months in 1933 only one physician had been present.[118] Schweitzer himself did not practice anymore. One doctor was responsible for European

---

115   Fernandez, *Bwiti*, 595; Mary, 'L'alternative de la vision et de la possession', 299; Swiderski, 'L'Ombwiri', 130.

116   Fernandez, *Bwiti*, 595–99; Swiderski, 'L'Ombwiri'.

117   The nurse Siefert also offers a detailed description, but focuses more on Schweitzer. Any further discrepancies between her account and that of Schweitzer's are minor. See: Siefert, *Meine Arbeitsjahre in Lambarene 1933–1935*, 56–60.

118   Ibid., 56. See also 'Statistique de l'Hôpital 1933', L – A – S2, AMS.

patients, psychiatric patients, urological cases and, most importantly, performing the main surgical work and keeping the pharmacy in order. Another doctor focused on cases of leprosy, sleeping sickness, tuberculosis and foot ulcers, while additionally overseeing women in childbirth and patients requiring regular injections. The third doctor also carried out surgery and supervised all bandaging procedures and dysentery patients.[119] These roles were not fixed, but flexibly assigned to the doctors present according to their abilities and preferences and in view of the diseases that were most prevalent at any given time. A close reading of Schweitzer's account reveals that the doctors' roles varied even within the same week. For example, each doctor was responsible for the pre-breakfast rounds on different days.[120]

According to Schweitzer's ideal schedule, the day would continue with consultations and new registrations from 8 a.m.[121] Each doctor, who would be accompanied by an interpreter, would summon their patients from the outside waiting area. A compulsory one-hour siesta followed the lunch break. Afternoons were ideally reserved to treat critically ill patients. Doctors were encouraged to discuss their work extensively amongst themselves and thus, when possible, joined their colleagues on their evening rounds. At 7 p.m. all Europeans dined together, after which prayers were held. One and a half hours later, the evening bell signaled silence for the rest of the night. This brief overview suggests that a collegial atmosphere and mutual understanding among staff, what we call 'Lambaréné Spirit', was essential.[122]

All European nurses were female until Schweitzer's death. From 1925 to 1965, roughly 20 percent of all physicians were women.[123] Initially, Schweitzer considered European women to be unfit for equatorial conditions, but soon changed his mind. He claimed that 'Blacks are at their command'; they were 'under the spell of female kindness', which nurses 'united with male knowledge'. Hence, they served them 'out of a desire to demonstrate their dedication to them'.[124]

---

119   Schweitzer, 'Briefe aus dem Lambarene Spital November 1935', 5.

120   Ibid., 2.

121   For the whole account, see: Schweitzer, 'Briefe aus dem Lambarene Spital November 1935'.

122   Mabika Ognandzi, Steinke, and Zumthurm, *Schweitzer's Lambaréné: A Hospital in Colonial Africa*.

123   These rather tentative calculations and observations are based on the following list of employees. However, this list is undoubtedly imprecise and incomplete: http://schweitzer.org/2012/de/lambarene/mitarbeiter-1913-1965 (This site no longer exists. The author possesses a copy of the list). The table lists forty-one doctors for the period from 1925 to 1965.

124   Albert Schweitzer, 'Le secours médical aux colonies', *Revue des Deux Mondes September 1931*. Cited in: Sorg, *Schweitzer, le médecin*, 34.

Schweitzer's confidence in his female staff was so great that, during the dry season of 1931, Dr. Anna Schmitz and Emma Haussknecht were sent on a 'medical excursion in jungle and savannah'. Guided by ten African porters, they visited approximately 200 villages, covering 300 kilometers on water and 800 kilometers on foot over a period of two months.[125] Swiss doctor Karl Hediger went on a similar but smaller tour in 1929, treating roughly one hundred patients.[126] Schweitzer had long envisioned having an itinerant doctor on constant duty in the surrounding regions in order to see patients in their villages.[127] However, besides the occasional visit on lumber camps and mission stations these plans were never realized, with those tours remaining exceptions.

Three of the eight nurses performed only medical duties. Flexibility and adherence to the Lambaréné Spirit were expected from nurses too. One worked in the operating theater, sterilized dressings, and monitored the African washwomen. A second nurse also assisted the surgeons, bandaged patients who had undergone operations, and cared for European patients. A third nurse worked in the consultation room, distributed medication, and was responsible for the care of mothers and newborn children as well as critically ill patients across all quarters. A fourth nurse dressed ulcers, cared for psychiatric patients, supervised African women who manufactured palm oil, and was in charge of the purchase and distribution of food. The other four nurses were responsible for housekeeping and food preparation, including one who mainly oversaw workers in maintaining the plantations.[128]

The same individuals could take on more than one of these roles during their time in Lambaréné. Throughout the study period, staff had to be highly flexible, both within and outside of the medical domain. The nurse Gertrud Koch, for example, was disappointed when she was assigned the role of working in the kitchen in 1929.[129] Later, she received the additional task of looking after European patients. This must have satisfied her as she returned to Lambaréné four times until 1952.[130] The nurse Emma Ott arrived in January 1937. In addition to kitchen and gardening duties, she also had to take care of the chickens and ducks. She was one of the few staff to voice dissatisfaction with her role. 'Because I don't know anything about it, I have no love for it', she wrote.[131]

125 Schweitzer, 'Briefe aus dem Lambarene Spital November 1931'. This volume is dedicated solely to the tour.
126 Hediger to Schweitzer, 9 August 1929, AMS.
127 Schweitzer, 'Neues von Albert Schweitzer März 1925', 2.
128 Schweitzer, 'Briefe aus dem Lambarene Spital November 1935', 6.
129 Koch, 'Lieber grand Docteur!', 165.
130 Schweitzer, 'Briefe aus dem Lambarene Spital März 1930', 4.
131 Ott, 'Kleine Steine im grossen Mosaik', 106.

It is important to underline once again that this organizational structure was an ideal. In practice, the hospital was run on a much more flexible basis, and the composition and number of personnel varied greatly. For the staff, flexibility remained one of Schweitzer's most persistent demands. In Chapter 3, I discuss how this influenced the recruitment process for both African and European obstetric personnel. In general, however, there was a trend towards specialization at the hospital. In the 1960s, nurses were tasked with a less diverse range of duties and were responsible for more specialized units, such as psychiatry or pediatrics, which until the late 1950s had often been one of the many responsibilities for an individual nurse. However, personnel still had to display a high degree of flexibility. They were often moved around between different roles and had to be willing to work in non-medical domains.

Before they started their work, new staff were rather informally shown around the different wards and given a taste of the various tasks that needed to be completed at the hospital, a process that could last up to a week.[132] They were then introduced to their specific role, usually by their predecessors.[133] Thereafter, they enjoyed considerable freedom in the performance of their duties. They could improve their wards according to their own ideas and were normally successful in acquiring any materials that they thought were missing if they showed some initiative. Allusions to this relatively independent working environment emerged more frequently in the interviews than in the written sources.

The Swiss nurses Marianne Stocker and Hedwig Schnee are only two of many examples that illustrate the above points. At the beginning of her stay in 1961, Stocker, who was trained in pediatrics, was given the job of spring-cleaning the pharmacy and distributing donated clothes. Then, she was occupied for five days with repacking multivitamins sent from the USA.[134] Even after she began her regular duty of nursing children, she was still responsible for sewing curtains[135] and continued to distribute food three times per week for some time.[136] She was also supposed to assist the surgeons and care for patients who had recently undergone operations, tasks which she refused because she did not feel sufficiently qualified.[137] Stocker initiated pre- and postnatal counselling during her second stay, which she commenced in 1965.[138]

---

132   Munz-Boddingius, 'Meine Chance und Freude, Hebamme in Lambarene gewesen zu sein', 65; Group Interview Speicherschwendi.
133   Group Interview Speicherschwendi.
134   Stocker, 'Diary 1961–63', 12–16.
135   Ibid., 51.
136   Ibid., 36.
137   Ibid., 50.
138   Interview Marianne Stocker.

Schnee was relocated frequently during her almost three-year-long stay and performed numerous tasks. She administered injections, distributed and manufactured medications, and assisted with anesthetics. Schnee helped to establish a ward comparable to an intensive care unit, which they named 'Case Japonais' to honor the donors from Japan. Schnee monitored patients in this ward and even buried deceased ones.[139] She acquired cortisone for the Case Japonais for patients suffering from allergic reactions. When she required infusion stands or a cupboard for storing drugs, Schnee recalled simply going to the carpenter and ordering them there without asking for anyone's permission.[140]

European staff followed different trajectories in coming to work in Lambaréné. Walter Munz answered a job advertisement in the 'Schweizerische Ärztezeitung', the professional magazine for physicans.[141] He was interviewed to Basel by Dr. Hermann Baur, then president of the Swiss association supporting the hospital. As all staff did, African and European alike, Munz received a modest salary as well as free board and lodging.[142] Stocker wrote to the same association, with which she was familiar through her mother, who used to donate bedding and similar items to it. Her contact person there was Anita Dinner, who sent her to Gunsbach, where her state of health was examined and she was interviewed by Emmy Martin, Schweitzer's administrator in Europe.[143] Another option for finding work at the hospital was through acquaintances; Schnee, for example, was invited by Munz.[144] These brief examples highlight the importance of Schweitzer's personal network of people he trusted. They served as his gatekeepers in Europe. They ensured that a candidate was not only in good health and sufficiently qualified, but also compatible with the 'Lambaréné Spirit', which demanded, among other things, that processes and people at had to be simple and natural, proficient and undemanding.[145]

When interviewed, nurses fondly recalled their often scarce free time. During communal dinner, a wide range of issues would be discussed, including medical matters.[146] The seating arrangement represented the hospital hierarchy: towards the end of their stay, staff sat closer to Schweitzer and his most

---

139   Interview Hedwig Schnee, Speicherschwendi.
140   Ibid.
141   Interview Munz and Munz. According to Munz, desired qualifications were two years of surgical experience, fluency in French, unmarried status, and a commitment to work for 32 months. The original advertisement could not be found.
142   Even among the same group, i.e. African assistants, not everyone received the same salary.
143   Interview Marianne Stocker.
144   Group Interview Speicherschwendi.
145   Mabika Ognandzi, Steinke, and Zumthurm, *Schweitzer's Lambaréné: A Hospital in Colonial Africa*.
146   Interview Ursula Bunch.

loyal personnel, who might offer their spot to important visitors.[147] Africans were present only as servants.[148] Staff members were generally satisfied with the food that they received; the fruit and vegetables from the hospital plantations are a happy memory.[149] When everyone had finished eating, Schweitzer would read from the Bible and play the piano, while staff members would sing together. Attendance at these gatherings was voluntary, but normally everyone participated.[150] Thereafter, there was time for staff members to write letters, converse with each other in their rooms, or, less frequently, to listen to records.[151] In general, former staff members described and remembered the communal aspects of life at the hospital in a positive light, although some complaints about a lack of privacy were raised.[152]

Typically, each member of staff enjoyed a day off on every second Sunday. On this free day, they would often go on an excursion. They ventured, for example, to one of the nearby mission stations to spend time with fellow Europeans and play pétanque.[153] Several interviewees also remembered visiting neighboring villages, where they were joyfully welcomed by former patients or employees. Pirogues were bought or rented and rowers hired for these journeys. According to some nurses, Schweitzer did not approve of such trips or even prohibited them.[154] However, the ban was not too strictly enforced.[155] Schweitzer also discouraged swimming in the river, but this did not prevent everyone from doing so.[156] Stocker wrote in her diary that she stole away one Saturday to attend a 'dance' in nearby Adouma. Other nurses reported similar occurrences.[157] This partly contradicts the observation made by Fernandez on the lives of European employees at the hospital at the time, namely that the majority 'had only left the hospital to go to Lambaréné town and then only

---

147   Zumthurm, 'Food at the Albert Schweitzer Hospital'.

148   Barthélemy, *Wie ich Lambarene erlebte*, 25; Fernandez, 'The Sound of Bells in a Christian Country', 543; Füllemann, 'Aus jüngster Zeit', 162.

149   Group Interview Speicherschwendi; Interview Ursula Bunch. During the dry season, a wide variety of European vegetables were grown there. An important component of every breakfast was quinine.

150   Group Interview Speicherschwendi; Interview Ursula Bunch; Interview Munz and Munz.

151   Interview Ursula Bunch; Interview Marianne Stocker; Interview Hedwig Schnee.

152   Interview Elisabeth Anderegg; Interview Ursula Bunch.

153   Interview Elisabeth Anderegg.

154   Ibid.; Group Interview Speicherschwendi.

155   During her time at the hospital, Schweitzers daughter Rhena lent a boat to a newlywed couple and Dr. Müller owned a motorboat. See: Interview Ursula Bunch.

156   Interview Elisabeth Anderegg; Interview Marianne Stocker.

157   Stocker, 'Diary 1961–63', 18; Interview Elisabeth Anderegg; Group Interview Speicherschwendi. See also Chapter 5.

once or twice. They were eager to hear of the life of their patients in the village, which they knew next to nothing about'.[158]

6   African Staff: Versatile Training and Reliable Service

Typically, nurses who were new to the job were introduced to their roles by African auxiliaries who had long been stationed in their respective wards; nevertheless, most nurses report that they themselves were also responsible for training new African personnel.[159] African auxiliaries had worked for Schweitzer since his initial arrival in Lambaréné. In his 1935 report, he only wrote that there were eight auxiliaries, who were assigned their tasks for the day by a nurse before breakfast.[160] Four years earlier, he had listed five: Mendoume and N'Gema dressed ulcers and cared for patients with dysentery or mental illnesses; Boulingui for whom Schweitzer was full of praise, had been employed in the surgical service since 1924; Arthur looked after the critically ill; and Nyama worked in the consultation room, administered injections, and prepared the necessary solutions.[161] In 1938, Schweitzer employed twelve Africans, including one woman.[162] They were all under the constant supervision of a doctor or, occasionally, a nurse.[163] Some of these auxiliaries were in almost lifelong service at the hospital. Jeannette Siefert, who had worked as a nurse at the hospital in the 1930s, visited it again in 1960 and noted that Nyama and Mendoume were still employed there.[164]

The story of Joseph Ndolo, as told by himself in a book edited by Munz, provides an idea of an auxiliary's responsibilities.[165] It remains one of the few written accounts by African personnel or patients. Ndolo, son of a 'healer', began working in 1954 at the age of twenty-two and remained in his position until 1987. Unlike most of his peers, he did not have any relatives who were already employed there.[166] He showed initiative and convinced Schweitzer to engage

158   Fernandez, 'The Sound of Bells in a Christian Country', 542f.

159   Group Interview Speicherschwendi,; Interview Elisabeth Anderegg; Stocker, 'Diary 1961–63'.

160   Schweitzer, 'Briefe aus dem Lambarene Spital November 1935', 2, 8.

161   Schweitzer, 'Briefe aus dem Lambarene Spital Pfingsten 1931', 9.

162   Schweitzer to Morel, 28 August 1938. Published in: Bähr, *Albert Schweitzer: Leben, Werk und Denken*, 153.

163   Schweitzer, 'Briefe aus dem Lambarene Spital November 1935', 5.

164   Siefert, *Meine Arbeitsjahre in Lambarene 1933–1935*, 180.

165   Munz, *Albert Schweitzer im Gedächtnis der Afrikaner und in meiner Erinnerung*, 97–103.

166   On the recruitment of personnel, see Chapter 3.

him. At first, his duties included packing drugs, cleaning and sterilizing medical instruments, and distributing medication. After three months, Ndolo was given the responsibility of performing laboratory analyses alongside Joseph Bissangoy, who had been in the role for years, and was also taught to give injections. These remained Ndolo's two primary tasks until his retirement.[167]

Ndolo lists his twenty-nine colleagues, as of 1964, by name and role. This allows for a tentative comparison with auxiliaries' responsibilities in the 1930s. In 1964, five of the auxiliaries were interpreters, two more than thirty years earlier. Seven assisted the surgeons and four cared for patients recovering from operations, whereas in the 1930s Boulingui alone had been responsible for both tasks. In 1931, two auxiliaries were supposed to share the task of dressing ulcers and caring for patients with dysentery or mental illness; over thirty years later, only Marcel Poungui was tasked with bandaging, Jean Mendoume and Samuel Lane looked after patients with mental illness, and dysentery ceased to have been a constant threat. By 1964, Nyama had received a colleague to assist the nurse in the injection room, which Schnee compared to a chicken coop annexed to the Grande Pharmacie. She claims to have administered the shots herself, while Nyama had been reported to do them in the 1930s.[168] Besides Evangéline Ebako and Véronique Mabwe in the maternity ward, there were only two other female auxiliaries in 1964: Annemarie Babalou in the operating theater and Mama Hélène, who assisted Alain Douviogou in the leprosy settlement. Ndolo additionally mentions Noel Ndoung who distributed medication, Kwamba who maintained the fire used for sterilizing instruments, and Pierre Ndounge who was responsible for preparing beds and food.[169] The auxiliaries did not occupy leading positions in these domains. Instead, they performed tasks that in European hospitals would have been fulfilled by the nurses supervising them in Lambaréné. The actual degree of responsibility and autonomy that these auxiliaries enjoyed differed considerably, as will become clear in the analyses of the different wards.

In 1964, Ndolo initiated informal anatomical and technical training for African auxiliaries, which was given by the European doctors.[170] The on-the-job training that the auxiliaries had had hitherto received had already been the subject of much criticism during Schweitzer's lifetime. Dr. Louis Paul Aujoulat, who would later open a hospital in Cameroon, first visited Lambaréné in 1935. At the time, he advised Schweitzer to open a school to train African nurses and,

---

167   Munz, *Albert Schweitzer im Gedächtnis der Afrikaner und in meiner Erinnerung*, 97–103.
168   Interview Hedwig Schnee.
169   Munz, *Albert Schweitzer im Gedächtnis der Afrikaner und in meiner Erinnerung*, 100.
170   Ibid., 100–102.

at a later stage, doctors too. He recalled Schweitzer's reaction: 'Schweitzer listened to me with infinite patience; he contradicted me, of course, and in the end, he interrupted me in my enthusiasm and said: "Have you come here to seek advice or to give it to me?"'[171] Dr. Clement Chesterman made the same suggestion almost twenty years later. Schweitzer replied, more concretely now, that he had too many other things to do and that he considered this to be the government's responsibility.[172]

Several of my Gabonese interviewees considered the training that their parents or grandparents received at the hospital to have been highly valuable. They did not differentiate between European and African personnel, using the French 'infirmier' or 'infirmière' for any nurse. They insisted that Schweitzer 'trained' and 'formed' his own nurses.[173]

7 Staff in Comparison

Historical research on African medical assistants in neighboring Cameroon, for example, has emphasized their peculiar position. On the one hand, they were suspected to benefit from 'the extraction of body substances' or saw themselves confronted with witchcraft accusations; on the other hand, they 'drew considerable social prestige and economic opportunities' from their positions.[174] In any case, they held a central role as translators of biomedical understandings of health and disease and as mediators between patients and doctors. Our case shows that even beyond these issues they were crucial in the daily routines of the hospital.

In China and India, mission stations started to train local Christian converts to staff their hospitals in the late nineteenth century.[175] In South Africa, formal nursing training for Africans was initiated in 1906, based on previous

171   Aujoulat, 'Albert Schweitzer, médecin de brousse', 222–23. For more on Aujoulat, see: Lachenal and Taithe, 'Une généalogie missionnaire et coloniale de l'humanitaire'.

172   Schweitzer to Chesterman, 24 March 1953, AMS. During the 1920s, Chesterman had worked for the Baptist Missionary Society in Yakusu near todays Kinsangani in the DRC. He was in constant contact with Schweitzer and would later become a director of the supporting foundation of the hospital in England. For more on his time in the Congo, see: Hunt, A Colonial Lexicon.

173   Interview Jacques Boucah; Interview Léontine Nsowe; Interview Jacques-Adrien Rolagho.

174   Lachenal et al., 'Neglected Actors in Neglected Tropical Diseases Research', 3, 10. Their analysis draws from the research of Cameroonian historian Wang Sonné, whose work I was not able to access.

175   Hardimann, 'The Mission Hospital', 207–9.

experiences in what is today Malawi.[176] In colonial Uganda, a medical service consisting of African officers was established in 1914.[177] The French government medical school in Dakar, Senegal, opened its doors to Africans two years later.[178] The British in colonial Ghana had established a training program for Africans by 1920.[179] Many of these programs would lead to a recognized diploma. It remains to be examined in greater detail, however, what exactly was taught in these programs and how they differed from Schweitzer's on-the-job approach to training. Rita Headrick writes that in the case of training programs for African nurses in AEF 'doctors, the health reports, and the nurses themselves all agreed that, with few exceptions, nurses were badly trained and incompetent at all but a few tasks'.[180]

European nurses, numerous and prominent in our case, have received increasing research attention. It has been argued that globally their qualifications tended to be assessed 'in terms of character rather than intellect'.[181] This was especially applicable in the colonies,[182] as indeed can be observed at Schweitzer's hospital. Nurses aspired to serve in the colonies due to the desire for more personal and financial independence, and greater professional responsibilities.[183] Catholic missionary nurses in particular were further driven by their faith and the wish to 'make a difference in the world by moving beyond the domestic realm'.[184] Similar motivations prompted women to seek employment at the Albert Schweitzer Hospital.

Colonial doctors have been more thoroughly researched. For example, Anna Crozier has published a detailed study on British doctors in colonial East Africa. As in other colonial services, interpersonal networks, mutual favors and patronage formed important elements of the recruitment process, as did the assessment of a prospective doctor's character.[185] Doctors maintained a distinct

---

176   Digby, *Diversity and Division in Medicine*, 243–44; Parle and Noble, 'The Hospital Was Just Like a Home', 192–93.
177   Lyons, 'The Power to Heal', 206.
178   Cole, 'Engendering Health', 119.
179   Patterson, *Health in Colonial Ghana*, 16–17.
180   Headrick, *Colonialism, Health and Illness in French Equatorial Africa*, 251.
181   Rafferty, 'Nurses', 520.
182   Headrick, *Colonialism, Health and Illness in French Equatorial Africa*, 247; Nestel, '(Ad)Ministering Angels', 262, 265.
183   Nestel, '(Ad) Ministering Angels', 263; Schweig, *Weltliche Krankenpflege in den deutschen Kolonien Afrikas*, 14–15, 37.
184   Wall, *Into Africa*, 30.
185   Crozier, *Practising Colonial Medicine*, 32.

group culture,[186] but had diverse career motivations.[187] Typically, they were politically conservative and of upper-class origin, but enjoyed a lower social and financial status than other colonial officials.[188] Almost all were men: less than 3 percent of all physicians having practiced in East Africa prior to World War Two were women.[189] Headrick notes a similar gender imbalance in the case of AEF.[190] Africa was considered particularly unsuited for women, an assessment with which Schweitzer apparently did not agree. In India, in contrast, more than half of all medical missionaries in 1900 were female.[191]

Mabika underlines the diverse class origin of doctors in Gabon. Those he interviewed were motivated primarily by the sense of participating in a 'civilizing mission' or a desire to serve France, but scientific curiosity and aspiration, as well as a yearning for adventure, were also mentioned.[192] Headrick highlights the 'esprit de corps' shared by doctors in AEF. She argues that this sense of fellowship was particularly well articulated there due to the low standing of a colony in which 'the administrators were newcomers, or mediocre, or known failures, and where most missionary doctors were more interested in religion than in medicine'.[193] Schweitzer had created an equivalent at his hospital with the 'Lambaréné Spirit' already referred to.

According to Headrick, the government doctors in AEF were usually young, of low social class, and prone to the worrying changes in personality so often described in novels on Europeans living in colonial settings.[194] Balandier's government doctor in Lambaréné, who has been introduced in the Introduction, appears to have undergone a similar transformation. He was sent home after imitating William Tell by shooting empty water bottles off the heads of his servants. Balandier concedes that this story sounds extraordinary, but argues

---

186 Ibid., 119.

187 A doctor's salary in East Africa was moderate, but comfortable; entry conditions were easy; and the social prestige and benefits were considerable. The region offered a promise of adventure in the form of hunting and other leisure activities. The East African climate was considered comparatively healthy. Many doctors already had a mentor in the area or were following the precedent of a friend or relative. Others were motivated by religion or humanitarianism. Professional motivations included the opportunity to become an expert in an emerging field or acquire knowledge in other natural sciences; the diverse nature of a local doctor's duties; and the chance to gain personal and professional independence. See: ibid., 47–68.

188 Ibid., 106.

189 Ibid., 98.

190 Headrick, *Colonialism, Health and Illness in French Equatorial Africa*, 261.

191 Hardiman, *Missionaries and Their Medicine*, 141.

192 Mabika Ognandzi, *Médicaliser l'Afrique*, 153–56.

193 Headrick, *Colonialism, Health and Illness in French Equatorial Africa*, 240.

194 Ibid., 45–50.

that it was indicative of Gabon's particular 'natural and human milieu'. This, according to him, differed significantly from that of the neighboring French Congo, the other colony that he had researched:

> It shows how quickly Gabon can use up the men at its service. It takes a particularly well-armed personality, or powerful material interests, to rise up against a natural and human milieu that possesses an astonishing capacity for annihilation and also has the benefit of being oversized and excessive.[195]

In this light, Schweitzer's enduring positive attitude and his quasi-immunity to tropical diseases are remarkable. Such self-control was strongly connected to 'other-control', as Johannes Fabian reminds us.[196] This partly explains Schweitzer's careful selection of hospital personnel and strict organization of their busy working lives. He was successful in minimizing Gabon's negative effects, as described by Balandier, on his staff. Stories similar to that of the government doctor at Lambaréné have not emanated from the Albert Schweitzer Hospital. Although most of the European staff would ultimately complain of tiredness, especially towards the end of their stay, accounts of them drifting into a state of mental decline similar to those described by Balandier or Joseph Conrad are absent.

8   Infrastructure: Necessity and Maintenance

Table 1 summarizes the growth of the hospital. The most significant period of growth occurred in the late 1950s, when, alongside an influx of patients, the number of staff rose appreciably. Most notable is the increase in African auxiliaries. The presence of more patients and staff at the hospital invariably required the construction of more buildings. By 1965, the main hospital premises

---

195   Balandier, *Afrique ambiguë*, 219.
196   Fabian described nineteenth-century explorers in Central Africa as follows: 'Typically, the traveller was depicted as an individual, often solitary, agent, full in control of himself and others. Psychologically, morally, and intellectually, he was equipped to carry out the assigned task, unless impeded or prevented by persons, events, or conditions beyond his control. Self-control required "other-control", which above all meant maintaining distance from the country to be explored and its people'. Fabian, *Out of Our Minds*, 7. This description offers undoubted parallels to the way in which Schweitzer understood his role in Lambaréné.

TABLE 1   The growth of the hospital

	Early 1930s to mid-1950s	1960s
Inpatients	150–250	290–390 (+ ca. 150 leprosy patients)
Doctors	3–4	4–6
Nurses	7–8	11–16
Auxiliaries	6–9	16–30
Buildings	20–30	ca. 70

contained as many as seventy structures,[197] as opposed to twenty to thirty in the 1930s. A number of new wards were established in the 1960s, such as a building specifically for children or an intensive care unit.[198]

After the hospital's relocation in 1927, Schweitzer left for a longer stay in Europe to accumulate more substantial funds, returning in early 1930. The nurse Marie Woytt-Secretan, who accompanied him on his return, recalled that the hospital consisted of seven buildings at the time. When she left Lambaréné in 1932, she counted thirty-two buildings, although she may have included annexes and other smaller structures.[199] In his 1933 annual report, Schweitzer listed sixteen buildings plus 'buildings necessary to house indigenous staff'.[200] The spatial core of the hospital was the Grande Pharmacie, a large building of 180 square meters that contained an operating theater, a consultation room, a bandaging room, a laboratory, a washhouse, a room for urology, and a small pharmacy for storing and one for producing basic medication. European patients were housed in their own building, which consisted of six rooms, each with two beds. Africans stayed in five different buildings with pallet beds, which housed a total of 216 patients. Unlike the majority of the other sleeping quarters, their windows were not equipped with mosquito nets.[201] There were also two storehouses, two buildings for European personnel, and

---

197   As estimated by: Harris, 'The Allure of Albert Schweitzer', 816. A rough map produced in 1966 suggests a similar number of buildings. See: 'Lambarene 1966 – Statistiques', L – A – S3, AMS.

198   Group Interview Speicherschwendi.

199   Woytt-Secretan, 'Souvenirs d'une infirmière', 32.

200   'Statistiques de l'Hôpital 1933', L – A – S2, AMS.

201   Schweitzer, 'Briefe aus dem Lambarene Spital November 1935', 15.

various quarters to isolate patients suffering from leprosy and other contagious diseases or mental disorders.

During the early 1930s, the hospital was modernized in various ways. In 1935, a European patient donated a powerful petroleum lamp that made it possible for doctors to perform emergency surgeries at night, a frequent enough occurrence.[202] In November 1933, an engine-driven refrigerator, which had been donated by an Alsatian doctor, was installed. They would keep certain drugs therein. In addition, Schweitzer was happy to report that the hospital could now store leftover food and further rejoiced that 'only those who have lived in equatorial primeval forest lowlands can appreciate what refreshment the glass of cool water, which we now receive at 10 a.m. and at 4 p.m., means to us doctors and nurses'.[203]

Water supply was a major concern throughout the study period. Pumps, first installed in 1927, frequently did not work and often had to be replaced.[204] The reservoir, built four years later, only provided water during the rainy season.[205] Recurring reports tell of patients and staff who were forced to drink water from the river.[206] This was a significant health concern, as will be shown in Chapter 4. In the 1960s, staff was still boiling river water for human consumption.[207]

In the early 1960s, after Gabon had gained its independence, criticism of Schweitzer's work in Lambaréné increased, as we have seen in the Introduction. The main critique was that the hospital still operated from a backward ideological perspective and was insufficiently modern in terms of its medical equipment and practices, issues that Gabonese evaluated much less disapprovingly.[208] However, many European visitors and staff who returned to the hospital on more than one occasion commented on its stagnation. When Aujoulat returned to Lambaréné in 1952, seventeen years after his first visit, he noticed no changes. Indeed, his only criticism of Schweitzer was that he did

---

202   Schweitzer, 'Briefe aus dem Lambarene Spital Juni 1935', 4. The introduction of new lighting and other technologies is a central focus of Chapter 2.

203   Schweitzer, 'Briefe aus dem Lambarene Spital Februar 1934', 8.

204   Schweitzer, 'Briefe aus dem Lambarene Spital Pfingsten 1931', 3.

205   Haussknecht, *Emma Haussknecht, 1895–1956*, 88.

206   Schweitzer, 'Briefe aus dem Lambarene Spital März 1938', 6; Interview Hedwig Schnee; Haussknecht, *Emma Haussknecht, 1895–1956*, 88.

207   Anderegg recalled that each drop of river water was boiled. See: Interview Elisabeth Anderegg. Margrith Stark-Bernhard, who was tasked with domestic duties from 1962 to 1964, wrote that one of her daily responsibilities was to supervise the boiling of river water. Thereafter, the water was filtered and then offered to the staff as drinking water. See: Stark-Bernhard, 'Waschfrauen, Büglerinnen, Schneider und Matratzenmacher', 28.

208   Emane, *Docteur Schweitzer: une icône africaine*, 32, 92–93.

not attempt to adapt to changing circumstances in the wider world.[209] Three years later, a visiting surgeon from South Africa reported that 'the consulting or outpatient department is exactly as it was built over 30 years ago, and looks rather like a film setting of the old fashioned wild-west saloons'.[210] Dr. Markus Lauterburg-Bonjour, who in 1925 was the third doctor to arrive at the hospital, returned in 1961. Stocker noted his casual observation in her diary: 'Actually nothing has changed [...] there are more people, more houses, but otherwise it is not much different'. Stocker was undecided as to whether this should be understood as a compliment.[211]

A number of visitors commented on the lack of up-to-date equipment at the hospital. Fernandez argued that 'Schweitzer's resistance to modernization (*was*) a resistance very likely to impersonal organization'.[212] The Alsatian organist Edouard Nies-Berger, who stayed in Lambaréné in the early 1960s while working with Schweitzer on a publication on J.S. Bach, is more outspoken. According to him, Schweitzer's 'well-known obstinacy had become a curse', and his 'reluctance to cope with modern needs' was shared by many of his longtime collaborators.[213] Such assessments surely depend on the observer's point of view and Schweitzer's standing certainly provoked its own criticism. Nevertheless, the persistence and regularity of these complaints and comments, and the fact that they came from visitors and collaborators alike, demonstrate that a conservative atmosphere pervaded most parts of the hospital.

Electricity was restricted to the operating theater and the radiology room. This power was produced by a diesel generator, a complex machine that was installed in 1951. It had to be turned on by the hospital mechanic, who needed to be ready to do so at any time in case of emergencies.[214] The hospital could have been connected to the public power supply network towards the end of the 1950s, but Schweitzer refused to allow this, possibly because he feared a loss of independence.[215]

---

209 Aujoulat, 'Albert Schweitzer, médecin de brousse', 223–24.
210 Penn, 'A Visit to Albert Schweitzer', 164.
211 Stocker, 'Diary 1961–63', 24.
212 Fernandez, 'The Sound of Bells in a Christian Country', 557. Italics mine.
213 Nies-Berger, *Albert Schweitzer as I Knew Him*, 108. Here, Nies-Berger explicitly identifies Mathilde Kottmann and Ali Silver. The former offered her services to Schweitzer as a midwife in 1923, while the latter arrived as a nurse after World War Two. Both rose in the ranks to take responsibility for administrative tasks and enjoyed a high position in the hospital hierarchy by 1960.
214 Interview Munz and Munz; Interview Elisabeth Anderegg; Interview Ursula Bunch.
215 Scholl, *Von der Ehrfurcht vor dem Leben zur transkulturellen Solidarität*, 103.

X-ray equipment was installed in 1954 after Emeric Percy, a Hungarian doctor who served two terms in the 1950s, had convinced Schweitzer to buy it, because it drastically improved a doctor's ability to diagnose tuberculosis. Percy had to undergo special training in order to guarantee the smooth running of the machine, also in case of defects.[216] As of 1965, the X-Ray room was the only room equipped with air-conditioning.[217] In the kitchen, petroleum-driven refrigerators were still in use. As their spark plugs were susceptible to failure and had to be exchanged several times a week, nurses who worked in the kitchen acquired some of the basic skills needed to fix them.[218] Because refrigeration was limited, a considerable quantity of drugs was stored in basements where they were protected from the sun.

A large number of these drugs, and other objects, had to be thrown away, because they were either badly packed and did not endure the heat and humidity or were invaded by ants.[219] Jacques Boucah, whose mother would work in the maternity ward, arrived at the hospital in 1956 at the age of nine years. One of his summer jobs was to identify and burn pharmaceuticals that had expired or spoiled.[220] Gerald McKnight, one of the hospital's first and most well-known critics, argued that no one at the institution could keep track of the incoming supply of drugs and suspected that pharmaceutical companies were using it as a dumping ground.[221] We do know, however, that doctors, together with some nurses, were responsible for ordering medication and must therefore have had at least some idea of what was missing.[222] Some medications were also produced on site, including all saline solutions.[223] Also to be found in the basements, occupying valuable storage space, were a large variety of objects with little practical value, from ties to pepper casters, which had been donated from overseas.[224] In order not to upset Schweitzer, employees secretly disposed of some of these items by burying them or throwing them

---

216   For a detailed discussion on the acquirement of the X-ray equipment, see: Mabika Ognandzi, Steinke, and Zumthurm, *Schweitzer's Lambaréné: A Hospital in Colonial Africa*.

217   According to Walter Munz, Dr. Rolf Müller found this air-conditioning unit in a basement. They both assumed that Ali Silver had stored it there without informing anyone else after it had been donated to the hospital. Arguably, Silver shared Schweitzer's distaste of new machinery. See: Interview Munz and Munz.

218   Füllemann, 'Aus jüngster Zeit', 163; Group Interview Speicherschwendi.

219   Cousins, *Dr. Schweitzer of Lambaréné*, 103.

220   Interview Jacques Boucah.

221   Gerald McKnight, *Verdict on Schweitzer*, 35f.

222   Interview Elisabeth Anderegg; Interview Hedwig Schnee.

223   Interview Marianne Stocker; Interview Hedwig Schnee.

224   Group Interview; Stocker, 'Diary 1961–63', 16.

into the river.[225] These accounts convey an image of abundance that differs from the typical one of a colonial health facility that is in constant shortage of supplies.

When Norman Cousins toured the hospital in early 1957, he noted that 'the sanitary facilities were at an absolute minimum. There were only two outhouses, one for each sex'.[226] European staff, for whose use they were reserved, detested the place and referred to it as 'Hinter-India'.[227] There were no sanitary facilities whatsoever for African patients. They were thus forced to relieve themselves in the open, the river being a preferred location.[228] Two showers, each in reality a bucket with holes attached to a rope, were located in a hut next to the dining room; only European staff knew where to find the keys.[229] Padlocks were a feature throughout the hospital, especially in the kitchen.[230] There was, like in the surrounding region, a widespread fear of theft, including among Africans.[231]

Another feature that added to the hospital's insanitary appearance were the free-roaming animals. In 1924, Kottmann wrote of two goats as well as some chickens that refused to lay eggs.[232] In 1933, Schweitzer claimed that 20 percent of the hospital's required milk came from its own goats.[233] In the early 1960s, goats were reportedly entering the Grande Pharmacie.[234] In addition to this subsistence livestock, a great variety of animals lived freely on the hospital grounds. A pelican, for example, gained considerable fame when Schweitzer published a whole book written from its perspective in 1950.[235]

---

225 Interview Ursula Bunch.

226 Cousins, *Dr. Schweitzer of Lambaréné*, 92.

227 Interview Hedwig Schnee; Interview Munz and Munz.

228 A remark made by numerous observers; see, for example: Cousins, *Dr. Schweitzer of Lambaréné*, 71; Fernandez, 'The Sound of Bells in a Christian Country', 544; Emane, *Docteur Schweitzer: une icône africaine*, 97.

229 Stocker, 'Diary 1961–63', 33; Interview Ursula Bunch.

230 Fernandez, 'The Sound of Bells in a Christian Country', 544; Oermann, *Albert Schweitzer 1875–1965*, 250.

231 Intrerview Ursula Bunch; Stocker, 'Diary 1961–63', 12. See also: Arnold, 'Vous les noirs, nous les blancs', 433. Arnold claims that fetishes protecting against theft were very common in the region. Fernandez underlines that for the Fang, 'thievery is one of the greatest evils, for it is an obvious and direct threat to the integrity of each social unit'; Fernandez, 'Christian Acculturation and Fang Witchcraft', 250.

232 Schweitzer, 'Neues von Albert Schweitzer Oktober 1924', 7. For a more detailed discussion about the role of animals at the hospital, see: Mabika Ognandzi, Steinke, and Zumthurm, *Schweitzer's Lambaréné: A Hospital in Colonial Africa*.

233 Schweitzer, 'Briefe aus dem Lambarene Spital Juli 1933', 7.

234 Interview Hedwig Schnee.

235 Albert Schweitzer, Richard Meiner, *Ein Pelikan Erzählt Aus Seinem Leben*.

Stories of nurses raising gorillas or chimpanzees abound.[236] In 1961, Stocker wrote in her diary that she was the only nurse who did not have a pet to look after in her room and complained of dogs entering the consultation rooms.[237] During the early 1960s, rats were considered such a pest that the legs of the tables in the kitchen were placed in buckets of kerosene in an attempt to keep the rodents away from edibles.[238]

While they acknowledged at least some of these shortcomings, the overwhelming majority of former staff whom I interviewed believed that the basic medical care provided at the hospital was of a high standard.[239] This is an opinion shared by many visitors.[240] In the latest biography of Schweitzer, Nils Ole Oermann comes to a similar conclusion. To further support this argument, he points to the fact that many Europeans preferred to be treated at Schweitzer's hospital than at the government clinic.[241] Jacques Bessuges, the colonial government physician in Lambaréné during the early 1950s, offers a different interpretation. He claims that some European residents in Gabon favored Schweitzer's hospital as a result of its glamorous atmosphere and because it looked impressive as a place of birth on their child's birth certificate. According to Bessuges, they were less positive about the conditions that they found there. He reports that one patient had exclaimed: 'What is so extraordinary about this Doctor Schweitzer? What a hospital, his hospital! It is shameful!'[242] Bessuges maintained good relations with Schweitzer, as we will see in Chapter 2. Indeed, his overall assessment of the level of service and the conditions at the hospital was not overly negative. In the hospital's defense, he contended that, considering the difficult circumstances in which it operated, it was not particularly unhygienic. He also sensed that staff and patients were happy there, whereas he complained about the depressing atmosphere and filth of his own workplace.[243]

---

236   Haussknecht, *Emma Haussknecht, 1895–1956*, 64; Sixt, 'Krankenschwester bei Albert Schweitzer', 62; Group Interview Speicherschwendi.

237   Stocker, 'Diary 1961–63', 17.

238   Group Interview Speicherschwendi. Schweitzer mentioned a rat problem already in 1937. In: 'Briefe aus dem Lambarene-Spital Mai 1937', 6.

239   Interview Munz and Munz; Group Interview Speicherschwendi; Interview Ursula Bunch; Interview Elisabeth Anderegg.

240   Cousins cites Dr. Cyrille Coulon, who, having worked as an itinerant doctor in South Africa, was impressed by the equipment that he found in Lambaréné in 1956. See: Cousins, *Dr. Schweitzer of Lambaréné*, 138. Dr. Lavdris Christensen concurred some two years later, adding that local conditions could and should not be compared with those of contemporary European hospitals. See: Østergaard Christensen, *At Work with Albert Schweitzer*, 66.

241   Oermann, *Albert Schweitzer 1875–1965*, 243–53.

242   Bessuges, *Lambaréné à l'ombre de Schweitzer*, 125.

243   Ibid., 54, 72, 125–26.

The presence of animals on the grounds of colonial hospitals was not unprecedented.[244] Backwardness and insalubrity were regular criticisms leveled against many healthcare institutions in various colonies.[245] This is not surprising given that hygiene was so central to the discourses of most colonial missionaries and physicians alike.[246] However, accusations against Schweitzer and his hospital were and remain especially persistent.

Colonial hospitals' access to equipment varied greatly, both within colonies and across the colonial world. For example, the first X-Ray equipment in what is today Malawi was installed in 1927 at the Livingstonia Medical Mission, but other mission hospitals in the same colony never acquired one.[247] The mission hospital at Agogo in colonial Ghana meanwhile, had acquired a radiography machine by 1938.[248] Schweitzer thus acquired his own radiography equipment comparatively late, but missions in India, for instance, received theirs even later.[249] A similar point can be made for electricity. In 1924, Chesterman wrote to Schweitzer from Yakusu in the Belgian Congo, reporting that he had equipped the whole hospital with electric lights.[250] In contrast, the general government hospital in Brazzaville did not acquire electricity in the 1920s.[251] Similarly, the government hospital in Libreville, for which electric equipment was planned for 1933, had to wait at least a further two years before being electrified.[252] Gabon's second most important city, Port-Gentil, and its hospital were only electrified in 1950, almost ten years after Schweitzer had electrified sections of the Grande Pharmacie.[253]

The reasons why any hospital might be equipped with comparatively few technologies were often economic, especially in the colonies, as Joel D. Howell reminds us. He also insists that, at the same time, cultural factors should not be

---

244 Hardiman, *Missionaries and Their Medicine*, 204; Headrick, *Colonialism, Health and Illness in French Equatorial Africa*, 195–96.

245 Eckart, *Medizin und Kolonialimperialismus*, 543; Kalusa, 'Christian Medical Discourse and Praxis on the Imperial Frontier', 256; Patterson, *Health in Colonial Ghana*, 19.

246 Bruchhausen, 'Practising Hygiene and Fighting the Natives' Diseases'; Lachenal, 'Le médecin qui voulut être roi', 139–40; Ombongi, 'The Historical Interface between the State and Medical Science in Africa', 356; Ratschiller, 'Kranke Körper'.

247 Good, *The Steamer Parish*, 402.

248 Schmid, 'Mission Medicine in a Decolonising Health Care System', 295.

249 Hardiman, *Missionaries and Their Medicine*, 209.

250 Chesterman to Schweitzer, 2 November 1924, AMS.

251 Headrick, *Colonialism, Health and Illness in French Equatorial Africa*, 194–97. It is not clear from the book precisely when Brazzaville's hospital was electrified.

252 See the Conclusion in: 'Rapport Annuel du Service de Santé de la Colonie Du Gabon 1932'. ZK 005-127, SHD. No references to electricity could be found in the 1933 and 1934 annual reports. Subsequent reports are missing.

253 Mabika, 'Médicalisation de l'Afrique centrale', 224. No information on the electrification of the government hospitals in Libreville or Lambaréné could be found.

neglected, positing that 'the belief that excellence in health care is machine-dependent may be less important in some parts of the world'.[254] For South African hospitals, Anne Digby concludes that in the period from 1930 to 1950, superior healing rates do not necessarily correlate with better or more modern facilities, or even a high standard of clinical care. Her case studies suggest that patients' attitudes and the geographical accessibility of healthcare institutions are significantly more important.[255] Terrence Ranger has observed this tension in the case of Tanzania, where it was widely acknowledged by the 1930s that 'mission medicine had not been triumphant after all'; in response, whereas the European clergy proposed simpler forms of treatment, medical personnel pressed for modernization.[256]

Schweitzer seems to have followed the logic of the theological personnel of missions, refusing to modernize his hospital on a large scale. However, he did not share the common missionary approach to medicine that often targeted

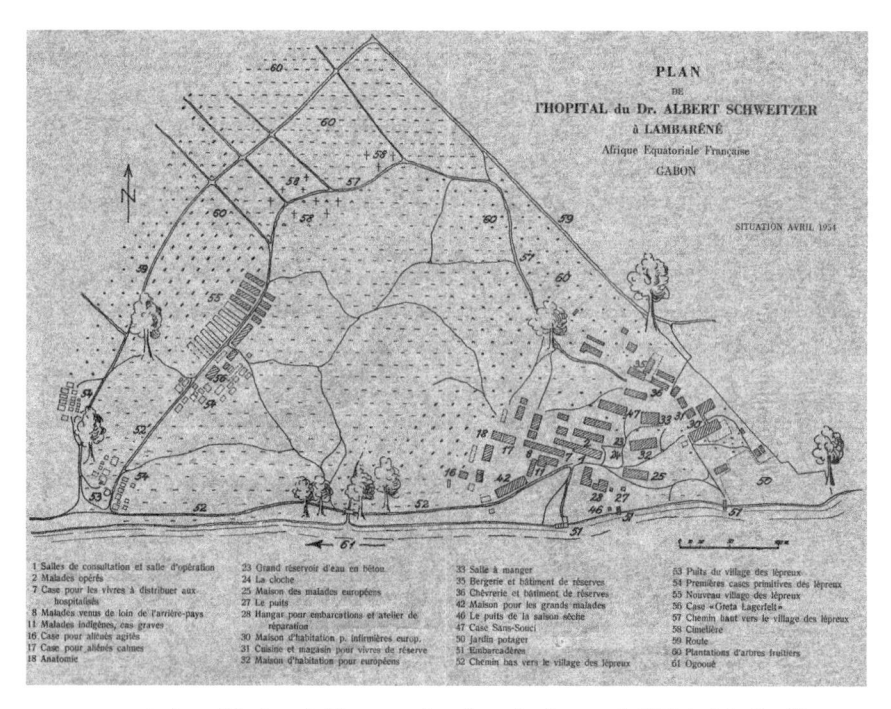

MAP 4   A plan of the hospital in 1954, taken from the 'Lettres de l'Hôpital du Dr. Albert Schweitzer à Lambaréné' (No. 14, 1954)

---

254   Howell, 'Hospitals', 513.
255   Digby, *Diversity and Division in Medicine*, 127.
256   Ranger, 'Godly Medicine', 273–74.

the community at large and aimed at transforming it. Schweitzer's ideology in this respect resembled that of biomedical practitioners, with their strong focus on the individual. Having said that, it has to be mentioned that this distinction was never unequivocal, and much of the work that missionary doctors undertook was targeted at the individual, not at the wider community.[257] Schweitzer believed that the medical services offered by his hospital (Map 4) were simply that: a service that any individual reaching for it would receive.[258]

9   Conclusion

When highlighting changes and continuities at the Albert Schweitzer Hospital in Lambaréné, the most obvious development was the institution's growth in all respects: in 1965, it had more patients, more doctors, more nurses, more auxiliaries, and more buildings than thirty years earlier. The most significant changes only occurred in the late 1950s, probably the result of new political dynamics in many areas of public service shortly before Gabonese independence, including in the health sector.

In reconstructing the routines of hospital life interviews were particularly valuable, as interviewees often recalled them in vivid detail. Interviews were less fruitful for recapitulating specific medical practices, as we will see in the following chapters, which rely more heavily on written sources. Furthermore, interviews were crucial in illuminating differences of opinion between Africans and Europeans, such as on the question of payment for treatment or on that of the training of local staff.

Schweitzer envisaged his hospital as a highly ordered space in which all staff had a specific role to play. On closer examination, however, his management style was very pragmatic. Doctors, nurses and auxiliaries were all required to switch between responsibilities throughout their stay and be highly flexible in the execution of their daily duties. On the other hand, a strong hierarchy prevailed; moreover, all staff had to adhere to a normative set of values, the 'Lambaréné Spirit'. Their willingness to do so as well as their personal contacts within Schweitzer's vast transcontinental network of supporters were decisive factors in whether potential personnel were hired.

Until the Great Depression, the vast majority of patients also made their way to the hospital via a network in its own right, the web of lumber camps

---

257   Jennings, 'Healing of Bodies, Salvation of Souls'.
258   This argument is further developed in: Mabika Ognandzi, Steinke, and Zumthurm, *Schweitzer's Lambaréné: a Hospital in Colonial Africa*.

in the surrounding region. After 1931, patients' origins diversified, but loggers remained a well-represented group. All patients were permitted, indeed expected, to bring *gardiens*, who were to provide basic care for their ill companions and contribute their labor to the hospital. This practice also occurred at other hospitals on the continent and was consistent with wider healing practices in the region. The Albert Schweitzer Hospital was successful in carving out a role for itself in this pluralist setting. Once there, patients had to follow a seemingly set and ordered routine that was, in reality, implemented in a more pragmatic manner. However, patients still had to submit to constant supervision in many aspects of their lives.

CHAPTER 2

In and Out of Control: Technologies and Patients in Surgery

In a letter to the German journalist Werner Gauss dated 7 July 1952, Albert Schweitzer complained that his surgical team often lacked an assistant who knew how to work with chloroform or ether. Moreover, the 'natives' considered general anesthesia 'something scary' and would therefore favor being subjected to other methods of anesthesia, the most frequent being infiltration anesthesia, a technique developed by the German surgeon Carl Ludwig Schleich in the 1890s. A photograph of Schleich hung on the wall of the operating theater in Lambaréné, because Schweitzer wanted his patients to meet their 'great benefactor from face'. He elaborated on this in a passage worthy of being quoted at length:

> When I operate myself, there is a ceremony of gratefulness at the end of the intervention when the patient is dressed, but before he is brought away. I insist that the natives are trained towards an appreciation of gratitude. The ceremony goes as follows: 'Say thank you, dear Dr Schweitzer'. The native responds: 'thank you dear Dr Schweitzer' – 'Say: thank you dear Miss Maria' (the nurse assisting in the operation room) 'thank you dear Miss Maria' – 'Say thank you Piere Piebé' (the black auxiliary in the operation room who is also assisting) 'thank you, Pierre Piebé' – 'And now finally say: thank you Monsieur Schleich' 'thank you Monsieur (and now something that very remotely sounds like Schleich is being articulated)' Because the Natives cannot pronounce Sch.[1]

How are we to understand such episodes in the context of surgical practices at the Albert Schweitzer Hospital, in Africa more generally, and indeed in the wider contemporary world? The passage illustrates common peculiarities of the doctor-patient relationship; it implies the importance of technology in surgical practice, in this case anesthesia; it hints at surgery's need to control procedures and all involved parties; and it evokes questions on how individuals understand the body. Technology, control, and the human body are common concerns for historians of medicine and the African continent alike. This chapter combines

---

1 Schweitzer to Gauss, 7 July 1952, AMS.

a Colonial Studies framework with one from Science and Technology Studies, merging different notions of control to assess the role and place of technology and patient agency in the hospital. Examining routines in and around the surgical ward, it illuminates an area that has, surprisingly, received only limited attention in both fields.

1   Surgery, Technology, and Control

The rise of surgery and the rise of the modern hospital are closely intertwined. Both built upon the scientific reasoning that had penetrated most domains of Western societies by the second half of the nineteenth century. Medical practices as well as administrative procedures and decision-making processes were reshaped according to these scientific norms.[2] Hospitals reflected these developments by becoming 'models of cleanliness, efficiency, and expertise' as well as of 'control and organization'.[3] Such principles were similarly crucial for the emergence of surgery as a medical practice. Indeed, according to Thomas Schlich, surgery can be understood as a network of control, with the latter defined as 'the power and ability of an individual to make a thing or an individual perform in a predetermined way'.[4] For this purpose, phenomena have to be predicted and quantified. Through such processes, control becomes strongly connected to technology. As in any operating theater, doctors at the Albert Schweitzer Hospital were very concerned to exert this sort of procedural control.

When focusing on medical practices, it is important to retain a broad and flexible definition of technology that is difficult to separate from science and that stresses the interaction and agency of objects, individuals, and society.[5] At least three meanings of the term 'technology' can thus be identified: 'physical objects or artefacts, [...] activities or processes, (and) what people know as well as what they do'.[6] In surgery, these correspond to instruments, lights, and tables; anesthesia and asepsis; and the anatomical atlas as well as surgery itself. As this chapter shows, surgery as a technology is sometimes difficult to differentiate from individual technologies in the narrower sense, which are usually

---

2 Donzé, *L'ombre de César*; Granshaw, 'The Rise of the Modern Hospital in Britain'; Howell, *Technology in the Hospital*; Schlich, 'The Days of Brilliancy Are Past'.
3 Stevens, *In Sickness and in Wealth*, 18.
4 Schlich, 'Surgery, Science and Modernity'. Schlich takes this definition from Levin, who in turn borrows from Blaise Pascal. See: Levin, 'Contexts of Control', 22.
5 This view is influenced by actor-network-theory. See: Latour, *Reassembling the Social* see Chapter 4 especially. See also: Pickstone, *Ways of Knowing*, 15.
6 Bijker, Hughes, and Pinch, 'The Social Construction of Technological Systems, Introduction', 4.

conceived as tools to uphold procedural control.[7] Since the hospital as an institution provided a more favorable environment to achieve this, these technologies accelerated surgery's move away from the home of the patient to what Sally Wilde describes as the doctor's 'territory'. This shifted the balance of power away from the patient and his or her relatives to the surgeon.[8] Another significant by-product of the increasing use of technologies was that medical treatment became more impersonal, to the extent that Joel D. Howell could term hospitals 'repair shops'.[9] This alienation was enabled through specific biomedical conceptions of the body as an individual site of intervention distinct from the patient's self.[10]

The introduction of new medical technologies depended on such shifting conceptions of the body, as well as on practical considerations and the broader social and political context. Anesthesia, a key technology of surgical control, eventually became standard in surgical wards, not only because it suppressed pain, but also because it produced a 'tranquilly pliant' patient, as Martin S. Pernick has shown.[11] Asepsis, the other main surgical technology that emerged in the late nineteenth century, has its theoretical foundations in germ theory. Pasteurian principles were fundamental for medical scientists and surgeons alike. As the former wanted to control organisms in laboratories in order to examine or manipulate them in a systematic way, the latter sought to control the patient's body.[12] Pasteurism, which views health as a social concern, also significantly shaped France's 'civilizing mission'.[13] Through science, control

---

7   On this point, see also: Schlich and Crenner, 'Technological Change in Surgery'.

8   Wilde, 'The Elephants in the Doctor-Patient Relationship', 2. See also: Tröhler, 'Surgery (Modern)', 995.

9   Howell, 'Hospitals', 511. It has long been observed that the use of technology in diagnostics estranged doctor and patient. See: Reiser, *Medicine and the Reign of Technology*, 230. This view has been challenged, see for example: Stanton, 'Innovations in Health and Medicine, Introduction', 3.

10 The sociologist Stefan Hirschauer considers the administration of anesthesia as a separation of the patient's body from his or her person, thereby protecting the patient and the surgeon from guilt or shame. See: Hirschauer, 'The Manufacture of Bodies in Surgery'. The medical anthropologist Arthur Kleinman likewise underlines biomedicine's focus on the individual body, which renders the suffering experienced by patients or their families as subjective and therefore irrelevant. See: Kleinman, 'What Is Specific to Western Medicine'. The historian Schlich formulates a similar argument: by treating bodies as objects separate from patients, doctors turn problems of society into 'purely technical and individual problems that can be solved by intervening into the indvidual's body'. Schlich, 'The Technological Fix and the Modern Body'.

11 Pernick, *A Calculus of Suffering*, 84.

12 Schlich, 'Surgery, Science and Modernity'.

13 Chakrabarti, *Medicine and Empire*, 164. He takes from: Conklin, *A Mission to Civilize*.

was now to be extended to spaces beyond the laboratory and the operating theater: the hospital, the city, the colonial world. This chapter provides an example of technology playing a less central role in surgical control. Furthermore, it adds to the growing literature discussed below that provides a more nuanced picture of what has hitherto been regarded as total colonial control.

With their arrival in Africa, biomedical technologies in the broad sense expanded an 'existing medical market by additional concepts and means'.[14] Africanist historians have frequently examined how practitioners and patients alike reconfigured the meanings, practices, and functions of such technologies, how they offered 'alternatives to the dominant order of things',[15] and provided different conceptions of 'bodies and their place in the world'.[16] Paul S. Landau in his study of Christianity in colonial southern Africa gives an example. Medical missionaries there targeted individuals through surgical treatments and thus linked disease with personal wrongdoing. In this manner, they shifted illness from the broader social context, within which it was usually understood in African societies, to the realm of simple biology. Behind this process was the missionaries' desire to remove individual Africans from their communities and to control and ultimately convert them.[17]

On the surface, Schweitzer appeared to differ in this respect. Florence Bernault argues that his 'patronizing triumph of medical assistance is predicated on hegemonic exchanges carefully confined to the physical'; she thus conceives of his hospital 'as a locale where Schweitzer's treatment of ailing bodies can refrain from reaching out to the patients' inner self or cultural assets'.[18] A closer examination of surgical practices and technologies at the hospital and an analysis of control inside and outside the operating theater reveal a more complex picture.

Surgery was a central element in the practice of biomedicine in colonial Africa too.[19] Across the continent, surgery took some time before it found a

---

14 Bruchhausen, 'Medical Pluralism as a Historical Phenomenon', 104.

15 They did so by 'creating new relations between herbal medicines and scientific technologies, between ancestors and laboratories, cures for witchcraft and the efficacy of pharmaceuticals'. Langwick, *Bodies, Politics, and African Healing*, 237.

16 White, *Speaking with Vampires*, 5. According to White, 'new technologies and procedures did not have meaning because they were new or powerful, but because of how they articulated ideas about bodies and their place in the world, and because of the ways in which they reproduced older practices'.

17 Landau, 'Explaining Surgical Evangelism'.

18 Bernault, 'Body, Power and Sacrifice', 226.

19 Crozier, *Practising Colonial Medicine*, 24–26; Eckart, *Medizin und Kolonialimperialismus*, 250; Kalusa, 'Christian Medical Discourse and Praxis on the Imperial Frontier', 256; Lachenal and Taithe, 'Une généalogie missionnaire et coloniale de l'humanitaire', 52; Landau, *The Realm of the Word*, 117.

place for itself in the pluralist medical setting.[20] Intrusive local body practices, such as cupping or piercing, accelerated the acceptance of surgery.[21] Some missionaries, hoping to enhance the reputation of their respective denominations, invigorated the process of reinterpretation by attributing supernatural qualities to surgery,[22] while others distanced themselves from such practices.[23] Finally, it should not be overlooked that Africans 'assessed empirical evidence', as Sokhieng Au has insisted for the case of the Belgian Congo.[24] Statistics for AEF suggest that biomedicine was most sought after when healing was perceived to occur after a low number of consultations. It is thus unsurprising that surgical interventions were the most frequent treatment in hospitals of the colony, along with injections against yaws.[25]

Despite its centrality in medical practice, there are very few studies in African medical history that place surgery at the center of analysis. This chapter helps to fill this gap by linking what I have defined as procedural control with an Africanist understanding of control. Control is a frequently employed but rarely defined notion in Africanist medical historiography that is conceptualized either very broadly[26] or rather narrowly.[27] A recurrent theme is how 'epidemic control provided a rationale for social control'.[28] Case studies of

---

20   This was the case in Malawi until the early 1960s. See: Good, *The Steamer Parish*, 407. In south-eastern Tanzania, local residents were reluctant to undergo surgery in the 1930s. See: Ranger, 'Godly Medicine', 268. The same has been observed for Zambia. See: White, *Speaking with Vampires*, 105.

21   Bruchhausen, 'Heil und Unheil aus dem Leib'; Janzen, *The Quest for Therapy*, 216; White, *Speaking with Vampires*, 104.

22   Benedictines in Tanzania regularly incorporated prayers, benedictions and holy water into their medical practices. See: Bruchhausen, *Medizin zwischen den Welten*, 325–26. Catholic missionaries of Efok in northern Cameroon referred to surgery as a 'miracle'. See: Lachenal and Taithe, 'Une généalogie missionnaire et coloniale de l'humanitaire', 52. See also: White, *Speaking with Vampires*, 104.

23   In Tanzania, missionaries did so due to pressures from the metropole, where the introduction of a magical version of Christianity in Britian's African colonies was feared. See: Ranger, 'Godly Medicine', 280–81. In the Belgian Congo, Dr. Chesterman performed surgeries in public in order to prove that there was nothing supernatural about the practice. See: Hunt, *A Colonial Lexicon*, 120. In Uganda, surgeons did the same to demonstrate that no body parts were stolen or eaten during surgery. See: White, *Speaking with Vampires*, 110.

24   Au, 'Cutting the Flesh', 306.

25   Headrick, *Colonialism, Health and Illness in French Equatorial Africa*, 386.

26   Feierman, 'Struggles for Control', 75. Feierman highlights that control over healing signified control over practical matters. Healers had the power to determine what professional or family duties an individual had to meet. They also had control over ideologies by defining the causes of suffering.

27   Cooper and Stoler, 'Introduction Tensions of Empire'. Cooper and Stoler often focus on policing.

28   Malowany, 'Unfinished Agendas', 331.

anti-sleeping sickness campaigns in particular have underlined the coercive nature of colonial medical and social control.[29] In this sense, colonial control is more about *gaining* 'the power and ability [...] to make a thing or an individual perform in a predetermined way' rather than executing it. Control represented a precondition for surgeons to perform their job, while for colonial doctors and administrators control was an expected outcome of their jobs.

Jonathan Sadowsky has recognized that by focusing on colonial medical institutions, for instance, historians must nevertheless modify 'the grand theory of the nature of colonial power'. His study of Nigerian 'institutions of madness' shows that even though social control can be observed to a certain degree, what is more striking is the 'contradictory, half-hearted nature of the institutions for most of the colonial period'.[30] In her book on 'violence, remedies, and reverie in colonial Congo', Nancy Hunt similarly concludes that 'the nervous state was limited in its ability to understand, perceive, and control its colonial subjects'.[31] Hunt's state has a second 'mode of presence', a biopolitical guise 'that worked to promote life and health'.[32] Lynn Thomas has likewise stressed that colonial power sometimes operated 'through a political technology that promised life rather than threatened death'.[33] The limits of Foucauldian biopower in African history have been frequently discussed;[34] nevertheless, what Hunt and Thomas describe in their books resembles the kind of control patients experienced at the Albert Schweitzer Hospital, an institution that was atypical, but certainly not half-hearted. Being neither government- nor missionary-run, its primary goal was neither to convert Africans, nor to recruit them as laborers. While procedural control was clearly strived for, social control was of secondary concern only; the former contributed to a specific understanding of the body and intensified the latter by dispersing biopolitical promises.

2 Surgery at the Albert Schweitzer Hospital: Context and Development

Schweitzer repeatedly underlined the central status of surgery at the hospital. On arrival, he was surprised to find that the demand was so high that operations

---

29   Bell, *Frontiers of Medicine*, 161; Lachenal, *Le médicament qui devait sauver l'Afrique*; Lyons, *The Colonial Disease*, 201–3.
30   Sadowsky, *Imperial Bedlam*, 115.
31   Hunt, *A Nervous State*, 237.
32   Ibid., 8.
33   Thomas, *Politics of the Womb*, 176.
34   Cooper, 'Conflict and Connection', 1533; Vaughan, *Curing Their Ills*, 8–12.

could have been performed on a daily basis. Having believed that surgery would be rejected in equatorial Africa, he attributed the significant demand in Lambaréné to a military surgeon who had performed a number of successful operations in the area. 'I harvest what he has sown', Schweitzer wrote.[35] Together with his wife, who acted as an anesthetist, they offered surgical interventions only two to three times per week. As he did not want to neglect his other medical duties, they were left with little time to wash surgical instruments and cloths. Moreover, he admitted that he was not overly confident about his surgical skills: before each new intervention, he consulted a handbook to revise how to perform the upcoming operation properly. Despite this, all his surgeries ended successfully. 'This only increases the redoubtable confidence of the blacks in my abilities. It makes me tremble', Schweitzer commented on the effects of these successes.[36] In a more confidential report, he revealed that he was afraid of performing operations for fear of losing the trust of potential patients in case of failure.[37] These writings support the assumption that African patients chose to go to a hospital only when a specific curative treatment, such as surgery, had proven to be efficient and successful.

Shortly after Schweitzer returned to Lambaréné in 1924, he wrote to Pierre Stolz, Professor of Medicine in Strasbourg, about how he had to neglect surgical patients because he was too busy treating numerous cases of various skin diseases as well as performing frequent blood tests. Schweitzer regretted this and sought for a solution:

> This is a pity, because there would be a lot of surgical work. Hence, I decided to bring in someone for surgery. Can you find me in Strasbourg or somewhere else a young unmarried doctor, who has some experience in surgery, who would be tempted to spend a year in Africa? [...] He doesn't have to be a great surgeon; the most important thing is that he knows how to properly operate on hernias, because this is the big piece of our surgical work here.[38]

By asking for a surgeon, Schweitzer responded to both the local demand for surgery and his own limitations in surgical skill and confidence. Soon thereafter, the Alsatian doctor Frédéric Trensz, who served in Lambaréné in 1926–27, reported that the main reason for the popularity of the hospital was its surgical service.[39] After the hospital's relocation in 1927, a routine was established in

---

35 Schweitzer, *Zwischen Wasser und Urwald*, 65.

36 Schweitzer, 'Notes et Nouvelles de la part du prof. Albert Schweitzer. Deuxième rapport', 36–37.

37 Schweitzer, 'Bericht an das Strassburger Comitee', 15 December 1913, AMS.

38 Schweitzer to Stolz, dated in retrospect 1924, AMS.

39 Trensz, 'Le médecin', 211.

which surgery would assume a central role. Once again Schweitzer attributed the renowned reputation of the surgical services at the hospital to the excellent work performed by his surgeons.[40]

Surgery's central position among hospital services and its radiance were reflected in doctors' nicknames. For example, the Swiss physician Mark Lauterburg, who practiced at the same time as Trensz, was known as 'Tschinda Tschinda', translated by his wife, Elsa, as 'the man who cuts the belly with courage'.[41] The belly appeared in the expression because it was regularly cut at the hospital, hernias and hydroceles being the most frequent operations. In his German translation of the nickname, Schweitzer simplified it to 'the man who cuts boldly'.[42] This was further reduced in translation by Dr. Margrith Schroeder, who served at the hospital in the late 1940s, to 'the knife',[43] thereby rendering man and technology as one. This example thus demonstrates how the surgeon, the scalpel and the surgery procedure as a whole came to be seen not only as interconnected, but as almost inseparable elements of the same technological process.

Figure 5 compares the number of patients who underwent operations with the total number of inpatients at the hospital from 1926 to 1965.[44] Every surgical intervention was recorded in books. These operation protocols include basic information on the patient, surgeon, and assistants; diagnosis and method of executing the intervention; and type of anesthesia as well as occasional general comments (see Illustration 10). For reconstructing surgical practices, these records are of limited value. However, they are useful for compiling statistics and cross-checking data with other sources. Between 1926 and 1960, the number of doctors working at the hospital besides Schweitzer remained largely stable at two or three; Schweitzer himself, with the notable exception of during World War Two, no longer practiced during this period. Only after Gabonese independence did the number of additional physicians rise to as high as four, five, or six.[45]

From 1930 to 1932, a considerable and inexplicable rise in surgical interventions occurred; their number almost quadrupled without a corresponding increase in patient or doctor numbers. In the years that followed, the number of surgeries stabilized; approximately a quarter to a third of all inpatients at the

40   Schweitzer, 'Briefe aus dem Lambarene Spital 1931', 6.

41   Lauterburg-Bonjour, *Lambarene: Erlebnisse einer Bernerin im afrikanischen Urwald*, 13.

42   Schweitzer, 'Mitteilungen aus Lambarene: Zweites Heft, Herbst 1924 bis Herbst 1925', 124.

43   Schröder, 'On fait ce qu'on peut', 179.

44   The statistics relating to patients who underwent operations are taken from the operation protocols, in which each operation since 1926 had been recorded. See: L – P – O1-9, AMS.

45   This can be observed in the operation protocols, in various reports (see Chapter 1), and on http://schweitzer.org/2012/de/lambarene/mitarbeiter-1913-1965 (This site no longer exists.).

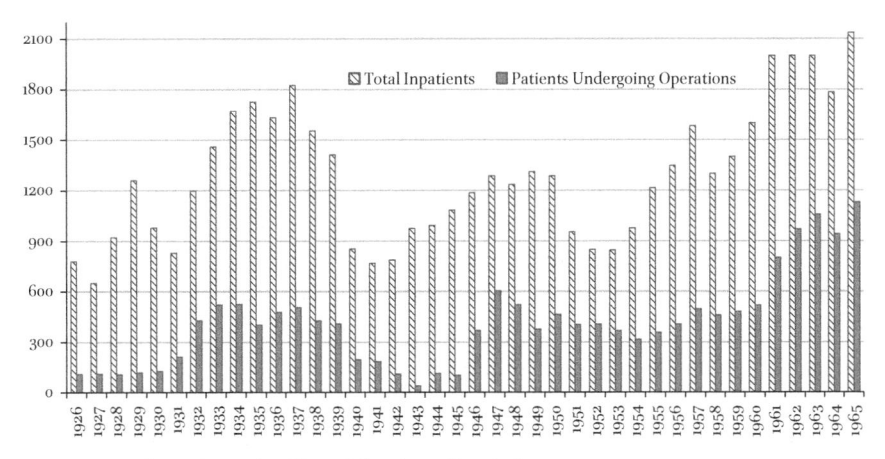

FIGURE 5   Surgeries at the Albert Schweitzer Hospital

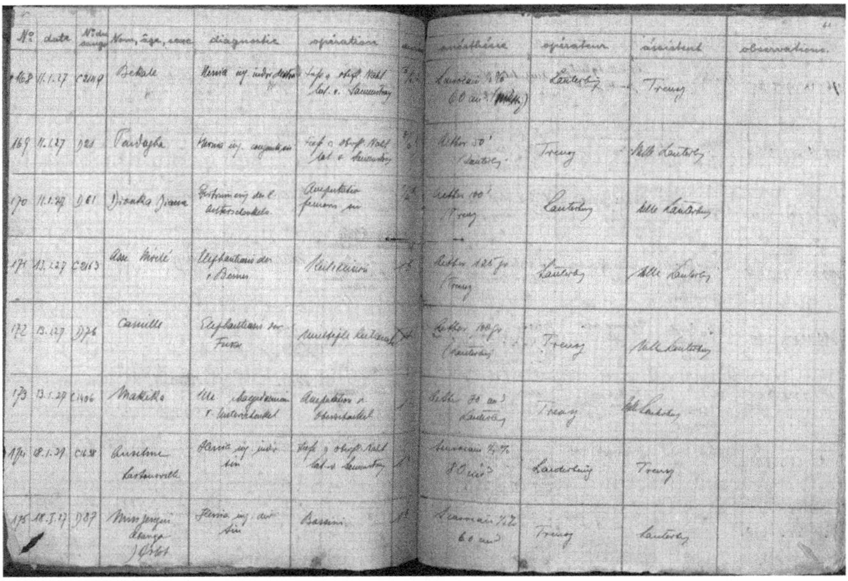

ILLUSTRATION 10   Operation protocols of January 1927, during the time of doctors Trensz
                    and Lauterburg
                    © ARCHIVES CENTRALES ALBERT SCHWEITZER GUNSBACH

hospital underwent operations. Typically, two of the three doctors were responsible for surgeries, while the third was often required to assist.[46] This was
sometimes to the detriment of other treatments. The Dutch physician Barend

---

46   Schweitzer, 'Briefe aus dem Lambarene Spital November 1935'.

Bonnema, for instance, complained in 1932 that he was forced to neglect treating very frequent ulcer cases because he had to perform so many operations.[47] Operations were scheduled for Tuesdays, Thursdays, and Saturdays. This timetable would be kept until Schweitzer's death, but was not overly rigid as emergencies or lengthy operations occurred regularly and surgical patients often came in waves.[48] In March 1934, for example, Ladislav Goldschmid, a Hungarian surgeon who served at the hospital three times until 1947, wrote of a 'surgical high season', in which operations were performed on a daily basis for a period of almost one month. He wanted to send patients home as soon as possible in order to minimize expenses for food.[49]

During World War Two, the proportion of patients who underwent operations dropped considerably to approximately 5 to 15 percent because the hospital did not have the capacity to do more. Schweitzer was required to participate in surgery again due to a lack of funding and qualified personnel. After the war, he quickly expanded the hospital's surgical services once more. The Swiss doctor René Kopp, who would serve in Lambaréné from 1946 to 1948 and again on several occasions after Schweitzer's death, learned that it would be 'useless for you to go to a school for colonial medicine. You work as a surgeon and you will be initiated into colonial medicine here on the spot'.[50]

The percentage of surgical patients had almost reached its pre-war levels by 1946. A year later, almost 50 percent of all inpatients underwent a surgical intervention, possibly to make up for the low number of operations performed during World War Two, as postponements were often feasible with hernias. Thereafter, the numbers stabilized to roughly where they had been in the 1930s. During the 1950s it appears that Schweitzer struggled to recruit surgeons,[51] even though his global reputation was growing rapidly at the time. He believed that eighteen months was too big a commitment for most surgeons, but considered this the required minimum in order to guarantee an efficient service.[52] A tentative count reveals that in the 1950s the number of doctors and

---

47   Bonnema to Schweitzer, 2 March 1932, AMS.
48   Schweitzer, 'Briefe aus dem Lambarene Spital November 1935', 8.
49   Goldschmid to Schweitzer, 7 March 1934, AMS. Dr. Bonnema reported the same surgical peak in: Bonnema to Schweitzer, 21 March 1934, AMS. The protocols support these claims.
50   Schweitzer to Kopp, 24 September 1945, AMS.
51   In 1951, Schweitzer approached the doctor at the government hospital of Lambaréné to request him to perform some surgeries, because he did not have enough personnel at the time. See: Bessuges, *Lambaréné à l'ombre de Schweitzer*, 92. In late 1958, a Danish doctor, who was visiting for three months reported that Schweitzer had claimed that he had not had a 'fully trained surgeon' for ten years. See: Østergaard Christensen, *At Work with Albert Schweitzer*, 13.
52   Schweitzer to Mellon, 7 July 1955. Published in: Schweitzer and Mellon, *Brothers in Spirit*.

the combined months that they served was only marginally lower than the corresponding figures for the 1930s.[53]

After Gabonese independence in 1960, the proportion of patients who underwent surgery at the hospital rose again to 40 and occasionally over 50 percent. One explanation for this is that state institutions faced a shortage of qualified personnel at the time.[54] In contrast, Schweitzer continued to employ new personnel and maintain his focus on surgery. In January 1961, Norbert Komora, assistant doctor in Bordeaux enquired if he might be allowed to work at Lambaréné. Schweitzer then wrote to Komora's superior to ask if he would allow his assistant to leave and if 'Mister Komora is capable of properly perform routine operations (hernias and others)? Hernias are our daily bread here. I have four physicians. Each of them has to know how to perform surgeries'.[55] Even though Komora would never come to Lambaréné, Schweitzer's questions illustrate the unceasing priority he assigned to surgery.

The information gathered for this overview indicates that surgery was the hospital's main service and that much organizational time and energy was devoted to it. Schweitzer did not perceive surgery as practiced in the colonies as essentially different from that practiced in Europe. Above all, he considered it to be the most important medical skill a physician needed to possess in order to practice at Lambaréné. As seen in Chapter 1, he had clear ideas about any prospective doctor's required competencies, medical and non-medical alike. In the area of surgery, this allowed Schweitzer to ensure procedural control, of which he had very specific preconceptions.

By far the most common surgical intervention during the whole study period was the repair of hernias.[56] Hernias were attributed to strenuous labor and

---

53   From 1930 to 1939, 15 doctors served for a combined total of over 370 months. From 1950 to 1959, 14 doctors served for a combined total of over 340 months. These figures are derived from the incomplete list on http://schweitzer.org/2012/de/lambarene/mitarbeiter-1913-1965 (This site no longer exists. The author possesses a copy of the list).

54   Mabika Ognandzi, *Médicaliser l'Afrique*, 235.

55   Schweitzer to Dubourg, 23 February 1961, AMS.

56   The 'Statistiques de l'Hôpital' provide the following numbers: In 1932, out of a total of 438 operations, 239 were hernia repairs and 38 were hydrocele surgeries. In 1937, there were 400 hernia repairs and 104 hydrocele surgeries in a total of 614 operations. In 1946, 186 hernia repairs and 43 hydrocele surgeries were conducted in a total of 360 operations. See: L – A – S2-3, AMS. For the years 1961 and 1962, Dr. Rolf Müller reported that 50.6 percent and 54.3 percent of all operations were to repair hernias and hydroceles respectively (see Müller, '50 Jahre Albert-Schweitzer-Spital', 16). This suggests a slight reduction in the relative frequency of these operations, probably due to the increasing number of women who visited the hospital and the resulting increase in gynaecological interventions.

were widespread throughout the region,[57] with Schweitzer having already reported the high prevalence of the condition during his first stay.[58] In 1933, Goldschmid repaired over one hundred hernias in the first eight months after his arrival.[59] Three years later, Dr. Heinz Barasch wrote to Schweitzer that he had performed a total of almost four hundred hernia operations in fifteen months. A hernia repair, he reported, would now take him no longer than thirty-five minutes, a pace which enabled him to conduct four instead of three repairs per operation day.[60] In August 1957, hernia operations alone were undertaken for a week to overcome a backlog of requests,[61] but a waiting list had developed once more just a month later.[62] In the 1960s, Tuesdays were reserved for hernia repairs. Using two operating tables, up to fifteen patients went under the knife per day.[63] This account clearly evokes the impersonal 'repair shop' invoked by Howell and cited at the beginning of this chapter. However, a closer examination of surgical practice and post-operative care at the Albert Schweitzer Hospital provides a slightly different and more nuanced picture.

Figure 6 is compiled from scattered and somewhat problematic records.[64] It compares the number of surgical operations performed at all government health facilities in colonial Gabon with the number of individual patients

---

57   In the Belgian Congo, hernias represented 50 to 80 percent of all major operations. Waiting lists of up to eight months were common for such interventions at mission hospitals. See: Au, 'Cutting the Flesh', 305. Mabika also refers repeatedly to hernias. See: Mabika Ognandzi, *Médicaliser l'Afrique*, 59, 249.

58   Schweitzer, 'Bericht an das Strassburger Comitee', 15 December 1913, AMS.

59   Schweitzer, 'Briefe aus dem Lambarene Spital Februar 1934', 2.

60   Barasch to Schweitzer, 3 June 1936, AMS.

61   Van der Kreek to Schweitzer, 18 August 1957, AMS. The protocols reveal that between 27 July and 29 August 1957, 44 of the 52 operations performed were hernias repairs. See: L – P – O6, AMS.

62   Friedmann to Schweitzer, 8 September 1957, AMS.

63   Müller, '50 Jahre Albert-Schweitzer-Spital', 16.

64   In the 1930s, there were three hospitals primarily responsible for surgical services: Libreville, Port-Gentil, and Oyem (the latter on an on-off basis). After 1950, a total of eight hospitals provided hernia repairs and other forms of surgery. See the annual reports of the Service de Santé for AEF and for Gabon: ZK 005-121(1934–35)/160(1940,1942–44)/089(1945–47)/093(1953)/016(1954)/095(1955–56), SHD; ZK 005-127(1925–33)/128(1950–51)/005(1957), SHD. Besides large and inexplicable fluctuations (from 1934 to 1935 or from 1953 to 1954), a major problem in compiling these statistics was the difference in categorising 'small interventions'. 'Abscess, caries, hydro adenitis, vaginal hydroceles, urethral stenosis, onychia, wounds, ulcers' were labelled as such and executed frequently, but they were not protocolled at the Albert Schweitzer Hospital. I have thus substracted those from the relevant government statistics. All records are rather inconsistent. The numbers should not be assumed to be complete, but serve their purpose of providing a general overview of surgical procedures.

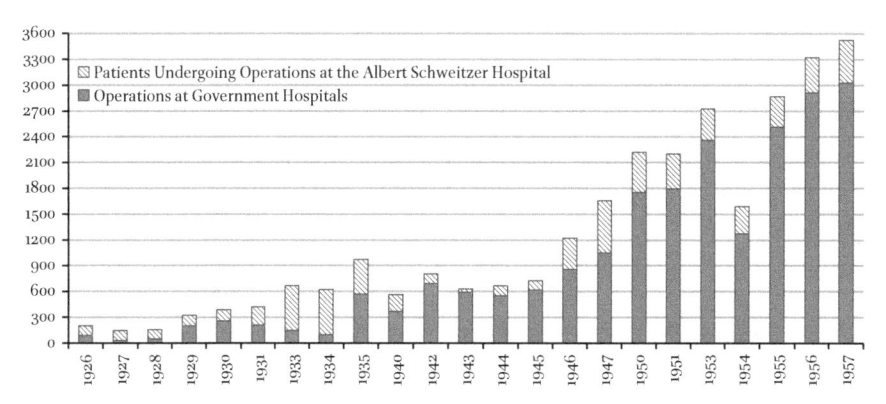

FIGURE 6   Surgeries in colonial Gabon

undergoing surgery at the Albert Schweitzer Hospital. During the interwar period, surgeons at the latter performed operations on at least as many patients as all those who underwent surgery at government institutions. Despite their superiors' suspicions about Schweitzer, touring government doctors or those from less well-equipped medical posts sent patients to his hospital.[65] Indeed, there are regular reports of people who came from over two hundred kilometers away to undergo an operation at the hospital.[66]

Immediately after World War Two, Schweitzer's surgeons still performed approximately one-third of all operations in the colonial territory of Gabon, but this proportion dropped below 15 percent by 1957. In the 1950s, a similar number of patients underwent surgery at the hospital as in the 1930s. While the population of Gabon is estimated to have remained more or less stable, more and more women started to come for treatment in the mid-1950s.[67] However, reports of surgical patients coming from afar diminish from 1945 onwards. This can be partially explained by the fact that during this period the French colonial government expanded its medical services by opening medical posts throughout Gabon, especially in the first ten years after the war, as

65   In 1932, Dr. Bonnema reported that a government doctor, who went on an anti-sleeping-sickness-tour, directed people with hernias and hydroceles to seek treatment at Schweitzer's hospital. See: Bonnema to Schweitzer, 29 May 1932, AMS. In 1936, Dr. Barasch performed an operation on a woman who had been sent to him by the government doctor in Mouila, which is almost two hundred hilometers to the south. See: Barasch to Schweitzer, 3 June 1936, AMS.

66   Hediger to Schweitzer, 18 May 1928, AMS. He mentioned people from Libreville and Fernan Vaz; Bonnema to Schweitzer, 10 April 1932, AMS. Bonnema reported of patients coming from Franceville.

67   As indicated in Chapter 1 and discussed in more detail in Chapter 3.

Hines Mabika has shown.[68] Some of these hospitals were also famous for conducting hernia repairs.[69] There is indeed a correlation between expanding government services and decreasing demand at Schweitzer's hospital, not only as a result of general trends, but also within individual years, such as 1935. This suggests, perhaps unsurprisingly, that patients tended to choose the nearest facility.

3   Controlling the Surgical Arena: Actors and Organization

The patient is physically at the center of every operation, but reports of surgery seldom focus on him or her. A close reading of the many reports of surgery at the Albert Schweitzer Hospital nevertheless allows for a tentative sketch of how patients went through it. Guy Barthélemy, a French forester who visited in 1951 while travelling through Africa, provided an especially detailed account.[70] On the day on which their operation was scheduled, patients moved from their sleeping quarters to the Grande Pharmacie, apparently without assistance from a nurse. There, they were made to wait in a designated area next to the operating theater. Here, Barthélemy takes up the already familiar thread of patients being policed. 'A black auxiliary guards them so that they do not disappear at the last moment or quickly take a big meal from their family to strengthen their courage', he wrote.[71]

During Barthélemy's visit, there were two mobile operating tables; while one patient underwent surgery on the one, another patient was prepared for his or her operation on the other. One nurse remained next to the patient for the duration of an operation to monitor blood pressure, pulse, and respiration.[72] Towards the end of the 1950s, surgeons at the hospital started to operate at two tables simultaneously.[73]

---

68   Mabika Ognandzi, *Médicaliser l'Afrique*.

69   Lavignotte, *L'évur: croyance des Fañ du Gabon*, 93. Lavignotte, a missionary, reported from Ovan in the north-east of the territory.

70   Barthélemy, *Wie ich Lambarene erlebte*. For Barthélemy's description of surgical practices, see pages 34f in particular. Barthélemy returned to Lambaréné towards the end of the decade to take charge of the hospital's maintenance. It was then that he met Dr. Greet van der Kreek, with whom he returned to France in 1960. After marrying each other, they opened a 'Village Albert Schweitzer' in Dordogne where they cared for mentally and physically ill patients.

71   Ibid., 34.

72   Ibid., 34–35.

73   Anderegg, 'Operationssaal und Sterilisation', 55; Müller, '50 Jahre Albert-Schweitzer-Spital', 16.

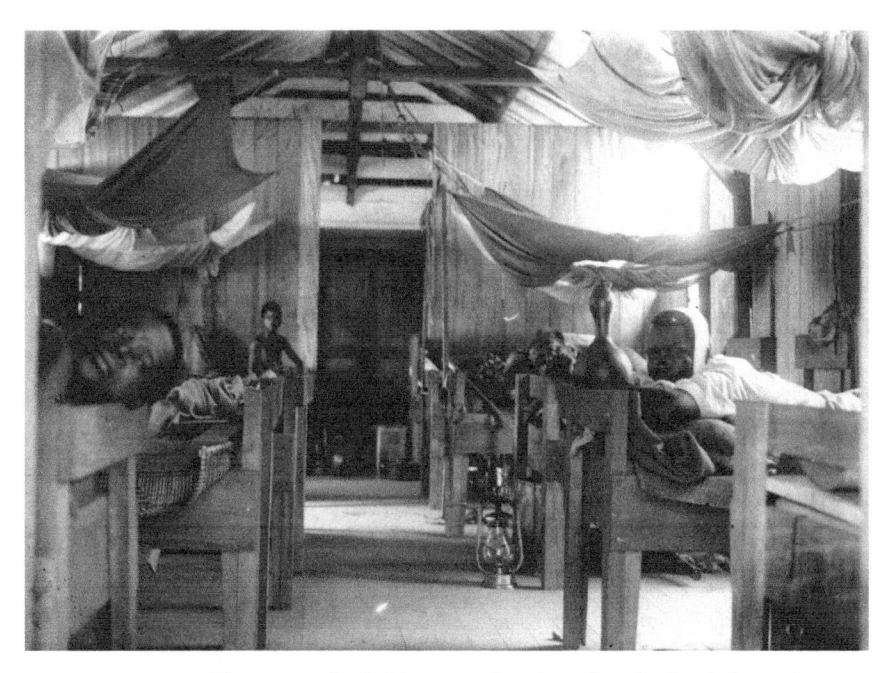

ILLUSTRATION 11   The quarters for freshly operated patients directly after their opening
                   in 1927
                   © ARCHIVES CENTRALES ALBERT SCHWEITZER GUNSBACH

Many reports describe in detail how patients who had just undergone surgery were moved back from the operating theater to their sleeping quarters (see Illustration 11). In 1925, patients were accompanied by the doctors themselves,[74] but they soon handed this task over. In the late 1920s, the auxiliary Boulingui was entrusted with the role of sitting next to the patient during an operation to monitor his or her vital signs. After the intervention, he then carried the patient 'on his arms' to the quarters for the recently operated.[75] In the 1950s, two helpers transported patients on a stretcher to the Case Bouka, the post-surgery ward named after Dominique, the long-serving African aide (see Illustration 12).[76] Here, patients were placed under the supervision of an African assistant and were visited daily by a physician.[77] In comparing these scattered accounts, a trend towards greater efficiency can be observed: from carrying patients by

---

74   Nessmann, *Avec Albert Schweitzer de 1924 à 1926*, 148.
75   Schnabel, 'Von ärztlichen Verrichtungen', 53–56.
76   Lehmann, 'Meine Erinnerung an das Frischoperiertenhaus', 59.
77   According to his long-term secretary Emma Haussknecht, it was Schweitzer himself who
      went on these daily rounds through the ward in the Case Bouka, at least until the late
      1940s. See: Haussknecht, *Emma Haussknecht, 1895–1956*, 113–14; Later, doctors wrote of

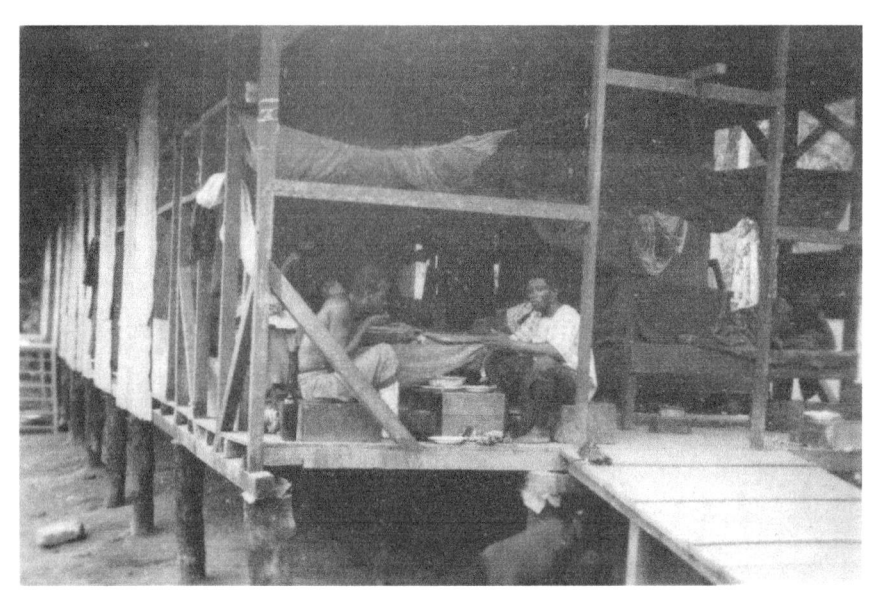

ILLUSTRATION 12   The same quarters, now called 'Case Bouka', at a later date
© ARCHIVES CENTRALES ALBERT SCHWEITZER GUNSBACH

hand to using a stretcher, or from performing operations one after the other to conducting two at the same time. Medical staff, rather than technologies, however, remained central to maintaining and controlling the surgical routine.

Schweitzer had a clear vision of how the hospital's surgical services should be run. In 1934, Goldschmid was happy to report that 'the surgical service is now provided according to your instructions'.[78] Over and above the organizational routine just outlined, Schweitzer provided a rigidly defined order for how surgical interventions themselves should be performed. Especially and unambiguously important to him was to be in control of the various personnel responsible for its execution. The recruitment process was a first step towards achieving this, but control continued to be exerted in Lambaréné. In 1947, Schweitzer wrote to Edward Hume, one of his most important supporters in the USA, that a new doctor would soon arrive from Switzerland, adding that

> I still insist on initiating them myself. Because you know well how necessary it is in medicine that new doctors conform to the traditions and

---

undertaking their own daily ward rounds in Schweitzer's absence. See, for example: Van der Kreek to Schweitzer, 27 October 1959, AMS; Percy to Schweitzer, 2 October 1955, AMS.
78   Goldschmid to Schweitzer, 22 August 1934, AMS.

spirit of the hospital in which they will work in order to assure that they do not introduce innovations there that have no reason.[79]

To his niece, Schweitzer wrote in a similar manner concerning his anxieties about novel staff introducing new practices that would run counter to the values and traditions of his hospital. He was nevertheless confident about his ability to control new personnel and convince them of the superiority of his specific approach:

> Dr. P and Dr. N. are hardworking and kind. They can be convinced to execute the service in my spirit and making sure that no innovations are introduced. This is the big danger for the hospital, because before having served for a year, the newcomers cannot really see its meaning as it is.[80]

In order to ensure that his surgeons practiced according to his wishes, Schweitzer often personally attended the first significant operations performed by recently arrived physicians. This was the case in 1925 with Dr. Lauterburg, a very experienced surgeon and the second additional doctor to arrive at the hospital: Schweitzer acted as an assistant in order to 'test the quality of surgery of the new doctor'.[81] Similarly, Dr. van der Kreek recalled that many of the approximately 2,000 operations that she performed from 1955 to 1960 were undertaken 'under his attentive gaze'.[82] These examples illustrate how the Lambaréné Spirit related to medical practice: besides a personable attitude on the part of his staff or their ability to engage in polite conversation at the dinner table, for instance, Schweitzer expected their full compliance with his medical ideals.

Schweitzer's desire to control the manner in which his employees practiced medicine is remembered explicitly by many of his former personnel. A case in point from the surgical domain can be found in a lively and engaging memoir by Dr. Edgar Berman. A surgeon from Baltimore, Berman visited Lambaréné for two months in the fall of 1960 and furnished an account of his stay replete with exaggeration and self-aggrandizement.[83] Schweitzer's controlling nature

---

79   Schweitzer to Hume, 8 November 1947, AMS.
80   Schweitzer to Oswald, 17 May 1950. Published in: Oswald, *Mein Onkel Bery*, 116–17.
81   Nessmann, *Avec Albert Schweitzer de 1924 à 1926*, 144.
82   Becht, 'Témoignage d'une chirurgien, Mme Le Docteur Greet Barthélémy', 170. Dr. Greet van der Kreek married Guy Bartélemy, thus explaining her change of name (see note 70).
83   Berman, *In Africa with Schweitzer*. Berman claims to have performed numerous operations at the hospital. In the protocols, he appears on 8 out of 21 occasions between 29 November and 17 December 1960, usually as an assistant and always working in cooperation with

occupies a central place in Berman's description of his first surgical intervention at the hospital, an intervention that cannot be found in the protocols. Two
hours after his arrival, Berman was asked to operate on a strangulated hernia.
He was assisted by three long-serving Gabonese aides: Joseph (Ndolo or Bissangoy), Pierre Piebé, and Ambroise Nyama. In addition, Schweitzer remained
in the operating theater for the two hours that it took to complete the procedure. Berman was certain that 'this case had purposefully been singled out to
test me'. After they agreed that the piece of bowel was beyond saving, Schweitzer
ordered a colostomy. At this point, Berman dared to disagree, explaining that
this method was no longer commonly practiced. Instead, he proposed to cut
out the diseased piece and sew the ends together. Schweitzer replied that the
hospital had achieved poor results with this method. Berman objected again
and then proceeded to perform the surgery in his preferred manner and
Schweitzer remained silent for the rest of the operation.[84] Although this story
is probably exaggerated or perhaps even invented, it does illustrate how even
short-term visitors were made to feel the constant presence of Schweitzer's
controlling gaze. Indeed, it was usually these very visitors who dared to describe it.

The colonial government doctor Jacques Bessuges performed a number of
surgeries at the hospital at Schweitzer's request in early 1950. He provided a
particularly detailed and more credible account of his first operation that ex-
pressly illustrates Schweitzer's desire for procedural control in surgical practice. During the three-and-a-half-hour intervention to repair an incarcerated
hernia, Schweitzer served as an assistant. In addition, Pierre Piebé and Ali Silver, who had both been at the hospital for years, were also present as assistants.
Schweitzer and Bessuges disagreed on a number of occasions during the operation. Bessuges assumed that the patient would receive a general anesthetic,
whereas Schweitzer proposed a local one. When Bessuges started connecting
the loose ends of the affected intestine by applying the usual French method of
'surjets', an overcast suture that he claimed would take only five minutes,
Schweitzer suggested the more reliable German method of 'points séparés', an
interrupted suture which took forty minutes to complete. Thereafter, Bessuges
wanted to end the operation so as not to place more strain on the patient and
to leave an opening in case of infection; Schweitzer, however, urged him to

---

another doctor. See: L – P – O6, AMS. In the preface to his book, he states that he was a replacement for the hospital's chief surgeon. It seems unlikely that this would have been the
case for such a short period of time given that the doctors Adler, Müller, Friedmann, and
Goldwyn were present during this period.

84   Ibid., 11–16.

perform the complete suture, which required another forty-five minutes' work. In all three of these differences of opinion, Bessuges ultimately surrendered to Schweitzer's authority and did as instructed.[85] Bessuges returned to perform surgery at the hospital regularly thereafter, but Schweitzer only assisted and supervised him on one further occasion. During these procedures, Bessuges was usually assisted by Piebé and Silver, or occasionally by Dr. Emeric Percy, a Hungarian who served two terms in the 1950s.[86] If not through his own presence, Schweitzer could thus ensure procedural control via that of his long-term employees.

All surgeons who describe surgical procedures at the hospital – from Ilse Schnabel in the 1920s and Bessuges in the 1950s to Rolf Müller in the 1960s – mention being assisted by at least one African and one European.[87] A glance through the protocols reveals that the names of African assistants were only recorded in some years of the 1950s. No clear pattern of surgical team-composition can be discerned for any period. The chief surgeon was sometimes assisted by an additional physician and two European nurses, sometimes by one European and one African nurse, or on other occasions by a single European or African assistant.

Unlike the majority of the European surgical personnel, who normally returned to their home countries after approximately two years, some African assistants served at the hospital for decades. Piebé started to work at the hospital in 1929. He had been a former surgical patient who went on to serve as a nurse in the post-surgery ward.[88] Here, his task was to ensure that patients would not eat, remove their bandages, or go for a walk or swim, all actions that were difficult to police. After World War Two, the nature of Piebé's duties changed (see Illustration 13). He now worked in the operating theater, where Dr. Jeanette Israël described him as 'very intelligent' with 'very fine hands'.[89] Dr. van der Kreek emphasized Piebé's value as a surgical assistant, underlining

85 Bessuges, *Lambaréné à l'ombre de Schweitzer*, 112–15.

86 According to the operation protocols, Bessuges had already performed two operations at the hospital two days before the episode described here, namely a simple hernia repair and a hydrocele procedure during both of which he was assisted by only Piebé and Silver. Thereafter, Bessuges performed eighteen further operations at the hospital, with his last on 14 February 1950. See: L – P – O5, AMS.

87 Schnabel, 'Medizinisches aus Albert Schweitzers Urwaldspital', 379–81; Bessuges, *Lambaréné à l'ombre de Schweitzer*, 100–116; Müller, '50 Jahre Albert-Schweitzer-Spital', 16–24.

88 Schweitzer, 'Briefe aus dem Lambarene Spital März 1938', 3. Piebé is on a 1962 'liste des employés les plus anciens, proposés pour une décoration' The list was found in a folder entitled 'affaires concernant le personnel indigene', within a box with the brief title 'divers', in the cellar of the AMS.

89 Israël, 'Schweitzer, le médecin que nous avons connu', 177.

his experience, which had equipped him with considerable confidence and even a certain authority over his chief surgeon, whom he occasionally corrected. She considered him 'irreplaceable' and recalled that he 'often gave peremptory suggestions and advice when we were hesitating'.[90] Echoing this sentiment, Schweitzer purportedly told Dr. Berman in 1960 that Piebé 'was rarely wrong in the operating room'. According to the American surgeon, whose assertions must be treated with caution, Piebé occasionally even operated on simple hernias himself.[91]

Another African assistant in the surgical ward was Boulingui, whom Schweitzer described in 1931. He highlighted the considerable surgical competence that his assistant had acquired:

> Bolingi, who has been with me since 1924, works in the operating theatre and the quarters of the operated patients. Since he has some judgement about the way a surgical intervention is performed from the many operations he has attended, he often acknowledges Dr. Schmitz with a word of appreciation if, in his opinion, she has completed an incarcerated hernia at a pleasing pace.[92]

In her characterization of Boulingui the nurse Elsa Lauterburg-Bonjour illustrates, albeit in a slightly mocking tone, the wide variety of tasks that auxiliaries had to perform. She wrote that Boulingui 'checks the pulse ('le moteur ça marche'), boils out instruments ('bouillir les sentiments'), opens ampules ('ouvrir la poule'), ignites the autoclave (an 'allumer l'esclave') and dresses the recently operated patients'.[93]

Lauterburg-Bonjour named Nyama as an important surgical assistant. Like Piebé and many others, he was a former patient at the hospital. For Lauterburg-Bonjour, Nyama was crucial as 'the right hand of the doctor'.[94] He was first mentioned in 1928 as an assistant in the pre-operation procedure.[95] By 1960, Dr. Berman claimed that Nyama 'ran the whole O.R. suite'.[96] Dr. Armin Rutishauser was similarly effusive in his praise of Nyama and other African aides in 1937, also mentioning their numerous and diverse tasks:

---

90   Becht, 'Témoignage d'une chirurgien, Mme Le Docteur Greet Barthélémy', 173.

91   Berman, *In Africa with Schweitzer*, 13.

92   Schweitzer, 'Briefe aus dem Lambarene Spital Pfingsten 1931', 9.

93   Lauterburg-Bonjour, *Lambarene: Erlebnisse einer Bernerin im afrikanischen Urwald*, 18.

94   Ibid.

95   Schnabel, 'Von ärztlichen Verrichtungen', 53.

96   Berman, *In Africa with Schweitzer*, 13.

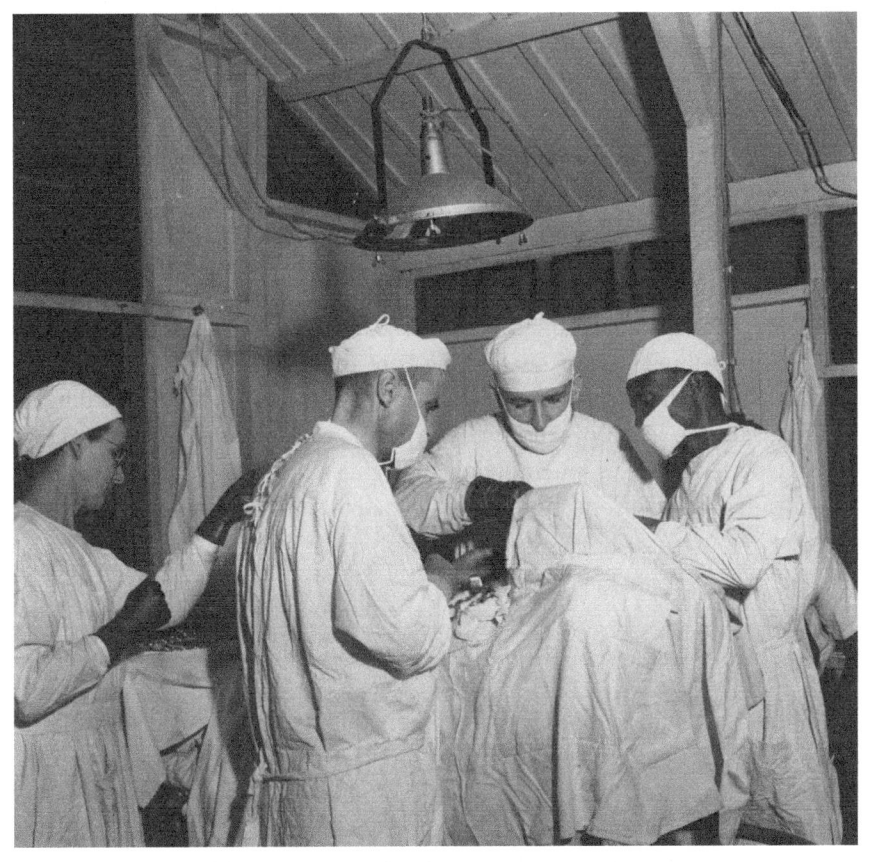

ILLUSTRATION 13   The nurse Maria Lagendijk, Pierre Piébé, and two doctors during an
operation, ca. 1950
© ARCHIVES CENTRALES ALBERT SCHWEITZER GUNSBACH

Nyama, our best, does intravenous injections like any white doctor, perhaps even better, since hardly anyone has as much practice as him, and it
is even more difficult to find a vein in Negroes than back home. He is also
the best in the surgical ward, besides he acts as an interpreter and other
things, although he can neither read nor write. What such auxiliaries do
is astounding. Year after year, day after day, from early in the morning to
late in the evening, always in a good mood, always helpful. You call the
name and he appears. Many barefoot, but cleanly dressed and washed.[97]

These examples show that when it came to concrete medical duties, especially
those relating to surgery, African staff at the Albert Schweitzer Hospital was
depicted as skillful and competent. This is a much more positive portrayal of

---

97   Rutishauser, 'Wie eine Insel', 131.

their ability than that we receive from more general sources relating to the hospital.[98] Even though the assistants had not been medically trained in the formal sense, they acquired a remarkable level of skill through their extensive on-the-job training, which demanded a high degree of flexibility and bestowed on them valuable experience. They combined competences in surgery assistance and nursing, enjoying considerable power and responsibility in the process.

African aides from the surgical ward helped to mediate between patients and doctors, but also functioned as middles for different types of control. They ensured procedural control by making sure that mistakes were minimized and that operations went according to plan – or, more precisely, according to Schweitzer's plan. Their proximity to the hospital's founder and their own levels of experience, often much higher than those of the typically young and recently graduated European surgeons, helped to secure their place within the hospital hierarchy.

4   Technologies of Control: the Example of Lamps

Schweitzer depended more on practitioners than technologies to implement and uphold his rigid vision of surgical practice. He ensured control over personnel working in the surgical ward by careful selection and via his own authority, which was often mediated through highly trusted long-term European and African employees. Nonetheless, technological artifacts played a significant role in surgical practices at the institution.

An important factor determining whether technological artefacts were introduced to the Albert Schweitzer Hospital was their cost, as is argued for other colonies.[99] In 1938, Schweitzer received a donation from European settlers living in the area to buy radiological equipment,[100] but with World War Two

---

98   As seen in the Introduction, Schweitzer and other European staff and visitors considered Africans as lazy and backward. Furthermore, a considerable number of reports did ascribe these qualities to the auxiliaries, but these mostly did not relate to those working in the surgical ward. These reports will thus be analyzed elsewhere, especially in Chapter 5.

99   Hardimann, 'The Mission Hospital', 204–5; Howell, 'Hospitals', 513. Yet, a shortfall of funding usually also implies a lack of will. In contrast, the Basel Mission's Agogo Hospital in the Gold Coast colony had a reputation for and self-perception of maintaining a high technological standard. The hospital was established in 1931, and less than ten years later already possessed state of the art surgical equipment, including X-ray machines. See: Schmid, 'Mission Medicine in a Decolonising Health Care System'.

100   Ott, 'Natur, Mensch und Tier', 110.

looming, he chose to spend the money on medication and rice instead.[101] When in March 1954 an X-ray apparatus was finally introduced, Schweitzer justified this not only with reference to the necessity for accurate tuberculosis diagnoses. He also emphasized that the machine had been especially designed by a Dutch manufacturer for use in the tropics and that Dr. Percy knew how to set it up and repair it.[102] This example suggests that Schweitzer was rather reluctant to introduce technical medical devices. He and other members of the hospital staff argued repeatedly that expensive machinery would be very prone to defects in the tropical climate and that it was difficult to repair easily and cheaply.[103] For Schweitzer, technological artefacts were thus perceived as operating outside of his own control; instead of ensuring procedural control they threatened the orderly functioning of hospital services.

The example of electric lights serves to illustrate this point more precisely. Lighting is one of the few aspects in which the agency of surgeons at the hospital becomes immediately visible. They took advantage of Schweitzer's regular leaves to Europe to improve the ward according to their own preferences. Lights were of considerable importance for visual control during surgery. Surgical interventions had to be regularly performed at night. In 1913, for example, Schweitzer performed an operation while using only a paraffin lamp for lighting.[104] The Swiss doctor Ilse Schnabel, who worked at the hospital from 1928 to 1930, recounted performing daring operations under makeshift lights:

> Operations in the dark require a great deal of time and effort. With the help of two large petrol lamps on stacked chairs or tables, the surgical area could be illuminated to a certain extent, but an electric torch had to be directed onto the areas to be made clearly visible and had to be held for hours during an extensive intestinal resection.[105]

In 1935, Schweitzer proudly reported that 'a grateful white patient has donated a big petroleum lamp with incandescent gas mantle, which gives wonderfully bright light'.[106] Apparently, these improvisations were sufficient until World

---

101   Schweitzer, 'Briefe aus dem Lambarene Spital März 1946', 2–3.

102   Schweitzer, 'Briefe aus dem Lambarenespital Oktober 1954', 17.

103   Lauterburg-Bonjour, 'Man stellt sich um', 164; Joy, Arnold, and Schweitzer, *The Africa of Albert Schweitzer*, 116; Taap, *Lambarener Tagebuch*, 65.

104   Schweitzer, 'Notes et Nouvelles de la part du prof. Albert Schweitzer. Deuxième rapport', 36.

105   Schnabel, 'Medizinisches aus Albert Schweitzers Urwaldspital', 379.

106   Schweitzer, 'Briefe aus dem Lambarene Spital November 1935', 4.

War Two. In 1941, Schweitzer ordered equipment for electric lightning from the USA. He justified its introduction not only with reference to the hospital's lighting challenges at the time – 'we need better lighting', as he wrote matter-of-factly – but also for its economic benefits; 'petrol is very expensive here', he explained.[107] It remains unclear when exactly the equipment eventually arrived, but three years later spare parts for a small engine that provided light in the operating theater had already been sent to Lambaréné.[108] In 1946, lighting equipment needed to be replaced. By then, operations took place regularly under electric light. Schweitzer now attributed this practice to the dim daylight in the equatorial latitudes.[109]

In July 1951, Dr. Percy informed Schweitzer that an engine had broken down and that the operating theater was without lights. Lighting had become essential for surgery, even during the day, and Percy went to great lengths to replace the defective engine. He retrieved an old engine and, with the help of a mechanic from a lumber company, worked for three days to repair it. Percy estimated that this makeshift solution would work for three months at the most and thus listed in great detail the properties that he thought a new engine should possess.[110] In the following months, Percy solved the problem and expanded their power system. In October he reported without providing details that 'everything is fine with the engines. [...] We supplied the whole central building with electricity; there are now lamps in all rooms except the delivery room'.[111]

The lighting situation, however, remained precarious. In September 1957, Dr. Richard Friedmann, who had arrived a year earlier, described to Schweitzer in a very detailed manner how the large operating lamp had been fixed. Its wires had been burnt through ostensibly due to a wet climate and previous inadequate repairs.[112] Eventually, in 1959, a powerful operating lamp was donated to

---

107 Schweitzer to Hume, 9 January 1941, AMS. Schweitzer rarely sent letters in English. When he did, he usually had these translated by a member of staff who could speak English.

108 Schweitzer to Hume, 27 August 1944, AMS. The digital file is falsely dated with 1942. Schweitzer attached a copy of a letter from the same date, which he sent to 'les Directeurs de la commission qui accorde la Licence d'importation pour l'AEF', in which he mentions the spare parts.

109 Schweitzer to Hume, 17 February 1946, AMS.

110 Percy to Schweitzer, 7 July 1951, AMS.

111 Percy to Schweitzer, 21 October 1951, AMS.

112 Friedmann to Schweitzer, 8 September 1957, AMS.

the hospital by the Prince of Monaco.[113] Subsequently, it appears that the surgeons were satisfied with the operating light.[114]

It was difficult to convince Schweitzer of the necessity to introduce novel technologies, whereas the surgeons demanded a steady improvement in the quality of lighting. Percy thus acquired new gear while Schweitzer was in Europe or Barthélemy brought surgical material from Paris 'while hiding myself'.[115] The frequent reports of electric lights that had to be repaired prove that they did not always operate smoothly, but visual control was a deeply rooted desire in the 1950s for the hospital's surgeons. Like the scalpel in Dr. Lauterburg's nickname, lighting is an example of the interconnectedness of object, technology and person: surgeons could not properly do surgery without adequate lamps.

5 Controlling Bacteria: Asepsis and Manual Labor

One of the most urgent practical concerns in surgical wards was and is bacterial control. Western operating theaters were specifically designed for enforcing asepsis, the state of sterility.[116] At the Albert Schweitzer Hospital a considerable amount of time and labor was dedicated to this quest. Surgeons described the disinfection of surgical instruments and body parts in great detail. It is difficult to tell if they were impressed or even surprised by the great care given to asepsis at the hospital, or if they wanted to underline that, even in more challenging circumstances, its surgical services operated in line with Western standards. Numerous reports allow us to outline how asepsis was enforced over the course of the study period and to recognize patterns therein. In 1928, Dr. Schnabel described the pre-surgical disinfection process as follows:

---

113 Anderegg, 'Operationssaal und Sterilisation', 55. Earlier in the decade, at the initiative of Barthélemy, the Prince of Monaco had already donated other surgical equipment, possibly including one of the above-mentioned lamps. See: Barthélemy, *Lettre à Albert Schweitzer*, 121. See also: Becht, 'Témoignage d'une chirurgien, Mme Le Docteur Greet Barthélemy', 174; Penn, 'A Visit to Albert Schweitzer', 174. A rather sophisticated lamp is prominent in Penn's photograph of the operating room.

114 This was stated explicitly by some. See, for example: Østergaard Christensen, *At Work with Albert Schweitzer*, 80; Müller, '50 Jahre Albert-Schweitzer-Spital', 17.

115 Barthélemy, *Lettre à Albert Schweitzer*, 121.

116 Schlich, 'Surgery, Science and Modernity', 231.

> When I enter the big room of the infirmary at ten past eight in the morning, three healing assistants are still gathered at the middle table, with spoon and fork in their hands. The first part of washing hands occurs in this room. My colleague and I put on a white cap, remove a sterile brush from the container that Nyama gives us, and wash our hands thoroughly with soap under running hot water. A Negress sits by the large container and lets the water run out of the tap as needed. [...] After this preparation, we move to the actual operating room. [...] On a long box, there is a basin with foaming lysol solution, into which we immediately dip our hands and continue washing them. [...] We receive sterile, perfectly white surgical gowns and the auxiliaries naturally assist us in putting them on. The gloves, however, meant a disappointment to me; we could not take them beautifully powdered from a gauze cover, as I had been used to, but from a pot filled with sterile solution, in which they were carefully piled up pair for pair by sticks of palm wood.[117]

Some twenty years later, Bessuges described a similar procedure: first the surgeons washed their hands in Cresyl water, before putting on coats and gloves and washing their hands again in alcohol (see Illustration 14). After having administered an anesthetic, they changed their gloves once more.[118] Almost ten years later, Berman reported that before entering the operation theater 'a native aide poured soapy liquid over my hands, then rinsed them with germ-free water – the excess running into a galvanized tub'. The surgical team received 'heavy rubberized aprons' and 'good modern O.R. gloves'. Berman also scrubbed himself a second time after administering an anesthetic.[119] These descriptions reveal that some innovations were introduced into the pre-operative asepsis process, as occurred, for example, through the provision of new gloves to increase surgeons' sense of touch and their manual control. However, the general sequence and extent of disinfection, as well as the sterilizing solutions used, remained very similar throughout the study period.[120]

The sheer physical challenge of performing surgical interventions in Lambaréné was a particular concern for surgeons practicing there. Dr. Jilek-Aall, a Norwegian physician who had previously worked as an itinerant doctor in Tanzania and for the United Nations forces in the Congo Crisis before practicing at the Albert Schweitzer Hospital in 1961, recalled that

---

117   Schnabel, 'Von ärztlichen Verrichtungen', 53–54.
118   Bessuges, *Lambaréné à l'ombre de Schweitzer*, 101–3.
119   Berman, *In Africa with Schweitzer*, 13–14.
120   Lysol and Cresyl were both brand names of disinfectants based on phenols.

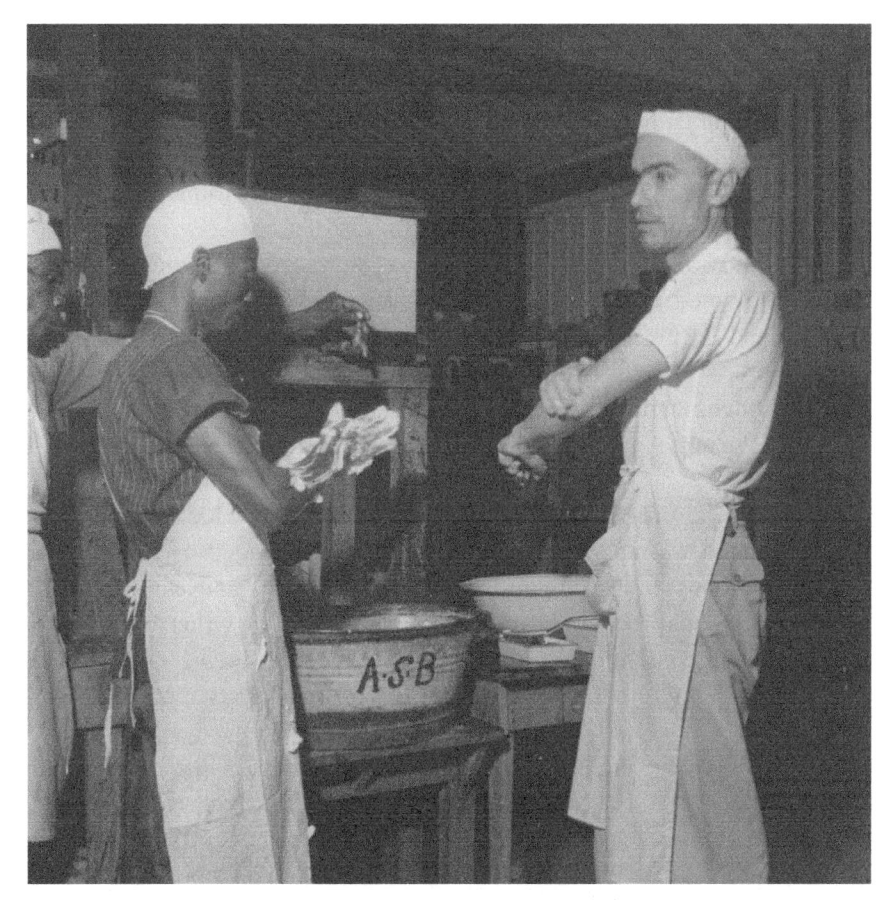

ILLUSTRATION 14 Pierre Piébé and Dr. Arnold Brack disinfect their hands, ca. 1947
© ARCHIVES CENTRALES ALBERT SCHWEITZER GUNSBACH

the ordeal of standing for hours in the humid, hot air, face mask, hair cover, heavy gowns, rubber gloves and all, was nearly more than I was able to endure. [...] The duty nurse had to constantly wipe our faces to prevent the sweat from dripping into the operating field. Sometimes when one of us was close to collapse she would quickly get us a cold drink.[121]

Jilek-Aall was not the only surgeon who remembered assistants having to wipe sweat from his or her face.[122] As was the case with the X-ray apparatus,

---

121   Jilek-Aall, *Working with Dr. Schweitzer*, 48.
122   Barthélemy, *Wie ich Lambarene erlebte*, 35; Berman, *In Africa with Schweitzer*, 14; Bessuges, *Lambaréné à l'ombre de Schweitzer*, 111.

Schweitzer did not want to install an air conditioning system, because he believed that it would soon break down and that there would be no one able to repair it. In the early 1960s, members of staff found an air conditioner in a basement and, without informing Schweitzer, installed it in the radiology room. When he discovered the machine, Schweitzer was 'furious', because his permission had not been sought.[123]

Medical instruments and cloths were other sources of infection. Sterilizing these was a time-consuming undertaking, much of which had to be done by hand. Indeed, during his first stay, Schweitzer could not satisfy the demand for surgeries precisely because there were not enough personnel to wash and prepare instruments and cloths.[124] Similarly, the Alsatian Victor Nessman, the first additional doctor to join Schweitzer in Lambaréné, complained in 1925 that

> the surgical procedure in Europe begins and ends with thorough and long hand washing. Here, contrariwise, it is preceded by sterilization preparations of instruments, gowns, sterile cloths and with the final washing of hands after the operation, it is not finished either. It is up to us to clean the instruments, boil them a second time, then grease them to protect them from the terrible humidity that ruins everything here.[125]

Soon thereafter, a nascent division of labor had emerged. In a 1926 report, Lauterburg-Bonjour listed the afternoon tasks of the African auxiliaries. They had to maintain a fire, boil water, degrease surgical instruments, and sterilize operating equipment in an autoclave that ran on a petroleum flame. Female relatives of patients, meanwhile, washed and prepared bandages and other cloths under Lauterburg-Bonjour's constant supervision.[126]

The development of these practices can be traced throughout the study period. In the 1930s, sterilizing surgical cloths, or supervising the Africans assistants responsible for this task, was a very time-consuming job for nurses on surgical duty.[127] The disinfection process was primarily undertaken using hot water (see Illustration 15). In the late 1940s, 'surgical instruments (were) boiled in pans, and kettles (were) kept steaming to provide sterile water of the operating room'.[128] Oxidation was also a problem. Dr. Schnabel wrote in 1936 that all

---

123   Interview Munz and Munz.
124   Schweitzer, 'Notes et Nouvelles de la part du prof. Albert Schweitzer. Deuxième rapport', 36.
125   Nessmann, *Avec Albert Schweitzer de 1924 à 1926*, 148.
126   Schweitzer, 'Neues von Albert Schweitzer Advent 1926', 3.
127   Schweitzer, 'Briefe aus dem Lambarene Spital März 1938', 2.
128   Joy, Arnold, and Schweitzer, *The Africa of Albert Schweitzer*, 140.

surgical instruments were stored in a layer of paraffin to prevent them from rusting; there was one set of stainless steel instruments reserved for emergencies.[129] A second was acquired over two decades later, as the Swiss nurse Elisabeth Anderegg, who served four terms in the surgical ward from 1958 to 1968, recalled. The other instruments continued to be disinfected in boiling water and soda in between interventions. For this purpose, the auxiliary Marcel Kwamba was given the task of maintaining a fire in a stone oven outside the Grande Pharmacie. As had been the case in the 1930s, the nurse responsible for the surgical ward was tasked with sterilizing surgical cloths on the three operation-free days per week.[130]

In the surgical ward, technological devices provided limited assistance for sanitizing cloths. In 1913, Schweitzer claimed to possess an autoclave for sterilizing bandaging material.[131] The next reference to a similar item dates from the late 1950s, when Anderegg wrote of a vapor autoclave that was used to disinfect rubber and plastic surgical material and to prepare two sets of surgical instruments on the night before an operation.[132] The nurse Hedwig Schnee remembers that in the 1960s there was an autoclave in the operating theater for cleaning dressing materials that could also be used by staff members from other wards.[133] Unfortunately, details of the size, structure, and workings of these autoclaves have not been provided.

What applies to the surgical procedure as a whole extends to the enforcement of bacterial control: people were more important than technological artefacts. With no air conditioning system, surgeons' sweat continued to be wiped from their brows by their assistants; instead of using a large autoclave, washerwomen were tasked with disinfecting cloths. Moreover, asepsis exemplifies how technology can be defined in different ways depending on the scope of analysis. All recognized meanings of the term have been raised in this discussion: 'physical objects or artefacts' – in the form of autoclaves or sterilized knives – have been used to sustain 'activities or processes', maintaining asepsis and executing the surgical intervention as such, – which are in turn dependent on 'what people know as well as what they do'.[134] This chain of action illustrates that asepsis, like surgery, only becomes operational when human beings who are in control of themselves and their environment become involved.

---

129 Schnabel, 'Medizinisches aus Albert Schweitzers Urwaldspital', 380.
130 Anderegg, 'Operationssaal und Sterilisation', 57.
131 Schweitzer, 'Notes et Nouvelles de la part du prof. Albert Schweitzer Lambaréné', 7.
132 Anderegg, 'Operationssaal und Sterilisation', 57.
133 Interview Hedwig Schnee.
134 Bijker, Hughes, and Pinch, 'The Social Construction of Technological Systems, Introduction', 4.

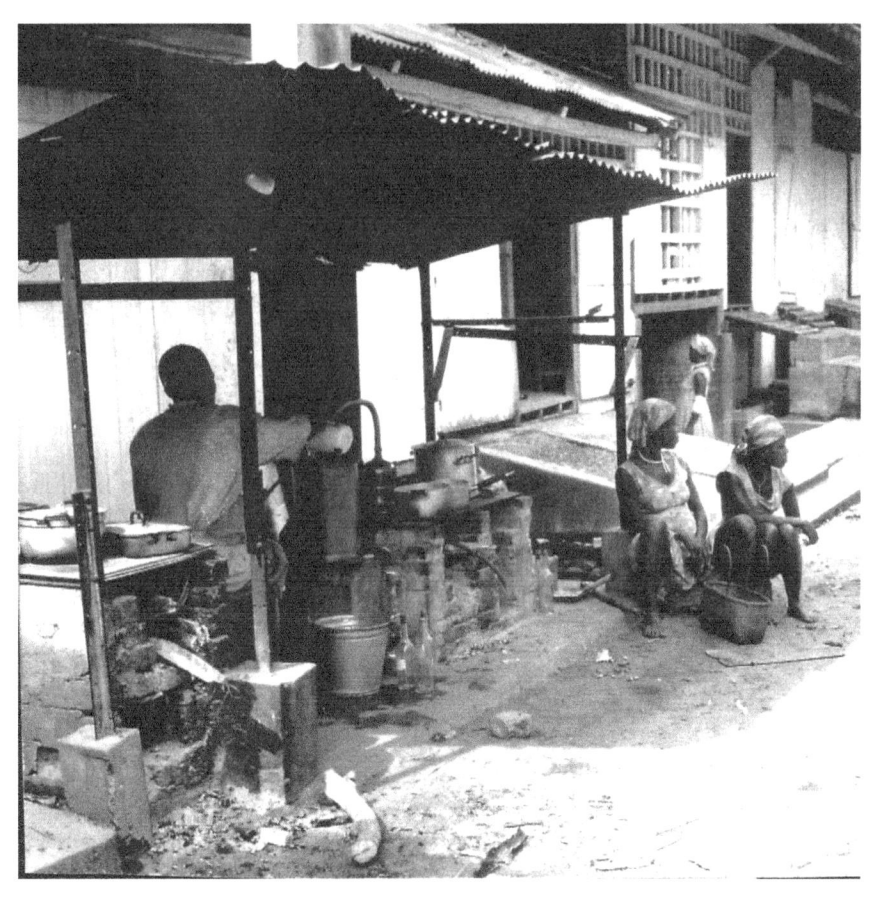

ILLUSTRATION 15   Sterilizing surgical instruments, probably late 1930s
© ARCHIVES CENTRALES ALBERT SCHWEITZER GUNSBACH

Animals, however, were less controllable. The operating theater at the hospital formed part of the Grande Pharmacie and, as such, was not hermetically enclosed. The floor and walls were wooden, while its finely gridded windows were built to keep mosquitos out and let air and light in. There are various anecdotes of unexpected guests arriving during surgery. For example, Jilek-Aall was assisting in an operation in 1961 when a lizard, seemingly dizzy from evaporating ether, dropped into the patient's open wound. This did not cause too much panic, she noted, as

> without a word, the surgeon took the forceps, fished out the lifeless animal, and threw it over his shoulder. He then sprinkled antibiotic powder

into the abdomen and continued the operation as if nothing unusual had happened.[135]

Dr. Berman wrote of a tarantula that suddenly appeared from a sterile pile of sheets as well as of a goat that knocked things down.[136] Two nurses confirm that goats and dogs roamed rather freely around the hospital grounds and were not a rare sight in the adjacent consultation rooms.[137] These reports may be exaggerated or even invented, but together they point towards one particular obstacle to ensuring bacterial control.

Despite such difficulties in maintaining asepsis, staff members claim that post-surgical infections were extremely rare.[138] In earlier years, they were referred to more frequently. Dr. Lauterburg reported in 1925 that patients would usually recover quickly after an operation, but added that 'the only danger is an infection, which occurs very easily here'.[139] In a 1932 letter, Dr. Bonnema explained to Schweitzer how surgeons tried to decrease such dangers:

> I have good news from the operating room. Miss Berthe had the good idea to prepare the patients for the intervention herself and to fix a strong cloth with cloth clips to the wound edges immediately after the skin incision, since we have been doing this even large hernias and Elephanitasis plastics heal primarily. Hopefully this will also prevent suppuration and the often lengthy after-treatment.[140]

In 1959, Dr. van der Kreek wrote to Schweitzer that no secondary infections had occurred, 'because we are very strict about sterility'.[141] The introduction of antibiotics at the beginning of the 1950s, after which reports of serious infections disappear, might have helped to lower the post-surgical infection rate. In 1957,

---

135 Jilek-Aall, *Working with Dr. Schweitzer*, 51.
136 Berman, *In Africa with Schweitzer*, 76–77.
137 Stocker, 'Diary 1961–63', 17; Interview Hedwig Schnee.
138 Interview Elisabeth Anderegg. Dr. Munz explained that constant micro-infections on his patients' feet from walking barefoot granted them some degree of immunity, in: Interview Munz and Munz. Reliable statistics on the post-operation mortality rate could not be found, but Dr. Berman placed it at 0.5 percent. See: Berman, *In Africa with Schweitzer*, 1986, 84. Dr. Goldwyn, who was present at the hospital at the same time, claimed that it lay at 0.88 percent. He also wrote of 85 'accidents' occurring during the 450 interventions that took place from June 1959 to June 1960. See: Goldwyn, 'Diary 1960', AMS, 32.
139 Lauterburg-Bonjour, 'Man stellt sich um', 31.
140 Bonnema to Schweitzer, 25 September 1932, AMS.
141 Van der Kreek to Schweitzer, 27 October 1959, AMS.

Dr. Friedmann calculated that half of the hospital's penicillin supply had been used in the Case Bouka, which at the time was not the only ward for recovering surgical patients. In his view, van der Kreek, who was responsible for the ward, had dispensed it far too liberally.[142] Intriguingly, antibiotics receive little attention in the primary sources.

6   Controlling Patients via Technology: the Example of Anesthesia

Another crucial aspect of surgical control is anesthesia, for which there were a variety of options at hand in Lambaréné. Ether was available, but difficult to control. In 1924, for example, Noel Gillespie, a chemistry student at the University of Oxford who accompanied Schweitzer on his second journey to Gabon, described how 'it was fiendishly hot in the theatre and the ether was all over the place – that's the main difficulty here – the ether vapourises so much in the heat that the operating staff risks being put to sleep'.[143] This difficulty was also mentioned by Dr. Schnabel in 1936, who added that 'ether becomes costly until it reaches the tropics'.[144] Another problem in controlling ether was its flammability, especially when used in proximity to paraffin lamps.[145] In 1934 Dr. Goldschmid reported to Schweitzer that he had used chloroform in two gynecological interventions that he had performed at night, because he 'did not dare to use ether with the open lights'.[146]

During Schweitzer's first stay in Lambaréné, most operations were performed using chloroform, which was administered by a missionary.[147] After the arrival of Dr. Nessman in October 1924, Joseph Azoawanié, who from 1913 had

---

142   Friedmann to Schweitzer, 8 September 1957, AMS. A degree of personal tension between Dr. Friedmann and Dr. van der Kreek is evident in their correspondence. Friedmann's letter is very interesting in regard to the use of antibiotics. He and Schweitzer had calculated earlier that year that the hospital, including the leprosy village, required 10–12 million units of penicillin per day. Shortly after Schweitzer left for Europe in July, Friedmann and Ali Silver discovered that, even without considering the leprosy village, the hospital used 20–25 million units daily. By the time Friedmann wrote the letter, this number had risen again to 60–70 million units per day (without specifying whether this included the leprosy village's usage).

143   Gillespie, 'With Schweitzer in Lambarene: Noel Gillespie's Letters from Africa', 181.

144   Schnabel, 'Medizinisches aus Albert Schweitzers Urwaldspital', 380.

145   Schweitzer, 'Briefe aus dem Lambarene Spital Juni 1935', 4; Berman, *In Africa with Schweitzer*, 84.

146   Goldschmid to Schweitzer, 21 December 1934, AMS.

147   Kik, *Beim Oganga von Lambarene*, 30.

been Schweitzer's first African assistant, was given this responsibility.[148] Thereafter, chloroform is rarely mentioned. In 1938, Schweitzer wrote to his pharmacist, Robert Weiss in Strasbourg, that the hospital would use it only for 'mixed anesthesia'.[149] As seen in this chapter's introductory quotation, Schweitzer justified his customary usage of infiltration anesthesia with reference to both a lack of competent personnel who could administer ether or chloroform and to the preferences of his patients.

All types of hernia, hydrocele, and elephantiasis procedures at the hospital were generally performed using infiltration anesthesia. This form of local anesthesia, which directly injects the sedating substance into the location of the operation,[150] was also standard for hernia operations in Europe at the time.[151] It appears that the technique was brought to Lambaréné in 1925 by Dr. Lauterburg, who was considered an experienced and distinguished surgeon by his colleagues and patients. He succeeded in convincing Schweitzer of the superiority of the method for the simple reason that 'this greatly diminishes the risks'.[152] This method was subsequently used as her standard approach by Dr. Schnabel, who reported that the anesthetizing procedure by infiltration was performed at the hospital in the same manner as it was in Europe.[153]

About a quarter of a century later, at the above-mentioned operation conducted by Dr. Bessuges, the French physician acknowledged that infiltration anesthesia would be sufficient for a simple hernia repair. For an incarcerated hernia, however, he considered general anesthesia necessary, because of the risk that the surgeon might have to make a very deep incision, for which the surrounding tissue would be insufficiently numb. The procedure could take so long that the patient would require a second narcosis before the closing of the wound. This disagreement can be interpreted as a clash of two preferences of control. While Bessuges ultimately did as he was instructed, the reasons behind

---

148 Nessmann, *Avec Albert Schweitzer de 1924 à 1926*, 155–56.

149 Schweitzer to Weiss, 31 January 1938, AMS.

150 According to the protocols, the hospital mainly used procaine anesthetics of the ester group. They preferred Scurocaine until World War Two when they switched to Novocaine. In the 1950s, the precise substance was rarely noted; instead, the records usually show only 'anes. loc.' (local anesthetic), with Novocain sometimes mentioned. See: L – P – O5-6, AMS. From 1964, Larocaine was the standard anesthetic. See: L – P – O8-9, AMS. All of these substances are said to be mood-enhancing, which may go some way to explaining patients' preference for them.

151 Friedl-Meyer, *Lehrbuch der Chirurgie für das Pflegepersonal*, 181. In her fourth edition (1969, 238), Friedl-Meyer continued to recommend infiltration anesthesia for hernias. See also: Vogeler, *Chirurgie der Hernien*, 26, 41.

152 Nessmann, *Avec Albert Schweitzer de 1924 à 1926*, 148.

153 Schnabel, 'Von ärztlichen Verrichtungen', 54–55.

Schweitzer's preference for infiltration anesthesia even in complicated cases remain unclear.[154]

Some experts claimed, however, that it did provide a sufficient degree of control for most interventions. During the late 1950s, a visiting doctor from Denmark reported that infiltration anesthesia was even used for very complicated hernias in Lambaréné and that there were 'no more narcosis complications than in Europe'.[155] Another visiting surgeon disagreed, arguing that 'anesthesia here is either too light or too deep'.[156] Dr. Rolf Müller, who served in Lambaréné from 1960 to 1964, explained to an expert readership in 1963 that local anesthesia for hernias 'has excellently proven itself'.[157] Barthélemy's explanation for this preference was similar to that given by Schweitzer: 'The doctors prefer, if possible, a local anesthetic to general anesthesia because it reduces the after-effects of the operation and is better tolerated by the natives'.[158]

We can now return to considering the introductory anecdote of this chapter. Firstly, it remains uncertain how often the ritual, as I want to call it, was actually practiced in Lambaréné. Schweitzer circulated the story quite widely,[159] but he only acted as a surgeon during World War Two, and no other physician mentioned it. How should the anecdote thus be interpreted in light of what has been revealed in this chapter about technology and control in surgical practice? Why did Schweitzer introduce a ritual that was seemingly foreign to the biomedical practices of surgery? How was it incorporated into the medical discourses and practices at the hospital?

At first glance, it appears that Schweitzer, like many biomedical practitioners, neglected the social context of his patients, instead choosing to invoke the legacy of a surgeon from a bygone era and a distant country. His motivations for the introduction of the ritual were in line with his thinking and it was an exception to his general reluctance to intrude into the manners of Africans. Following his conception of the 'civilizing mission', Schweitzer sought to provide his patients with a lesson in gratitude for and appreciation of his services.

---

154   Bessuges, *Lambaréné à l'ombre de Schweitzer*, 100–102.
155   Østergaard Christensen, *At Work with Albert Schweitzer*, 79.
156   Goldwyn, 'Diary 1960', AMS, 32.
157   Müller, '50 Jahre Albert-Schweitzer-Spital', 17.
158   Barthélemy, *Wie ich Lambarene erlebte*, 34.
159   The story has been published in slightly modified versions in: Kik, *Beim Oganga von Lambarene*, 36; Joy, Arnold, and Schweitzer, *The Africa of Albert Schweitzer*, 121. Additionally, it appeared in the Berlin or Viennese newspaper *Der Kurier* on Christmas Eve in 1953. A cut-out copy of the article was found at the AMS among the correspondence with Gauss. Schweitzer had contacted the journalist specializing in the history of Pomerania, where Schleich was born, to find out more about the German inventor of infiltration anesthesia.

Within the surgical service, this ritual represented an additional means of control, which was again to be exerted by people rather than technology. Schweitzer's patients were expected to perform, according to his own 'predetermined way'. In the process, he reached beyond the confined and controlled space of his operating theater, beyond his patients' bodies, to what Bernault terms their 'inner sel(ves) or cultural assets'.[160]

In this sense, the ritual can be read as one of submission: patients were expected to waiver to the authority of the medical staff and their technologies. From another perspective, however, this ritual did grant patients a certain presence that they would not have enjoyed under general anesthesia. They were more responsive than 'tranquilly pliant' patients and cared for in a more personal manner than bodies in a 'repair shop'.[161] Although the unequal power relations in the ritual are palpable, its interactive nature thus acknowledged the patient as an active participant within the surgical intervention.

The crucial question of how patients understood the ritual nevertheless remains. In the following subchapter, I address the delicate issue of the perspectives of African patients,[162] seeking to answer two key questions in the process. First, to what degree were European surgeons able or willing to control patients outside of their immediate territory, the operating theater? Here, I am especially interested in where, when, and how patients escaped this control. Second, I attempt to explain why patients were readily prepared to incorporate surgery into their quest for therapy and what the surgical process represented for them.

7   Beyond the Operating Theater: Limits and Implications of Control

Schweitzer effectively controlled the surgical procedure and the people responsible for executing it, namely the surgeons, nurses, and assistants. Patients, however, enjoyed considerable freedom.[163] There are numerous reports

---

160   Bernault, 'Body, Power and Sacrifice', 226.

161   Pernick, *A Calculus of Suffering*, 84; Howell, 'Hospitals', 511.

162   Flurin Condrau has discussed the complex nature of this task for medical historians. See: Condrau, 'The Patient's View Meets the Clinical Gaze'. I go some way towards enacting the solution that he proposes, namely to undertake 'carefully contextualised analyses of 'patients''' (536).

163   To remain coherent, this chapter maintains its primary focus on surgical patients. The inclusion of patients from other wards in this analysis would probably not render a manifestly different picture, although the use of some coercive measures against patients will be discussed in Chapter 4.

from European medical staff lamenting the undesired behavior of their patients. In a 1934 letter, the nurse Elise Stalder updated Schweitzer on a patient
who had just undergone an operation. Her statement is indicative of the difficult position held by African auxiliaries, who were required to act as mediators
between persons with unequal degrees of power, as well as between different
kinds of control. Stalder described how the African auxiliary Louemba

> had great difficulties in making him understand that he must not eat.
> Again and again the sick man made Palabres: he, Louemba, did not want
> to give him anything, while the doctor and I had supposedly agreed to do
> so. It is not always easy for Louemba either.[164]

Stalder's letter also shows that patients' diets were one of the many aspects of
patient care beyond staff members' control. According to the doctors, patients
often started to eat too soon after an operation.[165] There were other recurring
complaints about patients' non-compliance with doctors' orders. Staff members were irritated by patients' tendency to take the bandages off their recent
surgical wounds.[166] Another key issue was patient mobility. Barthélemy observed how recovering patients moved freely around the hospital to visit
friends in other wards, even reporting that some patients who had undergone
recent operations were going fishing.[167]

The reasons for the doctors' concerns were mostly medical, but they were
also upset by their inability to maintain control of their patients. Dr. Bonnema,
for instance, wrote in 1932 that

> a big hernia went for a walk a couple of days after the operation. Sud-
> denly, he felt very sick and soon he died. The dissection revealed an em-
> bolism. The fact that our patients always do what they are not allowed to
> do very much increases the risk of an operation here.[168]

---

164   Stalder to Schweitzer, 3 June 1934, AMS.

165   Schweitzer, *Afrikanische Geschichten*, 70–71.

166   Schweitzer, 'Briefe aus dem Lambarene Spital Juli 1933', 9; Joy, Arnold, and Schweitzer, *The
         Africa of Albert Schweitzer*, 123. The only explicit explanation offered by a European as to
         why patients may have done this is to be found in a children's book, according to which
         bandages were taken off to release pain as well as any evil spirits. See: Franck, *My Friend
         in Africa*, 63.

167   Barthélemy, *Wie ich Lambarene erlebte*, 50–51.

168   Bonnema to Schweitzer, 10 April 1932, AMS.

Stalder, on the other hand, was astonished at the lack of consequences for such premature exercise. She claimed that she had not witnessed any deaths from intestinal resection during her eighteen-month stay and was surprised that 'walks down to the landing place during their first night did not even harm'.[169]

A final recurring staff complaint was that patients frequently went for a bath in the river. Dr. van der Kreek recalled that the Gabonese 'wash very often, mostly in the river. And our concern [...] was to prevent the operated patients of going to soak themselves with their bandages from the day before in the nearby Ogooué'.[170] According to Schweitzer, this sort of bathing had occurred since the hospital's establishment.[171] Barthélemy assumed that patients believed this would accelerate the healing of their wounds.[172] Contemporary missionary and ethnographic writing supports the view that many Gabonese attributed healing powers to water.[173] Most of the staff did not seem interested in an explanation, or at least did not provide one, for this seemingly perplexing behavior among their patients.[174]

The fact that accounts of patients' supposedly ignorant behavior appear repeatedly throughout the study period indicates that Schweitzer tolerated their conduct intentionally. It also suggests that he either did not seek complete control over his patients or was willing to accept that this was not possible. Frederick Franck, a Dutch dentist who regularly visited the hospital in the late 1950s, observed how recovering surgical patients went fishing and visited friends. Exasperated, he asked a nurse whether they were 'allowed to get out of their beds?' She responded that there was 'nothing to allow, they just go. We can't have cops around here. It would not help anyway'.[175] Similarly, Anderegg recalled that she once asked Schweitzer why the surgical staff needed to be so careful in following disinfection procedures when their patients were allowed to swim in the river shortly after their operations. Her superior replied: 'Elisabeth, if you do not understand this, you are in the wrong place'.[176] Here, Schweitzer refrained from intruding into his patients' personal realm. He did not aim to change their habits, but nevertheless expected his staff to provide

---

169 Stalder to Schweitzer, 3 June 1934, AMS.
170 Becht, 'Témoignage d'une chirurgien, Mme Le Docteur Greet Barthélemy', 172.
171 Schweitzer, 'Briefe aus dem Lambarene Spital Mai 1937', 3.
172 Barthélemy, *Wie ich Lambarene erlebte*, 36–37.
173 Fernandez, *Bwiti*, 218; Grébert, *Au Gabon*, 136–41; Lavignotte, *L'évur: croyance des Fañ du Gabon*, 64.
174 The next chapter on obstetrics will explore such indifference further.
175 Franck, *Days with Albert Schweitzer*, 103.
176 Interview Elisabeth Anderegg.

them with the best possible service. This approach might have been motivated by an awareness that patients would be more reluctant to come to the hospital if they were forced to remain lying still for days after surgery. In another sense, this attitude conveyed an abdication of responsibility, a reading supported by Schweitzer's lack of involvement in public health measures.

As we have seen, one task assigned to the African assistants was to police patients in the post-surgery ward in order to ensure that they did not eat. However, the low numbers of assistants, the fact that Schweitzer and his other staff were aware of the close relationship that they enjoyed with their patients, and statements such as the ones just cited suggest that keeping patients under control was not the auxiliaries' primary duty.

Doctors had little control, if any, over when a patient sought hospital treatment. Doctors and prospective patients had drastically different conceptions of when it was appropriate to operate on a hernia. When Dr. Karl Hediger toured the surrounding region in 1929, he sent several of the approximately one hundred patients whom he examined to the hospital to undergo surgery.[177] Three years later, a government doctor on tour in the area, who was tasked with administering sleeping sickness prophylaxis, sent people to Schweitzer's hospital for surgery.[178] Hernias and hydroceles were conditions that allowed patients to choose their moment of entry. During the 1932 dry season, Dr. Bonnema reported that 'the hospital gets a little less crowded. I belief people prefer to go fishing and do not really have the time to have their hernias and hydroceles operated'.[179] There are frequent reports of patients arriving at the hospital too late for surgery; if a hernia was incarcerated, this occasionally resulted in the patient's death.[180] Other hernias simply became too large to be repaired.[181] Schweitzer was aware of this danger and attempted to 'let the whole region know' that hernias had to be operated upon as quickly as possible.[182]

Schweitzer believed that two of the main reasons for patients coming too late for surgery were that they and their relatives did not want to make the long journey to the hospital or that local healers had delayed them from making the decision to seek biomedical treatment.[183] In relation to the first of these claims, it is notable that accounts of patients arriving too late for hernia repairs

---

177   Hediger to Schweitzer, 9 August 1929, AMS.

178   Bonnema to Schweitzer, 29 May 1932, AMS.

179   Bonnema to Schweitzer, 3 July 1932, AMS.

180   Bonnema to Schweitzer, 3 May 1934, AMS.

181   Stalder to Schweitzer, 3 June 1934, AMS.

182   Schweitzer to Boyard, 18 August 1946, AMS.

183   Schweitzer, 'Briefe aus dem Lambarene Spital März 1938', 3; Schweitzer, 'Briefe aus dem Lambarene Spital Februar 1939', 2.

decrease significantly after World War Two, a period when the colonial government expanded its healthcare services. In connection to the latter, reports of prior treatment of hernias are scarce,[184] but a few exceptions from various phases of the study period offer some valuable insights.

Dr. Walter Munz asserts that most of his patients had seen a 'medicine man' before coming to the hospital, a claim that he deduced from examining their scarring.[185] Dr. Berman, who was in Lambaréné shortly before Munz's arrival, describes a surgery that he performed on a patient who had already undergone an intervention in which a fishbone had been used as a counter-irritant. According to Berman, no one at the hospital was willing to talk about the incident and the local treatment behind it.[186] In 1932, Dr. Bonnema examined two patients with incarcerated hernias, adding rather dispassionately, as was the manner of many of the doctors when they wrote to Schweitzer, that 'one of them, who had torn his intestines in two while trying to have it reduced in the village, has died'.[187] Ten months later, he wrote of a man who had cut open his own incarcerated hernia, adding in a similarly disinterested tone that 'there were still enough intestines to take over so I did not have to perform a resection'.[188] Even if some misunderstandings are contained these accounts, together they clearly suggest that hospital surgery was not necessarily the first choice of every patient.

Statistics do reveal, however, that a considerable number of Gabonese did seek surgery at the hospital. As I argued earlier in this chapter, the wider context had to be conducive for the introduction and broad acceptance of a technology like surgery. The question thus arises why they were willing to expose themselves to the knife in such great numbers. The obvious answer is that surgery offered 'a possibility for the treatment of ailments that were previously not effectively treated'.[189] This claim is difficult to dispute and must undoubtedly be taken into consideration; nevertheless, in other parts of Africa people

---

184   This could simply be a result of the limitations of the sources. It may also indicate a lack of interest in the matter on the part of Schweitzer and his personnel. Another possibility is that it was the product of a taboo at the hospital, possibly imposed by Schweitzer, that dictated that the local customs of patients should not be discussed. Whatever the cause, it comes as no surprise, since references to Gabon's wider medical, economic, social, or political context are unexpectedly rare in the sources.

185   Munz, *Albert Schweitzer im Gedächtnis der Afrikaner und in meiner Erinnerung*, 222.

186   Berman, *In Africa with Schweitzer*, 97. As always, Berman's accounts should be treated with some skepticism. It can be assumed, however, that they had some foundation in reality.

187   Bonnema to Schweitzer, 29 May 1932, AMS.

188   Bonnema to Schweitzer, 14 February 1933, AMS.

189   Au, 'Cutting the Flesh', 306.

were less satisfied with the results surgery produced and were much more reluctant to make use of it.[190]

In Gabon, surgery was consistent with local understandings of disease and
health, as well as with common conceptions of the body and practices related
to it. Cutting the body, for instance, was common during autopsies. These were
performed neither to acquire anatomical knowledge nor strictly to identify the
cause of death, but to locate what was typically referred by European observers
as a sort of parasitic being, the 'Evu' of the Fang language.[191] The *Evu* granted
those who hosted it enhanced and often destructive powers over others. Although hosting the *Evu* was considered essential for personal success, Gabonese felt very ambivalent towards it due to its aggressive potential to harm
others.

Some accounts of surgery at the Albert Schweitzer Hospital resonate with
the idea of *Evu*, even if they never explicitly refer to the concept as such. Joy
and Arnold, two important supporters from the USA who visited Schweitzer in
1947, for example, wrote that 'in the early years of the Hospital, relatives of a
patient insisted on standing over Dr. Schweitzer to make sure he took something out ('there goes the Evil Spirits') and did not put anything in'.[192] It is unclear if Schweitzer or his surgeons believed that patients thought that they
would extract something during surgery.

The vast majority of doctors did not discuss local conceptions of disease in
their writings, and their practices certainly did not reflect a special awareness
thereof. One exception can be found in Barthélemy's account of his stay at the
hospital. Visiting Lambaréné after the publication of Joy and Arnold's book, he

---

190   Good, *The Steamer Parish*, 407; Ranger, 'Godly Medicine', 268; White, *Speaking with Vam-
       pires*, 105.
191   Bernault writes of an 'organic/mystical substance' with 'divine agency'. In: Bernault, 'Car-
       nal Technologies', 178. Raponda-Walker and Sillans provide translations of the term for
       many other Gabonese languages, but the Fang's use thereof has been by far the most in-
       tensively studied. See: Raponda-Walker and Sillans, *Rites et croyances des peuples du Ga-
       bon*, 82–84. They further write that around 1900 almost all corpses underwent an autopsy,
       but that this practice had become uncommon by the mid-twentieth century (116). Con-
       temporaries provided anatomical-biomedical explanations for the Evu. The botanist and
       ethnologist Günter Tessmann claimed to have attended autopsies in which he had seen
       'Ewus', which he believed to be internal injuries. See: Tessmann, *Die Pangwe*, 2:129–33. The
       missionary Lavignotte wrote that 'each trace of tumour, ovarian or liver cyst, or syphilis on
       a placenta, internal bleeding, etc., is proof of the presence of the évur'. In: Lavignotte,
       L'évur: croyance des Fañ du Gabon, 53–54. According to anthropologist James Fernandez,
       autopsies 'uncover certain unnatural growths or formation (zi evu) which are said to be
       the seat of the evus'. In: Fernandez, 'Christian Acculturation and Fang Witchcraft', 247.
192   Joy, Arnold, and Schweitzer, *The Africa of Albert Schweitzer*, 124.

refuted their statement that the belief in spirits had been more widespread in the hospital's early years. Barthélemy explained that patients

> attach great importance to seeing the parts removed from their bodies later on, and after they have determined the removal of the bad pieces in this manner, they explain with a content expression that they now feel much better.[193]

Another reference to spirits can be found in a children's book published by Franck in 1960 in memory of his stays in Lambaréné the previous years. The protagonist is a local child who comes to the hospital to have an ulcer treated at the narrator's insistence. The boy reflects on surgery, thinking to himself how 'everyone knew that a knife was a powerful thing. So it must be the very best thing for cutting out the evil spirits that made a man sick'.[194] Through the eyes of a child, we thus return to the knife, the technological artefact that had become inseparable from the physician and the surgery process itself, a powerful technology of healing that could possibly even free spirits and *Evus*.

There is no evidence, however, to suggest that Gabonese viewed surgery in this way. The legitimacy of the above accounts is hampered by their lack of specificity; for example, what precisely did these authors mean by 'evil spirits'? It appears that they subsumed everything that they considered supernatural, including the *Evu*, under this term. These accounts are therefore perhaps best understood as colonial genre-writing, as discussed in the Introduction. Furthermore, some Europeans living in the region claimed that the *Evu* prevented Gabonese from seeking surgical care. The head of the Service de Santé observed that patients were reluctant to undergo surgery, because they feared that the *Evu* would be released.[195] The missionary Lavignotte asserted that local residents believed that European hospitals, including Schweitzer's, were powerless to treat diseases of the *Evu*.[196]

Contemporary ethnographers were a little more exact, both when discussing the causes of and the therapy for hernias specifically or the wider significance of surgery and its connection to the spirit world. In general, spirits were assumed to be able to cause disease, as we have seen in Chapter 1 in relation to

---

193   Barthélemy, *Wie ich Lambarene erlebte*, 36.

194   Franck, *My Friend in Africa*, 61.

195   Gaulene, 'Coutumes des races gabonaises'. In: 'Rapport Annuel du Service de Santé de la Colonie du Gabon 1932', ZK 005-127. SHD, 139.

196   Lavignotte, *L'évur: croyance des Fañ du Gabon*, 91.

the *Nganga*, who was required to perform a sort of 'exorcism' in response.[197] James Fernandez supposed that the main goal of such treatments was the 'voiding, actually or sympathetically, of the interior of the body'.[198] He described a 'water spirit' that caused 'afflictions of the stomach and bowels', especially 'watery bowels', which were treated with various plants.[199] Fernandez further alluded to 'demons' that caused 'blockages'. These were countered with 'running water and the flow of verbal confession'.[200] 'Exorcism', 'voiding', and 'blockages' could easily be linked to surgery; however, since the course of therapy depended to a large degree on the cause of the affliction, the question of how locals believed surgery acted to cure hernias is difficult to answer. A linguistic comparison connects hernias with neither cause nor therapy, but with form: in the Fang language they were known as the 'disease of the nut'.[201]

However, the *Evu* remains important to understand the willingness of Gabonese to undergo surgery. By being connected to a specific person and his or her body, belief in the *Evu* allowed for a conception of the individual body as both a seat of disease and a site of intervention, in the sense outlined by Landau.[202] The use of charms to improve personal fortunes, widespread in early colonial Gabon, illustrates this. Bernault explains how charms channeled the agency of the dead through the use of body parts from 'remarkable ancestors', whose agency was thereby rendered present in 'ritual experts' and 'political leaders' in the form of their *Evu*.[203]

---

197 Raponda-Walker and Sillans, *Rites et croyances des peuples du Gabon*, 137–41; See also: Gollnhofer and Sillans, 'Phénoménologie de la possession', 742.

198 Fernandez, *Bwiti*, 625.

199 Ibid., 598.

200 Ibid., 218.

201 A dictionary published in 1892 provides two Fang translations for the French 'hernie' or 'descente': 'Ethout' and 'Mbang'. Lejeune, *Dictionnaire français-fang*. The first of these terms could not be found in a dictionary published seventy years later by the Swiss missionary Samuel Galley. 'Mbañ' is translated therein as 'Fruit kernel, almond, etc.' and is also one of the words given for 'testicles' (Mbañ afam). Hernias, here specifically testicular hernias, were 'Ôkon Mbañ', with 'Ôkon' the term for 'sickness'. Galley adds: 'It is called that way, because what comes out looks like a nut'. He also provides a further translation for hernia: 'minsoñ', a plural noun for all kinds of worms, including intestinal ones. He insists, however, that for hernia, 'it's improper, the true word is mbañ'. Galley, *Dictionnaire fang-français et français-fang*.

202 At the same time, building on the work of Homi Bhabha, Landau cautions us that 'the very idea of the 'individual' was a particular European historical construct'. As this paragraph suggests, I retain my doubts about this claim. Landau, 'Explaining Surgical Evangelism', 279.

203 Bernault, 'Carnal Technologies', 178.

In the 1920s, the French colonial government imposed laws regulating the handling of corpses, which complicated the production of charms. Consequently, their trade grew more occult and their contents less specific.[204] In the next decade, wage labor, of which hernias were a painful reminder, and colonial head tax collection intensified.[205] Given these developments, it is unsurprising that in the years that followed Fernandez observed a growing importance being attached to the *Evu*, which now came to be viewed in a more positive light.[206] The contemporary sociologist Georges Balandier had already highlighted the *Evu's* individualizing aspects; from a social and political perspective, he interpreted the workings of this 'non-communal power for strictly personal purposes' as a 'radical form of opposition to the clan order; they represent its most individualizing part, the most revolutionary part of Fang magic'.[207] Taking into account the dynamic reciprocal relationship between technology, individual agents, and society at large, my argument can be stretched further. Hernia repair contributed to the growing sense of individualization in the region because it relied on existing individualistic conceptions of the body, disease, and power that it in turn further reinforced and diffused.

In addition, the above-mentioned accounts from the hospital, invoking powerful knives and relatives glancing over surgeons' shoulders, remind us of the 'work of the knife' in the Belgian Congo, the expression patients and their relatives used to refer to surgery. Dr. Clement Chesterman, encouraged the use of this term, which again blurred the boundaries between agents, objects, and technology. He staged surgical interventions as public events in order to increase local acceptance of surgery and demonstrate that there was nothing 'magic' about it. Nancy Hunt then conceives of missionary surgery, just like dining, as a performance.[208] The Albert Schweitzer Hospital also provided reasons to support such a reading.

Returning to the introductory anecdote of this chapter, Schweitzer continued his letter disclosing the performative aspects of surgery at his hospital. He described what happened before a patient entered the operating theater as follows:

> In the room where patients who were recently operated lie together with those to be operated soon, the ones who have already participated in the

---

204   Ibid., 181.
205   Gray and Ngolet, 'Lambaréné, Okoume and the Transformation of Labor'.
206   Fernandez, *Bwiti*, 209.
207   Balandier, *Sociologie actuelle de l'Afrique Noire*, 146–47.
208   Hunt, *A Colonial Lexicon*, 84, 117–20.

ceremony of gratitude, rehearse with those who still wait to be part of it. Mainly they articulate the difficult name of Schleich and are greatly amused when the really wild people from the interior are not able to stutter something like Schleich. When he is carried out for the operation, they call after him: 'say Schleich'.[209]

How can we relate what we have learned in this final subchapter to this ritual, a practice that can simultaneously be read as one of Schweitzer acknowledging the presence of the African patient and as one of the patient submitting to Schweitzer and his technologies? The patients' reaction, as described by Schweitzer, is thought-provoking. They rehearsed and joked, but then complied, turning the pre and post-surgical act into a theatrical spectacle, a performance (see Illustrations 16 and 17). We can only speculate as to why patients felt the need to comply with this ritual. Perhaps they believed that it was an essential step towards being healed by Schweitzer in particular. Another contributing factor may have been the relative freedom that they enjoyed elsewhere in the hospital, where they were less frequently subjected to such measures of submission and control. Perhaps they really wanted to express their gratitude and felt acknowledged; or possibly the answer is even more straightforward: namely, patients tend to do as doctors say in their presence. After all, the latter 'promised life rather than threatened death'[210] and hence followed the biopolitical logic. Whatever the patients' motivations, the story is an excellent illustration of the ambiguous interactions in the colonial medical sphere. It serves to broaden our understanding of medical and colonial control and the role played by technology therein.

8   Conclusion

There is every reason to believe that patients came to the Albert Schweitzer Hospital for surgery of their own volition. They wanted to see and experience the surgeons, the knives, and the lamps that repaired hernias and other conditions. Surgery did not upset their relationship with their own body, which they were able to conceive of as a site for individual medical intervention. This idea pre-dated Schweitzer's arrival in Gabon, and hence was a precondition for surgery's ultimate success in Lambaréné. During the study period, however, Gabonese expanded their conceptions of the individual, as tax-payer, convert, consumer, political participant, powerful person, and so on; simultaneously their

---

209   Schweitzer to Gauss, 7 July 1952, AMS.
210   Thomas, *Politics of the Womb*, 176.

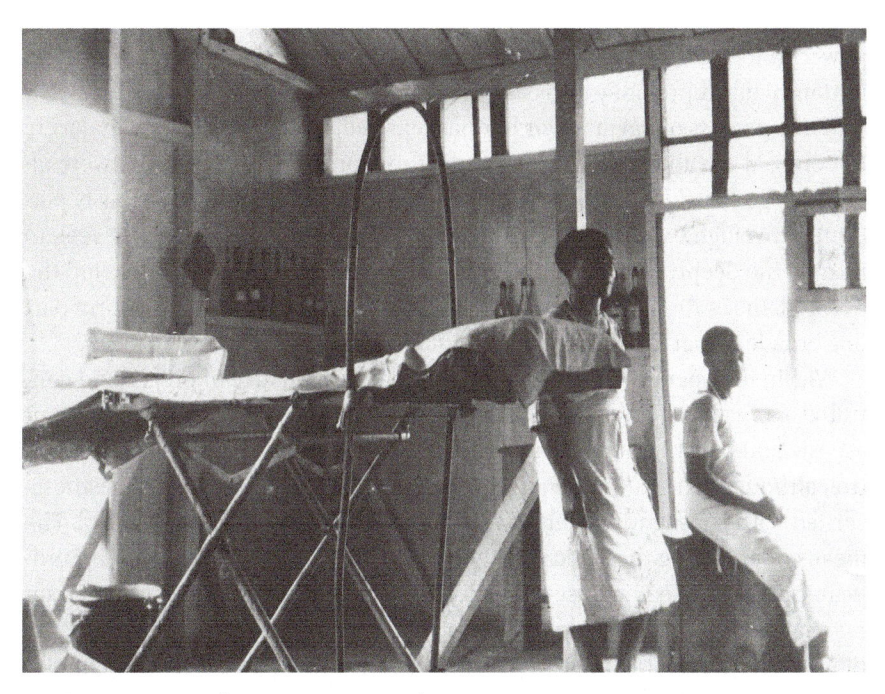

ILLUSTRATION 16   The operation room and two assistants in 1940
                    © ARCHIVES CENTRALES ALBERT SCHWEITZER GUNSBACH

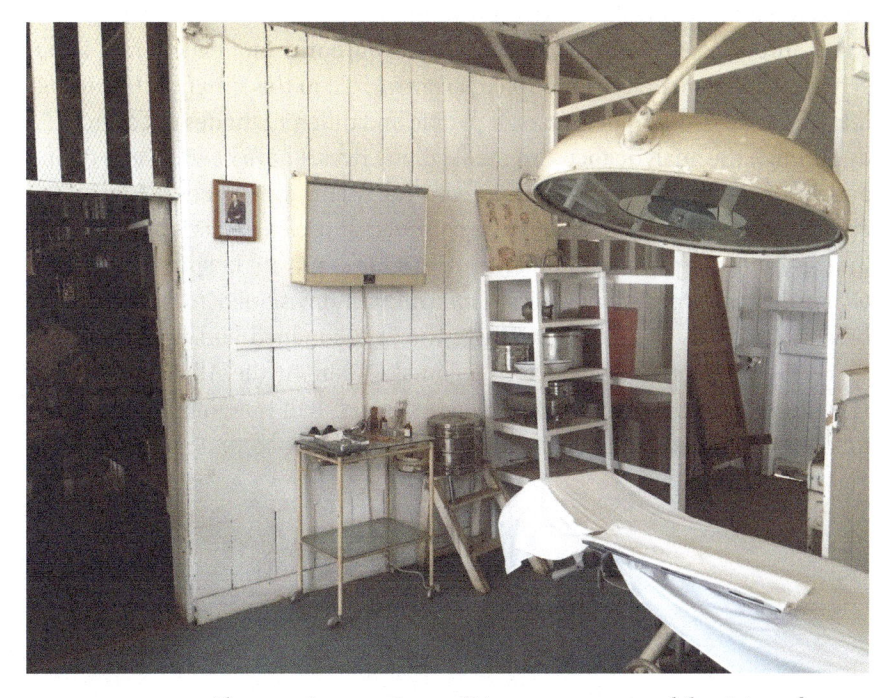

ILLUSTRATION 17   The operation room in 2015. It is now a museum and the picture of
                    Schleich still hangs there
                    PHOTOGRAPH BY HUBERT STEINKE

powerful individual force *Evu* grew in importance. Surgery drew from these notions while it probably also contributed to their broader acceptance.

In the process of having their hernias repaired, patients at the hospital were not obliged to submit themselves to doctors' complete control. They were allowed to go for walks, bathe, or possibly even fish. Schweitzer consciously permitted this high degree of personal freedom. He and his staff did not seek to intrude too deeply into the daily lives of their patients within and beyond the hospital. In Lambaréné, the practice of surgical biomedicine did not form part of a broader program of strict colonial social control.

Within the operating theater, however, the maintenance of procedural control was of central concern. In Lambaréné as elsewhere, the technologies of asepsis and anesthesia were unsurprisingly important in enforcing this control, although, due to the frequent use of the infiltration method, anesthesia carried with it a slightly different meaning with less emphasis on control. The means of enforcing these technologies of control were different than in European operating theaters. Asepsis relied less on technological devices than on manual work. The same is true for the whole surgical process; individuals, patients and medical staff alike, were controlled by other persons, with technologies playing a less influential role. There were exceptions, such as lamps, which posed considerable technical challenges. However, Schweitzer believed that he could remain in control – make things and individuals act in a predetermined way – through his own and others' personal authority and experience. Long-serving African auxiliaries occupied a central role in this order, acting as mediators between different groups of people and different modes of control.

Through the analytic focus on medical practices, I have been able to define and contextualize different layers of control. Medical procedural control occurs during specific instants only; the control that it then exerts is almost absolute, as our example of an operating theater in a private hospital in colonial Gabon has shown. Colonial social control was envisioned to be extremely broad, but it was not all-embracing, even in a confined and well-organized space such as a private hospital in colonial Gabon. At the Albert Schweitzer Hospital, both types of control on their own and their merging empowered a number of improvised reactions to counter or uphold them.

CHAPTER 3

Dimensions of Ignorance: Discourses and Practices of Obstetrics

Less than a year after Schweitzer's death, Guy Barthélemy published an extended 'letter' addressed to his former employer. In this thoughtful book, Barthélemy thanked Schweitzer for being an inspiration to him and recalled the following episode from a stay at the hospital in 1960:

> I remember that surreal night when, in the pharmacy, we watched a film on atomic war, while an operation took place in the next room. The coincidence was disturbing. From the United States, you had received a copy of the film 'on the beach', telling a story about the end of humanity following a nuclear conflict. A projector had been installed at one end of the room and the curtains of a consulting space served as a screen. [...] In the middle of the film, some members of the audience started to move around. A cesarean section had to be performed in the operating area next door. Greet and a nurse worked marching like ghosts in the glow of the projector, arms raised so as not to contaminate their sanitized hands. Each time, on their white backs, you could see for a few seconds a woman's face shaking or a submarine diving. It was much more hallucinating than the, still atrocious, subject of the film by itself. What was the sick woman in childbirth to be thinking, in the midst of those strange cries that resonated, two steps away, to announce the end of the world?[1]

This account raises key topics concerning maternity care and obstetrical practices at the Albert Schweitzer Hospital. It is an unusual description, for it places the act of giving birth, which received comparatively little attention in the daily work at the hospital, in the spotlight. Cesareans, however, were an area of significant discursive concern in the sources. They occurred relatively frequently in comparison to other hospitals in Gabon, but remained rare in relation to the number of births categorized as 'normal'. Unusually, the outside world, here in the form of the nuclear threat, intrudes on hospital life during this screening. While officials and missionaries in many colonies targeted mothers as key to solving the supposed wider societal issues of depopulation

---

1   Barthélemy, *Lettre à Albert Schweitzer*, 79–80.

and to reconfiguring conceptions of domesticity, doctors and nurses at Schweitzer's hospital generally ignored the concerns of these external actors.

Such dynamics of 'deliberate and inadvertent neglect'[2] are an excellent lens through which to study the hospital in the context of colonial medical trends and local practices alike. The analytical framework of agnotology, the study of ignorance, enables the historian to write about that which did not occur or which does not appear in the sources. It exposes the connections between in-attention and knowledge and how these influenced practices. An analysis of ignorance thus aids to understand why staff shaped obstetrical practice at the Albert Schweitzer Hospital to take on a, what they perceived to be exclusively medical, role as a curative service.

1 Depopulation, Domesticity, Ignorance: Framing Maternity Care in Colonial Africa

A number of practices around childbirth are common to all types of hospitals throughout colonial Africa. One that was popular with local residents was the distribution of extra-medical items, such as soap or clothing.[3] A more contested practice was the introduction of lying to replace sitting as the standard birth position.[4] As well as pre- and postnatal consultations, hospitals usually offered curative services. These treatments for mother and child were often the most in-demand services at maternity centers in Africa.[5]

Just as in most African societies, childbirth in colonial hospitals was a predominantly or even exclusively female domain. This was widely accepted by the parties involved in medical policy-making, including male and female colonial officials, medical personnel, and missionaries as well as local male leaders, midwives, and mothers.[6] In Gabon too, as the Service de la Santé's 1935

---

2   Proctor, 'Agnotology. A Missing Term to Describe the Cultural Production of Ignorance (and Its Study)', 8.

3   Some colonial women associations, often responsible for providing these services, even suspected that the gifts constituted the main reason why women chose to come to maternity centers. See: Hunt, 'Le Bebe en Brousse', 422; Hugon, 'La redéfinition de la maternité en Gold Coast', 157–58.

4   In colonial Ghana, this had been accepted by most local mothers by the 1940s. See: Hugon, 'Les sages-femmes africaines en contexte colonial', 186. In French West Africa, this was the case only from the early 1960s. See: Barthélémy, 'Sages-femmes africaines diplômées en AOF', 138.

5   Addae, *The Evolution of Modern Medicine in a Developing Country*, 230; Allman, 'Making Mothers', 32; Van Tol, 'Mothers, Babies, and the Colonial State', 122.

6   Thomas, *Politics of the Womb*; Bruchhausen, *Medizin zwischen den Welten*, 449; Kumwenda, *The Development of UMCA Medical Work in Northern Rhodesia*, 9.

annual report emphasized, 'each hospital has its own maternity ward with the female staff indispensable for its operation'.[7] This was also the case at the Albert Schweitzer Hospital; however, obstetrical encounters occurred exclusively at the clinic and never itinerantly in the wider community. Thus another typical feature of colonial maternity care is lacking: the interaction between a local birth attendant and a biomedically trained African or European midwife.[8]

Biomedical maternity care in colonial Africa has usually been understood in relation to one or two dominant discourses. The first played on a fear of depopulation and resulting economic inefficiency. Meredeth Turshen points out that in 'efforts to control rates of population growth', the disparate levels on which colonial policy operated can be observed. 'At one extreme were microlevel attempts to change breast-feeding practices, for example, and at the other extreme were macrolevel policies such as taxation', she notes.[9] Medical doctors were crucial in laying the groundwork for these measures. From the 1910s, physicians in different African colonies conducted interviews with mothers to find out more about the number and survival rate of their children. These surveys were often built on a weak scientific foundation, even by the standards of the day, but provided the basis of official demographic statistics.[10]

In France, officials had been concerned about depopulation since the start of the country's colonial expansion in the late nineteenth century.[11] In the interwar period, European powers believed that low fertility rates, poor maternity services, and emigration to neighboring territories had led to, among other challenges, a shortage of labor in many colonies.[12] The equatorial region spanning from Uganda to Cameroon was of particular concern in this respect.[13] French colonial documents from the 1920s relating to AEF 'are filled with impressions of population decline, high mortality, and impending demographic

---

7   'Rapport médical sur le fonctionnement durant l'année 1935 des services sanitaires et médicaux civils de l'Afrique Equatoriale Francaise'. ZK 005-121, SHD.

8   Hunt, *A Colonial Lexicon*, 157; Kalusa and Vaughan, *Death, Belief and Politics in Central African History*, 303; Hugon, 'Les sages-femmes africaines en contexte colonial', 187; Cole, 'Engendering Health', 114.

9   Turshen, 'Reproducing Labor', 231.

10   Coghe and Widmer, 'Colonial Demography'. For an example of such a survey, see: Hunt, *A Nervous State*, chapter 4.

11   Pedersen, 'Special Customs', 47.

12   Cordell, Ittman, and Maddox, 'Counting Subjects'. Current research suggests that anxieties about depopulation were exaggerated because 'African growth rates for the nineteenth and early twentieth centuries were lower than previously thought, with the result that African population in the nineteenth and early twentieth centuries were considerably higher than previously thought'. Manning, 'African Population', 264.

13   Hunt, *A Nervous State*, 12–14.

disaster'.[14] In the 1950s, the area around Lambaréné was considered to be particularly affected by these issues, with the blame placed on either 'the extreme simplicity of morals'[15] or venereal diseases.[16] Numerous local elders throughout the equatorial zone shared these concerns, including among the Fang in Gabon.[17] Schweitzer and his staff, however, displayed little awareness of these ongoing debates.

The second main discursive pillar of colonial maternity care envisioned a new domesticity for Africans. Colonial officials and missionaries aimed at redefining and expanding the role of African women as mothers and heads of the household. It was hoped that they could thus serve not only as advocates for better health by improving family hygiene and nutrition, but also as conveyors of Christian values and Western ideas about gender and domesticity. To this end, many of the services offered at infant and maternal healthcare facilities run by missions and colonial governments involved raising awareness about preventive healthcare.[18] These efforts culminated in a joint transnational government-missionary conference on the African child, which was hosted in Geneva in 1931. Participants 'avoided the obvious issues of economic exploitation and political expediency' and reassured themselves that 'social and educative solutions' worked best for the welfare of African women and children.[19] In Gabon too, missions prioritized the refiguring of local family structures and gender roles, making a pronounced effort to recruit girls for attending their schools.[20] Once more at the Albert Schweitzer Hospital, however, such issues were rarely addressed.

Colonial ideals of domesticity were connected to a belief in the superiority of European values. The supposed ignorance of local mothers was a recurring theme invoked to justify biomedical and pedagogical interventions all over

---

14 Cinnamon, 'Counting and Recounting', 131. See also: Headrick, *Colonialism, Health and Illness in French Equatorial Africa*, 104–5.

15 Sautter, *De l'Atlantique au fleuve Congo*, 800–801. Sautter, a geographer, found that women in the Lambaréné area had much fewer pregnancies than women in other parts of rural Gabon.

16 Fernandez, *Bwiti*, 163. In his endnote (621), Fernandez refers to a WHO research team that he met that had found 'evidence of venereal infection' in 30–40 percent of the population in northern Gabon.

17 Giles-Vernick, *Cutting the Vines of the Past*, 118. Songs from the region reflected these anxieties. See: Hunt, *A Nervous State*, 128. On the Fang specifically, see: Balandier, *Sociologie actuelle de l'Afrique Noire*, 90–91; Fernandez, *Bwiti*, 162.

18 Manderson, 'Women and the State', 171; Van Tol, 'Mothers, Babies, and the Colonial State', 124; Hugon, 'La redéfinition de la maternité en Gold Coast', 157–58.

19 Allman, 'Making Mothers', 25.

20 Mebiame Zomo, 'Le travail des missions chrétiennes au Gabon pendant la colonisation', 63–64; Mekodiomba, 'Rôle et influence des églises missionnaires dans la mission civilisatrice au Gabon', 88–89.

Africa and beyond.[21] Various scholars have drawn attention to the fact that very similar discourses on maternal ignorance were circulating in Europe from roughly 1900 to the beginning of World War Two,[22] which underlines that discussions on proper maternity care did not only circle around race, but also gender and class.

In order to further pursue this chapter's central focus on the production and accusation of ignorance, other key aspects of maternity care in Africa have to be neglected, most notably issues of medicalization and gender. Ignorance operates on a number of different levels. On the one hand European staff at the Albert Schweitzer Hospital blamed Africans for being ignorant of proper biomedical practices, an attitude that they shared with missionaries and colonial government officials. On the other hand, staff ignored not only the typical colonial discourses on maternity care outlined above, but also the circumstances and practices of local mothers. Constructing such arguments 'about who is ignorant of what' is problematic, yet unavoidable when studying ignorance.[23] This chapter also demonstrates how difficult it is for the historian to draw a clear distinction between 'intentional and unintentional not-knowing', a differentiation typically made in ignorance studies.[24]

The favoring of certain types of knowledge over others is a key feature of colonialism. Londa Schiebinger writes of 'a kind of cultured apathy or cultivated disinterest',[25] which Ann Laura Stoler terms 'the averted gaze'.[26] Wenzel Geissler has introduced the term 'unknowing' in the context of present-day North-South cooperation in scientific knowledge production. Field scientists practicing in the South, 'invest effort in "unknowing" difference'. They neither 'deny, hide, nor ignore' practices or realities that are strange or different in their view, but they refrain from establishing difference as 'explicit truth'. Such a process seems necessary to render scientific endeavors feasible.[27] Following Geissler's definition I retrace how biomedical personnel devoted effort to unknowing difference in order to practice their idea of medicine.

---

21 Greenwood, 'The Colonial Medical Service and the Struggle for Control', 94–95; Havik, 'Public Health, Social Medicine and Disease Control'; Jolly, 'Maternities and Modernities, Introduction'; Kanogo, 'The Medicalization of Maternity in Colonial Kenya', 85.

22 The key text being: Davin, 'Imperialism and Motherhood'. See also: Manderson, 'Women and the State', 174; Kalusa and Vaughan, *Death, Belief and Politics in Central African History*, 300; Van Tol, 'Mothers, Babies, and the Colonial State', 124.

23 Smithson, 'Social Theories of Ignorance', 210. See also: Groß and McGoey, 'Routledge International Handbook of Ignorance Studies, Introduction'.

24 Dilley and Kirsch, 'Regimes of Ignorance', 1. See also: Proctor, 'Agnotology. A Missing Term to Describe the Cultural Production of Ignorance (and Its Study)', 6–7.

25 Schiebinger, 'West Indian Abortifacients and the Making of Ignorance', 156.

26 Stoler, *Along the Archival Grain*, 255.

27 Geissler, 'Public Secrets in Public Health', 17.

Schweitzer and his staff followed the colonial logic by disregarding local maternity practices. However, while they simply ignored them, missionaries and colonial officials dismissed them as invalid or dangerous. Schweitzer and his staff intentionally refrained from participating in the colonial discussions on depopulation and domesticity because they were following a different agenda. Schweitzer did not intend to contribute towards ensuring an adequate supply of healthy laborers or educating a cohort of housewives, but instead envisaged the hospital as a shining example of his ethics. These motivations shaped the production of ignorance at the hospital and thus its medical practices. Murray Last has raised the question of 'how much people know, and care to know, about their own medical culture and how much a practitioner needs to know in order to practice medicine'.[28] He concludes that 'a segment of medical culture can flourish in seeming anarchy', in part because of 'people not knowing and not wishing to know'.[29] In at least the case of maternity care at the Albert Schweitzer Hospital, these observations are valid for patients and practitioners alike.

2   **Maternity Services in Colonial Gabon and at the Albert Schweitzer Hospital**

Infant mortality was the cause of considerable concern in Gabon. Europeans frequently blamed maternal ignorance for premature deceases. Nevertheless, as Rita Headrick writes, 'the problems of mothers and babies were not considered important enough for the government to divert resources from other areas. This responsibility could be left to colonial wives'.[30] In the 1930s, European women living in Libreville ran the privately financed 'Berceau Gabonais', which distributed soap, clothes, and canned milk among mothers-to-be. Together with a community health worker who was trained by the midwife in Libreville, they encouraged African women to undergo prenatal consultations and to deliver their babies at hospitals. Their efforts did not meet with much success; the most in-demand services offered by the Berceau were curative consultations for infants.[31] As late as in the mid-1950s, when the French colonial government increased its efforts to reduce child mortality in Gabon, officials still based their interventions on discourses that assumed ignorance among local mothers and families.[32]

---

28   Last, 'The Importance of Knowing about Not Knowing', 393.

29   Ibid., 403.

30   Headrick, *Colonialism, Health and Illness in French Equatorial Africa*, 151.

31   Ibid., 271; Mabika, 'Médicalisation de l'Afrique centrale', 339.

32   Tezi, 'Une approche socio-historique de l'avènement de la pédiatrie au Gabon', 114–18.

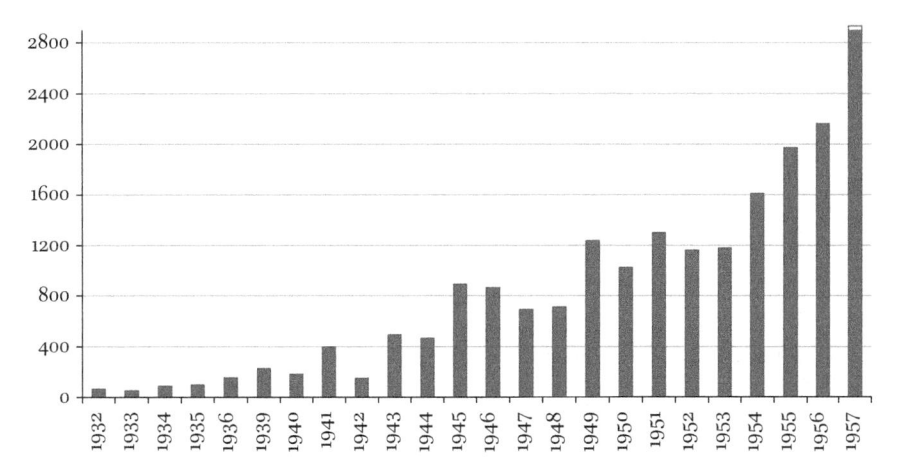

FIGURE 7   Deliveries at government clinics in Gabon

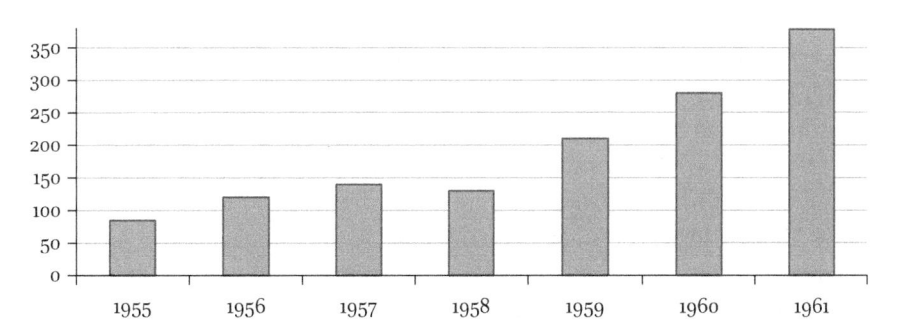

FIGURE 8   Deliveries at Lambaréné government hospital

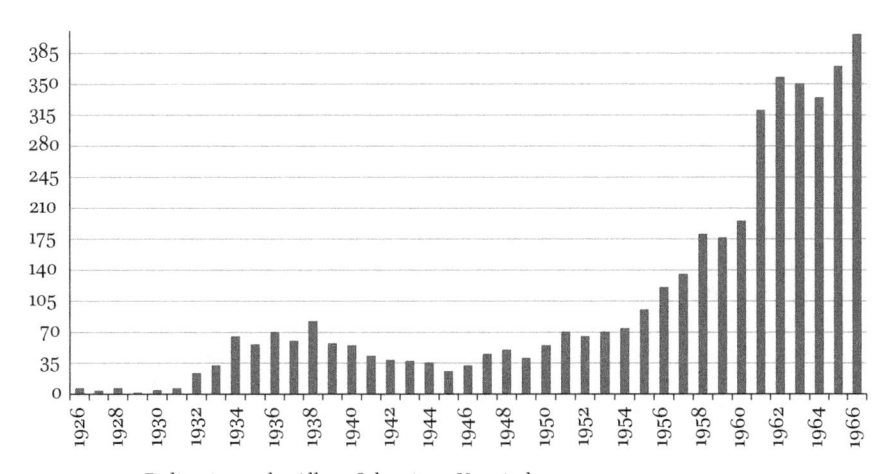

FIGURE 9   Deliveries at the Albert Schweitzer Hospital

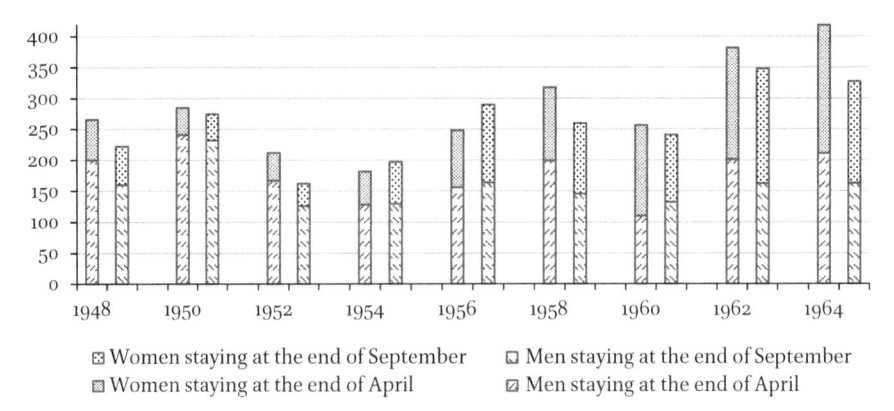

FIGURE 10   Gender ratio of inpatients at the Albert Schweitzer Hospital

The first maternity ward run by the colonial government in Gabon was established at the hospital in Libreville before World War One. It was usually
staffed by European midwives, and from 1938 also by African matrons. Until
1960, it had no doctor who had been trained in obstetrics.[33] In 1934, the hospital hosted sixty-two of the eighty-eight deliveries performed at all government health facilities in Gabon.[34] One year later, plans to improve maternal
and infant care while restructuring AEF's 'Assistance Médicale et Rurale' were
formulated, but these proved to be too ambitious and were never realized.[35]
Hines Mabika highlights that prenatal consultations in Gabonese hospitals
rose together with the number of deliveries from 1939 to 1941, but much less
drastically from 1943 to 1945 when the number of hospital births substantially
increased again.[36]

All the figures on delivery numbers contain considerable uncertainty and
only serve to provide a broad picture. Figure 7 illustrates the total number of
recorded deliveries at all government clinics in Gabon from 1932 to 1957.[37]
A sharp increase to almost 900 deliveries occurred in 1945, when there was a
total of eight maternity wards in Gabon. By 1951, there were twelve in the territory. Four years later, the number of deliveries had risen considerably again,
even though no additional wards had been opened; the existing units provided

33   Mabika, 'Médicalisation de l'Afrique centrale', 298, 323.

34   'Rapport Annuel du Service de Santé de la Colonie du Gabon 1934'. ZK 005-127, SHD.

35   Mabika, 'Médicalisation de l'Afrique centrale', 337–39.

36   Ibid., 325.

37   No data could be found for 1937 and 1938. See the annual reports of the Service de Santé
      for AEF and for Gabon: ZK 005- 121(1933–36)/160(1939–44)/089(1945–47)/091(1949–
      50)/092(1951)/097(1952)/093(1952–53)/016(1954–55)/095(1955–56), SHD; ZK 005- 127(1931–
      34)/128(1946–51)/005(1945, 1952–57), SHD.

a total of 177 beds.[38] It is unclear how many wards were in operation in 1957, when the colonial records end and a sudden rise in hospital deliveries occurred. One explanation for this increase is that in the course of the Service de la Santé's restructuring in that year, birth certificates became obligatory for all Gabonese newborns.[39]

The maternity ward at the government clinic in Lambaréné was established in 1945, twelve years after that at the Albert Schweitzer Hospital.[40] According to the calculations of the colonial administration, the demand for deliveries in the Lambaréné Subdivision was sufficiently high to support two maternity clinics. A 1956 evaluation concluded that an ideal maternity ward would host 90 to 240 births per year and serve an area with a twenty-kilometer radius and 3,000 to 8,000 inhabitants.[41] In comparison, the population of the Lambaréné Subdivision was an estimated 17,000 people at the time.[42] Figure 8 illustrates the numbers of deliveries at the government facility in Lambaréné for the period from 1955 to 1961.[43] Unlike in the rest of Gabon, there was no abrupt increase in births in 1957, which suggests that the legal requirement to obtain a birth certificate is not sufficient to explain African mothers' sudden motivation for delivering their babies at hospitals. The steep rise after independence, in contrast, parallels the trend at Schweitzer's hospital across the river, a fact which refutes simple explanations based on demand and supply, instead suggesting external push factors. The Gabonese state paid for hospital births in the early 1960s, something never referred to before.[44] During this short period of data overlap, approximately the same number of babies was delivered at the

---

38   Annual reports of the Sérvice de la Santé for Gabon, ZK 005-128 (1946, 1951), ZK 005-005 (1955), SHD.

39   Mabika Ognandzi, *Médicaliser l'Afrique*, 242–47. Mabika does not explicitly refer to the new birth certificate requirement, but outlines the restructuring of the service.

40   In the 1946 annual report of the Service de Santé for Gabon, Lambaréné is not included on the list of 'Maternités'. According to the 1951 report, the maternity ward there consisted of two structures with a total of five rooms for patients. The 1954 report states that the ward at Lambaréné hospital had been constructed in 1945 and comprised three rooms, each with four beds, ZK 005-128 (1946, 51), ZK005-005 (1954), SHD.

41   'Rapport Annuel du Service de Santé de la Colonie du Gabon 1956', ZK 005-005, SHD. The report also claims that women favored coming for pre- and postnatal consultations. The main aim of the report was to calculate the cost of a hospital birth for the state, which it estimated at 5,200 francs.

42   The 1953 Rapport Annuel du Service de Santé de la Colonie du Gabon lists the population at 17,249, ZK 005-005, SHD.

43   No numbers could be obtained for earlier years. The data is from the 1961 annual report of the Centre Médical de Lambaréné, PR(H), 1 H 226.1, ANG.

44   Müller, '50 Jahre Albert-Schweitzer-Spital', 26; Stocker, 'Diary 1961–63', 7; Interview Munz and Munz.

government hospital as at Schweitzer's hospital, but the numbers of surgical interventions were up to ten times higher at the latter.[45] The tempting argument that pregnant women only chose the Albert Schweitzer Hospital to give birth because it did not involve campaigns on how to be a good housewife and deliver more children is thus difficult to uphold.

Figure 9 illustrates the approximate number of deliveries by African mothers at the Albert Schweitzer Hospital.[46] Prior to 1932, no more than six children were ever born to African women in a single year. In that year, a drastic increase occurred, with twenty-three births recorded. Within the following two years, the number of deliveries almost tripled, possibly due to the newly built maternity ward established as a separate unit in 1933 (see Illustration 18). Previously, women in childbirth had been accommodated alongside surgical patients, whose numbers had also increased.[47] The eight beds in the small unit were well-occupied throughout the decade.[48] The head of AEF's Service d'Hygiène, who was otherwise rather hostile towards Schweitzer and his hospital, was impressed about the high number of childbirths there.[49]

Like overall patient numbers and the number of surgical cases, the number of deliveries dropped during World War Two; not until 1955, when fifteen beds were provided in the maternity ward,[50] did annual childbirths significantly

---

45   The government hospital performed 68 operations in 1960, while the surgeons at Schweitzer's hospital conducted 517. One year later, this ratio stood at 58:800. This data is from the 1960 and 1961 annual reports of the Centre Médical de Lambaréné, PR(H), 1 H 226.1, ANG.

46   The data for the years 1926–38, 1942–43, 1946, and 1966 are taken from 'Statistiques de l'Hôpital'. L – A – S1–3, AMS. Birth protocols are available for the years 1938–41, 1953–54, 1959–64. L – P – A1–8, AMS. The 1955 annual report is held at: PR(H), 1 H 235.4, ANG. Dr. Greet van der Kreek provides the number for 1956 in a letter to Schweitzer dated 18 July 1957 (held at AMS). The other statistics (for the years 1943–45, 1947–52, 1957–58, 1965) are taken from: Munz, *Mit dem Herzen einer Gazelle und der Haut eines Nilpferds*, 199. Munz provides a rather imprecise graph, the exact numbers in which are difficult to render. He claims to have taken these figures from 'patient records and operation books'. For the years for which I had data, my numbers correlated well with those provided by Munz. This was not the case, however, for the number of surgical operations, which he also lists in the same graph.

47   Schweitzer, 'Briefe aus dem Lambarene Spital Februar 1934', 4. The maternity ward at Schweitzer's hospital was not mentioned in the annual report of the Service de la Santé for 1932, but in that of the following year. It reportedly consisted of three rooms with two beds and two rooms with one bed each, ZK 005-127, SHD.

48   Schweitzer, 'Briefe aus dem Lambarene Spital Januar 1935', 3; 'Briefe aus dem Lambarene Spital Mai 1937', 3.

49   Goldschmid to Schweitzer, 10 October 1936, AMS.

50   This is indicated in one of the few annual reports (1955) sent by Schweitzer to the colonial administration after the outbreak of World War Two, PR(H), 1 H 235.4, ANG.

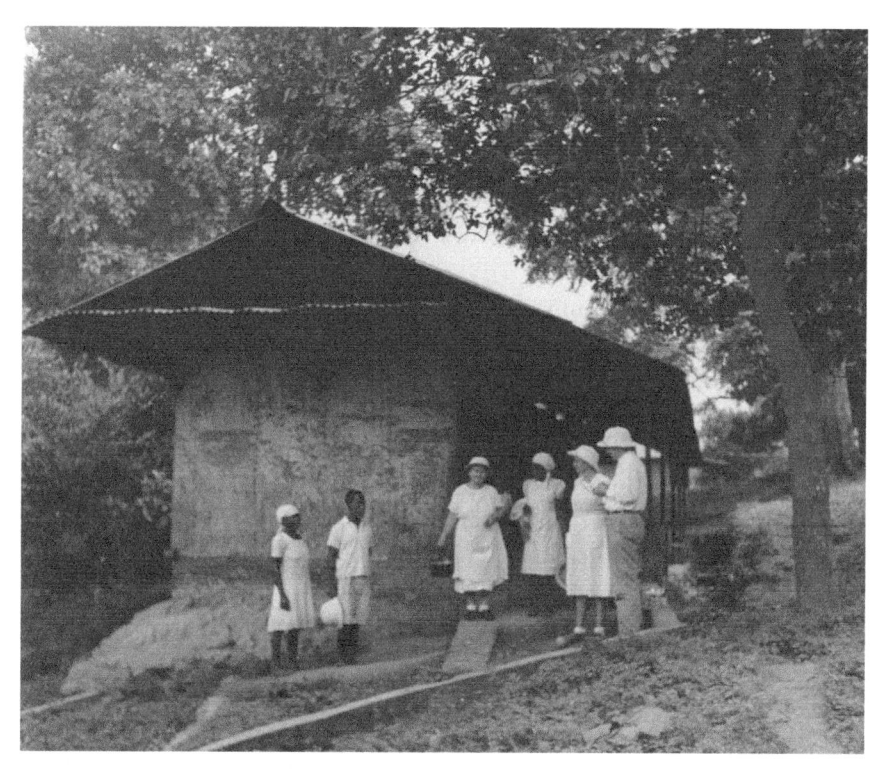

ILLUSTRATION 18   Staff in front of the hospital's maternity ward, ca. 1934
© ARCHIVES CENTRALES ALBERT SCHWEITZER GUNSBACH

outnumber pre-war levels. The increase in the following years is slightly delayed in comparison to the overall numbers for Gabon. After independence,
another significant rise correlates with an increase in overall admissions and
the growing number of deliveries at the government hospital. In 1960, a new
building was constructed with thirty-five beds for mothers-to-be.[51] The new
ward had 'a dirt floor' and, one year later, 'its aluminum walls (were) already
darkened from the smoke of cooking fires', as the visiting US American medical student Eugen Schoenfeld noted.[52]

   With the rise in births, the number of female patients at the hospital grew,
as Figure 10 demonstrates. In the mid-1950s, women accounted for approximately 25 percent of all inpatients. After 1960, half of them were female. On the

---

51   Siefert, *Meine Arbeitsjahre in Lambarene 1933–1935*, 178.
52   Schoenfeld, 'A Summer at Dr. Schweitzer's Hospital (Draft)', AMS, 7. A modified and con-
      siderably shortened version of this text was published in the *Journal of Medical Education*,
      Vol. 36, March 1961.

surface, it may appear that the rise in female patients was mainly due to the increasing number of babies being delivered at the hospital. However, the *appels mensuels* reveal that not only did births steadily increase, but so did 'gynecologic affections' in general. This was a minor category of illness in 1954, but in 1962 was the diagnosis most frequently given to inpatients after hernias and none at all.[53] Thus, more and more women attended the hospital to treat common afflictions.

Maternity care was of minor concern at the Albert Schweitzer Hospital, at least until the mid-1950s. As Figure 9 shows: before 1955, there had rarely been more than seventy births per year. When compared to surgery, the hospital's top priority, the number of deliveries had always been much lower, with the notable exception of during World War Two, when the number of births equaled the number of operations performed. Usually, the number of births was about five times less than the number of operations. However, after 1957, there were only four times more operations than births, and after 1961 the ratio was at roughly three to one.

Another manifestation of the marginal status of maternity care at the hospital in comparison to that of other services are the comparatively few references to it in the sources and the fact that the doctors did not find it worthy of more than passing mention it in their reports. While surgery, for example, frequently provided evidence of spectacular pathologies, deliveries – even when conducted by cesarean – seemed comparatively uninteresting. From the strictly medical perspective of Schweitzer and his staff, who did not attach any wider meaning to maternity care, obstetrics remained insignificant at the hospital until the number of deliveries increased. When Dr. Ilse Schnabel presented a portrait of the hospital in one of the main Swiss medical journals in 1936, over a quarter of her article focused on surgery, but she did not mention maternity services at all.[54] Her neglect of the topic is remarkable, because she wrote her article not long after the hospital's maternity services had been expanded for the first time. Twenty-seven later, Dr. Rolf Müller dedicated only three pages to obstetrics in a similar article, in comparison to almost ten on surgery.[55] Schweitzer himself considered obstetrics not worthy of a mention when he discussed the services offered at the hospital in 1948.[56] Although he and his staff may have thought it unnecessary to inform their readers about a fairly routine service such as maternity care, there is strong evidence to suggest that for hospital

---

53 Pregnancy was cited as the fifth most common reason for hospitalization in 1962.
54 Schnabel, 'Medizinisches aus Albert Schweitzers Urwaldspital'.
55 Müller, '50 Jahre Albert-Schweitzer-Spital'.
56 Schweitzer, *Das Spital im Urwald: Aufnahmen von Anna Wildikann*, 12–16.

staff, and perhaps especially for its director, maternity services were not a main priority.

3 Ignoring Training: Recruitment Priorities

While Schweitzer always aimed to ensure that qualified surgeons performed surgical interventions, he did not specifically require an obstetrician, gynecologist, or midwife to carry out deliveries. This could be left to general physicians or nurses. From a medical point of view, this made sense: surgeons usually have the necessary skills to perform a cesarean, whereas an obstetrician is seldom equipped with sufficient surgical knowledge to perform other operations.

The Albert Schweitzer Hospital thus contrasts other hospitals in Africa. Most of those expanded their maternity services in the 1920s, and, by the outbreak of World War Two, had employed at least one midwife. In many parts of the continent, African women were trained for this purpose.[57] In contrast, Schweitzer explained to Emmy Martin, in 1951 that 'as a midwife we need someone who at the same time does infirmary services'.[58] As seen at various points in this book, Schweitzer expected flexibility from his staff, a characteristic that he considered more important than the holding of a formal biomedical diploma in an obstetric specialty. Nurses responsible for the maternity ward had to carry out a range of other duties. They worked in the pharmacy, cared for women who had recently undergone surgery, administered injections, and assisted the physicians during consultations and even during the anesthesia process.[59] Most of these women had no special training in obstetrics; those who did also had to work outside of the maternity ward.[60]

---

57 Turrittin, 'Colonial Midwives and Modernizing Childbirth in French West Africa', 71; Bell, *Frontiers of Medicine*, 199; Summers, 'Intimate Colonialism', 804.

58 Schweitzer to Martin, 17 December 1951, AMS.

59 Martinelli-Stettler, 'Wie eine Insel', 122; Weber to Schweitzer, 13 November 1934, AMS; Lagendijk to Schweitzer, 14 January 1949, AMS; Lagendijk to Schweitzer, 14 September 1957, AMS.

60 Mathilde Kottmann arrived in July 1924 and became the second nurse, after Helene Schweitzer, to be employed at the hospital. As its secretary until Schweitzer's death, she would later hold a position that was crucial for the smooth running of the institution. She had some background in midwifery and/or the care of newborns. See: Munz and Munz, *Albert Schweitzers Lambarene, Zeitzeugen berichten*, 123; Woytt-Secretan, *Albert Schweitzer baut Lambarene*, 20–21. Another exception was Alice Schmidt who attended a midwifery school in 1936, before coming to Lambaréné after World War Two as a general nurse. See: Martin to Schweitzer, 14 December 1936, AMS.

Like the nurses, the doctors responsible for maternity care were required to perform numerous other tasks. In addition to supervising the maternity ward, Dr. Anna Wildikann, for instance, treated ulcers, performed operations, assisted at other surgical interventions, and provided dental services.[61] In the late 1950s, Dr. Greet van der Kreek was in charge of the maternity ward, but also had to look after some of the surgical patients.[62] In 1957, she remarked that 'managing deliveries has gradually become so much work [...], that it is almost a task in itself',[63] suggesting that caring for patients and new mothers had not been enough workload to fully occupy one nurse up to then. When South African midwife Olive du Preetz arrived in 1959, she was the first nurse to be given the space to focus entirely on maternity care, which included managing the nursery and looking after premature babies.[64] Jo Boddingius, a Dutchwoman who had also obtained her midwifery diploma in South Africa and who would later marry Dr. Walter Munz, took up the post in 1962, after the numbers of deliveries at the hospital had increased drastically. Although a European nurse, 'who had learned in Lambaréné how to supervise deliveries', stood in for her on two nights per week and on every other Sunday, she felt overwhelmed by the amount of work she had to carry out.[65]

From the 1930s, African women were given the role of looking after the hospital's newborns and orphans at its 'pouponnière', a unit in which children of staff members and orphans were accommodated (see Illustration 19). In the memoir of her stay in Lambaréné from 1933 to 1935, the nurse Jeanette Siefert recalled that Bike, the gardener's wife, assisted in bathing, feeding, and changing the diapers of infants. Unlike European medical personnel in other colonies and many of her colleagues at the hospital, Siefert had full confidence in African women's abilities to babysit. Describing Bike, she wrote: 'Like all black women, she was loving and indulgent to the children; she was patient, let herself be tyrannized by them'. Siefert then quoted a letter she had received from Schweitzer in which he acknowledged Bike's contribution and promised her a

---

61   See, for example, her letters to Schweitzer dated 15 December 1935; 25 March 1936; and 15 August 1936; these are held at the AMS. Wildikann first served in Lambaréné from 1935 to 1937 and was on very good personal terms with Schweitzer. She would return to the hospital during World War Two.

62   Van der Kreek to Schweitzer, 27 October 1959, AMS. As the letter continues, van der Kreek discusses various surgical challenges with which she was confronted. Maternity services, on the other hand, are not mentioned again.

63   Van der Kreek to Schweitzer, 18 August 1957, AMS.

64   Schoenfeld, 'A Summer at Dr. Schweitzer's Hospital (Draft)', AMS, 16.

65   Munz-Boddingius, 'Meine Chance und Freude, Hebamme in Lambarene gewesen zu sein', 65–66.

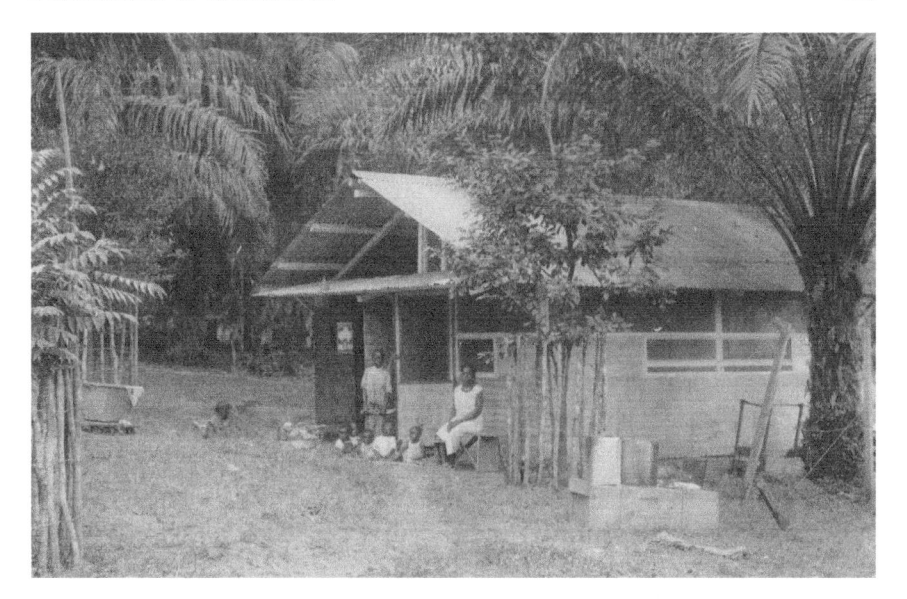

ILLUSTRATION 19   The 'Pouponnière', the hospital's day-care facility for children of staff and
orphans, 1935
© ARCHIVES CENTRALES ALBERT SCHWEITZER GUNSBACH

'beautiful present'.[66] This was rare praise, because later in the 1930s Schweitzer complained about the ignorance of African women in matters of childcare. By that stage, as he wrote, only N'Fagha, the widow of an auxiliary, 'fulfills her duties with great conscientiousness and with touching devotion she cares for the poor little beings entrusted to her'.[67] Judging from this small set of evidence, African personnel in the maternity ward were given specialized roles earlier than their European colleagues.

By the early 1960s, there were four African assistants in the maternity ward, all of whom were women.[68] One of these was Daudette Azizet Mburu, whom I interviewed in 2015. She gave birth to seven children at the hospital from 1951 to 1963. After her last delivery, Schweitzer offered her the opportunity to stay on and work as an 'infirmière accoucheuse', a delivery nurse.[69] Describing the tasks that African auxiliaries had to perform in the maternity ward, Mburu first recalled having to clean the unit. She also received the mothers-to-be and

---

66   Siefert, *Meine Arbeitsjahre in Lambarene 1933–1935*, 97.
67   Schweitzer, 'Briefe aus dem Lambarene Spital xx Mai 1937', 4.
68   Munz-Boddingius, 'Meine Chance und Freude, Hebamme in Lambarene gewesen zu sein', 65.
69   Interview Daudette Azizet Mburu.

cared for them until they were ready to deliver. When a woman went into labor, Mburu called for the nurse-in-chief. If a quick and unproblematic delivery followed, African auxiliaries could assist the mother without supervision of a European superior.[70] They were also indispensable for translating the numerous languages spoken by patients.[71] Given the general tendency not to mention Africans in most contemporary sources, including in the surgical protocols, it comes as no surprise that the role played by African auxiliaries was usually not noted in the birth protocols that were maintained in the ward.[72]

Clémentine Boucah's story, as told by her children Marie-Joséphine and Jacques, provides us with an example of how African assistants were recruited.[73] She began serving at the Albert Schweitzer Hospital as an *infirmière accoucheuse* after the death of her husband in the mid-1950s, having been invited to do so by her uncle, who already worked at the hospital. The institution had required assistance in the *pouponnière,* which was under the supervision of Suzanne Awo, who had worked at the hospital since at least 1947 and was frequently referred to as Mama Suzanne in the sources and the interviews I conducted (see Illustration 20).[74] Clémentine Boucah, who was assigned to assist her, was trained on the job. At that point, this involved assisting during deliveries, which were performed by Awo and the on-duty European nurse.

Other children of African employees recount similar stories. Albert Bouassa's father came to work at the hospital in the early 1930s, joining his brother, who was already employed there. Anne-Marie Padje-Poabalou, who started to work at the hospital in 1967, was the daughter of the long-serving auxiliary Ambroise Nyama.[75] Positive references and personal connections, especially kinship ties, were a great asset for those who sought employment at the Albert Schweitzer Hospital. This also applied for European personnel.

When a prospective employee showed an interest in serving at the hospital, Schweitzer or Emmy Martin would request information about the person from trusted sources. Formal biomedical qualifications were of secondary interest, as various examples from the maternity ward illustrate. Maria Lagendijk, who

---

70   Ibid.

71   Munz-Boddingius, 'Meine Chance und Freude, Hebamme in Lambarene gewesen zu sein', 66.

72   The first African auxiliary mentioned in the birth protocols was Boyé Suzanne in September 1961. L – P – A4, AMS.

73   Interview Marie-Joséphine Ndiaye-Boucah; Interview Jacques Boucah.

74   Awo's grandson claims that she started to work at the hospital in 1935. Interview Jacques-Adrien Rolagho. A 1962 'list of the longest-serving employees, proposed for a decoration' lists her year of arrival as 1947. She is the only woman on the list, in which she bears the title of 'aide-infirmière'. The list was found in a folder entitled 'affaires concernant le personnel indigene', within a box with the brief title 'divers', in the cellar of the AMS.

75   Interview Albert Bouassa; Interview Anne-Marie Padje-Poabalou.

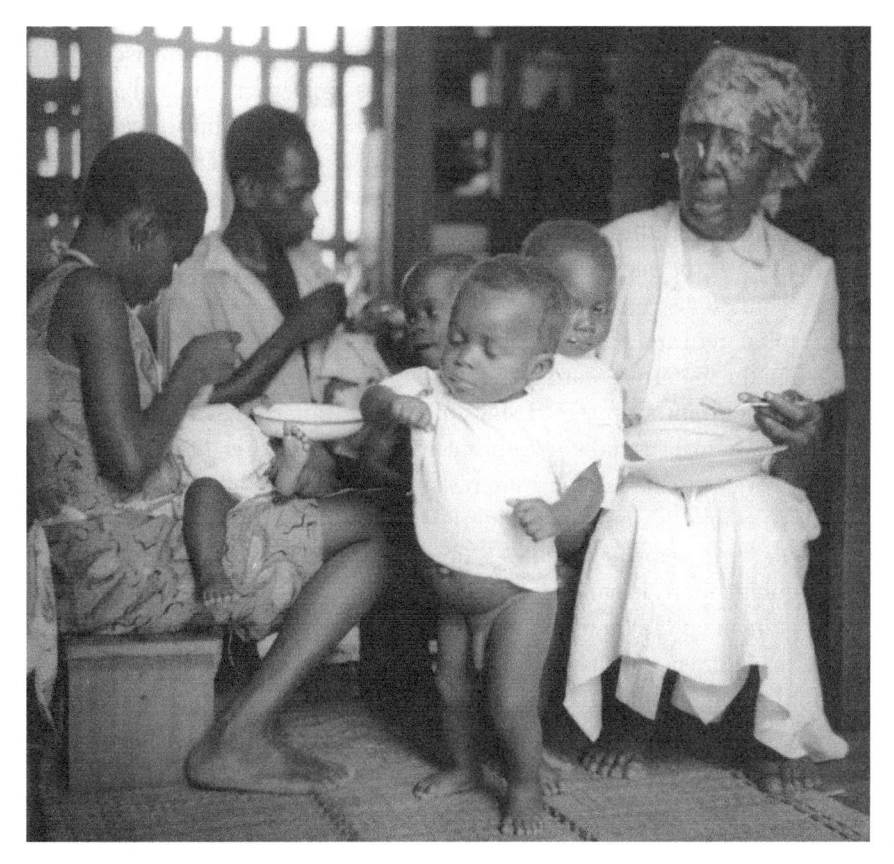

ILLUSTRATION 20   Suzanne Awo and unidentified nurses or parents feeding babies, mid-1950s
© ARCHIVES CENTRALES ALBERT SCHWEITZER GUNSBACH

would return to serve in Lambaréné on several occasions until after Schweitzer's death, had obtained a midwifery diploma in Britain and was able to 'independently lead deliveries', as Martin added in brackets in her letter presenting Lagendijk to Schweitzer in August 1938. However, this was not the main reason for employing her; Martin instead underlined that Lagendijk 'doesn't have to take care of anyone. Impression very kind and fine. [...] The medical report is good. [...] I made inquiries about her, they were good, too. Analysis very good'.[76] The final point refers to handwriting analysis, a test which Schweitzer routinely had done for each candidate by a specialist in Paris.

From this analysis, Schweitzer expected to gain insights into the applicant's personality, the favorable assessment of which represented a key precondition

---

76   Martin to Schweitzer, 11 August 1938, AMS. Like other prospective employees, Lagendijk was sent to two doctors – one in Alsace, one in Rotterdam – for medical examinations.

for being hired. Schweitzer looked for characteristics that were consistent with the 'Lambaréné Spirit'. For example, the results for Devika Frankenbach were 'not brilliant' – he suspected that she was a 'housemaid' – but since she was described as 'willing to work' and 'reasonable' he made further enquiries.[77] After learning that Frankenbach was a nurse, Schweitzer ordered that she should be 'be instructed in all areas of medical operations so that she can be deployed anywhere'.[78] At the beginning of her stay in 1957, Frankenbach was found to be 'too nervous' to distribute medication,[79] but she ultimately found her place at the hospital, returning for a second stay in the early 1960s, during which she worked in the maternity ward.[80]

More important than the findings of handwriting analyses were personal references. In 1939, a midwife from near Gunsbach with eighteen months of work experience expressed an interest in serving in Lambaréné. Martin rejoiced: 'Of course, it would be wonderful to have someone from here and even a midwife'.[81] After further inquiries, however, the candidate's superior gave a 'unfavorable report', leaving Martin to conclude that 'she has a bad character, so she's not an option for us'.[82] The Swiss nurse Sonja Müller, who would serve two terms in the maternity ward in the 1950s, had worked as a nurse in Conakry, but had undergone no formal training as a midwife.[83] Her personal references were so convincing that Schweitzer employed her in 1955 without waiting for the results of a handwriting analysis.[84] By recruiting staff that he thought would adhere to the 'Lambaréné Spirit', Schweitzer ensured that they ignored, or at least quietly accepted, local delivery practices. This careful selection of personnel thus contributed to processes of unknowing and to the hospital's guiding vision of healthcare provision.

4   Giving Birth at and Outside the Hospital

In order to understand Gabonese women's motivations for choosing hospital births and their experiences thereof, it is useful to compare the delivery

---

77   Schweitzer to Martin, 1 August 1956, AMS.
78   Schweitzer to Martin, 25 November 1956, AMS.
79   Van der Kreek to Schweitzer, 18 August 1957, AMS.
80   Stocker, 'Diary 1961–63', 3; Schoenfeld, 'A Summer at Dr. Schweitzer's Hospital (Draft)', AMS, 17. It remains unclear if Frankenbach attended some form of obstetrical training before returning to Gabon.
81   Martin to Schweitzer, 4 April 1939, AMS.
82   Martin to Schweitzer, 6 May 1939, AMS.
83   Schweitzer to Martin, 15 March 1955, AMS.
84   Schweitzer to Martin, 25 March 1955, AMS.

process in a biomedical ward with that which typically occurred in the settlements of Gabon. A considerable number of ethnographies provide information on the latter; however, they often did not report in detail on the act of giving birth itself. Instead, they focused on aspects that were ignored or did not occur at the Albert Schweitzer Hospital, such as post-delivery rituals concerning the placenta or the umbilical cord. It is unclear whether it was the African informants, the mothers, or the ethnographers themselves who were more interested in discussing these customs than the actual delivery process.

A period of seclusion after childbirth, during which the mother was not allowed to leave the hut in which she had given birth, was customary among the Fang of Gabon.[85] At the Albert Schweitzer Hospital, mothers were also kept in a maternity ward for some time, where they were looked after, hidden from the male gaze. However, the degree of privacy and silence afforded to the mother was quite different in these two settings. Ethnographers from different periods generally agree that the delivery of the baby and the postnatal seclusion happened in the village of the new mother's own mother.[86] Reasons for this move were not given, but can be understood in two ways in relation to hospital births. The more straightforward interpretation is that this habit hindered hospital births. However, it is also plausible that this passage was not about soil or place, but leaving the environment of the father's family and passing through a symbolic voyage into the mother's family and an all-female environment. Since her mother and other female relatives could accompany a pregnant woman to Schweitzer's hospital, its maternity ward can thus be interpreted as representing a setting as suitable for childbirth as the maternal village.

Some oral testimonies assert that a woman would come to the hospital in the eighth month of her pregnancy.[87] In contrast, Azizet Mburu reports that

---

85 Ethnographers have not agreed on how long this period normally lasted. In the early twentieth century, Tessmann described how mothers would stay in the hut in which the birth had occurred for eight to ten days. Another month to two months would pass before they would be allowed to take up their regular duties once again. See: Tessmann, *Die Pangwe*, 2:276. Fernandez, who conducted his fieldwork in the late 1950s, wrote that mothers would remain in the hut together with the baby for up to one month. See: Fernandez, *Bwiti*, 115.

86 Tessmann, *Die Pangwe*, 2:274–75; Alexandre and Binet, *Le groupe dit Pahouin*, 91; Fernandez, *Bwiti*, 115. Henri Trilles, in contrast, reported that the mother-in-law played the key role in the birth ritual, which took place in the husband's home village and saw the participation of all local women. See: Trilles, 'Les rites de la naissance chez les Fang', 405. Other parts of Trilles' work, notably his theories on the origins of the Fang, have been rejected by the majority of anthropologists and historians. See: Cinnamon, 'Missionary Expertise, Social Science, and the Uses of Ethnographic Knowledge in Colonial Gabon', 430.

87 Emane, *Docteur Schweitzer: une icône africaine*, 124. Some of my interviewees recalled the same. See: Group Interview Port-Gentil; Interview Marie-Joséphine Ndiaye-Boucah.

there was no firm rule in this regard: some women arrived shortly before delivery; others had already been coming for regular consultations for months.[88] According to Jo Munz, the ideal scenario was for a woman to come for prenatal consultations as soon as she suspected a pregnancy. She would then be asked to return to the hospital two weeks before the anticipated date of birth.[89] In 1961, the nurse Marianne Stocker recorded in her diary that a pregnant woman would come to the hospital 'a few weeks before the delivery' and stay there until her baby weighed more than three kilograms and its umbilicus was dry.[90] Jo Munz reported that the latter typically occurred three weeks after the birth.[91] According to Azizet Mburu, mothers usually left the hospital after eight days, if the doctor who had visited them daily permitted them to do so.[92] These differences in medical guidelines reflect the piecemeal nature in which the hospital was run. They also underline the agency of mothers, an agency similarly observed among surgical patients in the previous chapter.

To gain more insight into how childbirth occurred at the hospital, an entry from Stocker's diary for 22 April 1961 can be compared to other accounts from the same period. Stocker usually worked as a pediatric nurse and was not required to perform midwifery duties, but on this particular night her assistance was requested by the on-duty nurse in the maternity ward.

> A birth under petroleum light. Everything was a bit more primitive but not unclean. Mother and grandmother held the head and hands of the woman giving birth. Other family members waited in front of the building. From time to time we hear them sigh and sometimes laugh. A strong, rosy girl was born. She screamed and kicked her legs. 'A girl, you are rich', said the black aide. 'Thank you thank you', laughed the grandmother and pranced around in the room, humming a monotonous melody. Evangeline bathes the child, dresses her and puts her in a liana basket. [...] Mother and child remain in the delivery room for two hours. Then the woman who has recently given birth walks into her case on foot. The grandmother follows, carrying the little basket with the child on her head.[93]

In this passage, instead of discussing the baby's delivery, Stocker focuses on the presence and behavior of family members and on the postnatal mobility of the

---

88   Interview Daudette Azizet Mburu.
89   Interview Munz and Munz.
90   Stocker, 'Diary 1961–63', 7.
91   Interview Munz and Munz.
92   Interview Daudette Azizet Mburu.
93   Stocker, 'Diary 1961–63', 6–7.

mother. She does not specify if the birth occurred with the mother in a lying or sitting position. According to both Jo Munz and Azizet Mburu, lying was the standard birth position used at the hospital.[94]

Azizet Mburu, however, disagrees with Stocker on whether relatives could be present during the birth, recalling that they were made to wait outside the delivery room. Schoenfeld reported that the mother of a woman in labor would usually wait at her daughter's bedside while five to six other family members waited outside.[95] He did not mention any dancing or singing, a vivid memory of the dentist Frederick Franck, who had his dentistry next doors.[96]

Like Stocker, the visiting pediatrician Hermann Mai was struck by how quickly new mothers regained their mobility. In his diary, he noted that 'on the day of her child's birth I saw the mother carrying buckets of water on her head. She got up after the removal of the placenta and walked away as one gets up from eating (or the opposite!)'.[97] On this point, Schoenfeld disagreed slightly, reporting that a new mother typically 'walked to a wooden stretcher and was carried to the cottage. She was usually out of bed the following morning'.[98]

These diverse reports from the same time period illustrate that very few strict rules were enforced during childbirth, in complete contrast to the processes prior to and during a surgical intervention; less control was deemed to be necessary during the delivery process (see Illustrations 21 and 22). Still, women were made to give birth in a room in the Grande Pharmacie, some distance away from their sleeping quarters. Schweitzer wanted medical procedures to take place at a central location, where he could easily oversee and control them. Recurring reports of babies being born elsewhere on the hospital grounds suggest that this was not as easy to ensure in the delivery room as it was in the surgical ward. Protocols list deliveries taking place on pirogues, in the sleeping quarters for pregnant women, or on a sandbank in the river in front of the hospital.[99]

European medical personnel at the Albert Schweitzer Hospital were remarkably ignorant of local birth practices and the significance that local residents attached to these. The nurse Elisabeth Anderegg, for example, recalled a

---

94   Munz-Boddingius, 'Meine Chance und Freude, Hebamme in Lambarene gewesen zu sein', 68; Interview Daudette Azizet Mburu.

95   Schoenfeld, 'A Summer at Dr. Schweitzer's Hospital (Draft)', AMS, 17.

96   Franck, *Days with Albert Schweitzer*, 100.

97   Hermann Mai's diaries are held at the AMS. This entry is from 1958.

98   Schoenfeld, 'A Summer at Dr. Schweitzer's Hospital (Draft)', AMS, 18.

99   L – P – A2–5, AMS. For the pirogues: April 1959, October 1959, April 1962, January 1964; for the sleeping quarters: January 1959, March 1962, August 1963; for the sandbank: September 1963.

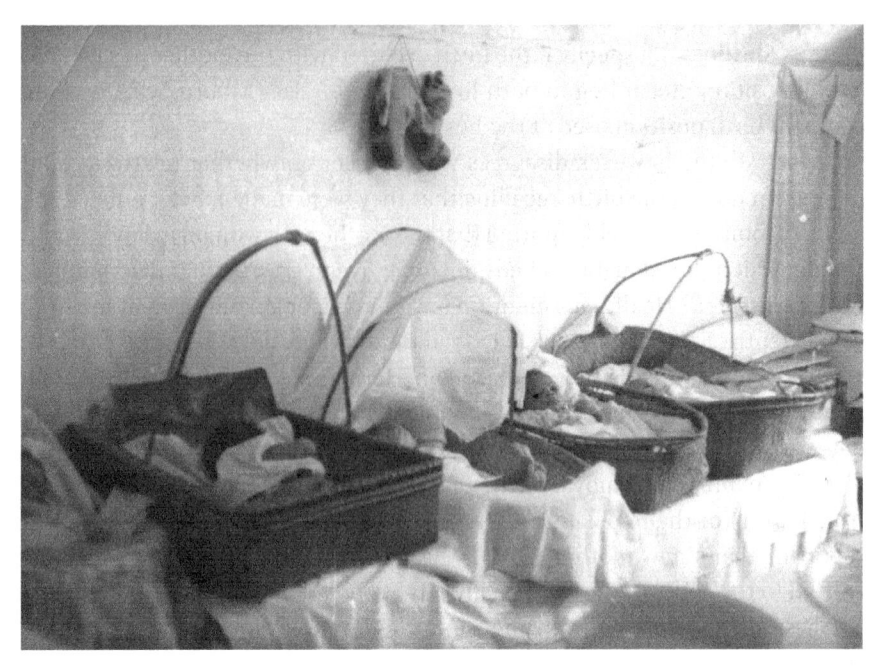

ILLUSTRATION 21   Accommodation for babies, undated
© ARCHIVES CENTRALES ALBERT SCHWEITZER GUNSBACH

woman who arrived at the hospital with a piece of rock attached on a liana to the umbilical cord with which to extract the placenta. Anderegg commented this episode as follows: 'we couldn't understand it. The way they treat … in these villages'.[100] In various accounts, staff members proclaimed the outlandishness of Gabonese practices from their biomedical point of view. These descriptions are important because they prove that staff were confronted with different childbirth practices and that knowledge about these circulated among them. They illustrate how ignorance functioned on many dimensions at the hospital. Narratives of childbirth blur the question of who is ignorant of what, as the following examples demonstrate.

In 1949, Joy and Arnold reported a number of pregnant women who had come 'to get hospital care before and after childbirth but, fearing that a male doctor may help in the delivery, steal off into the bush and then carry the crying infant into the Hospital'.[101] Yet, similar occurrences were recorded in the birth protocols even when a woman was in charge of the maternity ward. This

---

100   Interview Elisabeth Anderegg.
101   Joy, Arnold, and Schweitzer, *The Africa of Albert Schweitzer*, 132.

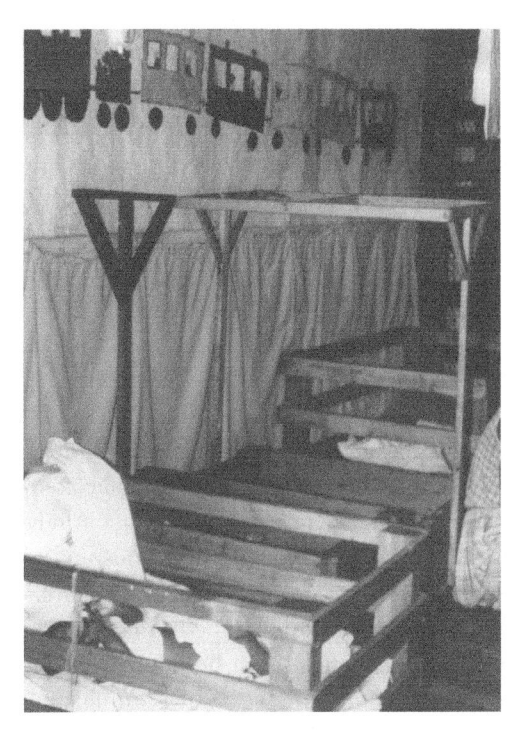

ILLUSTRATION 22   Another accommodation for babies, also undated
© ARCHIVES CENTRALES ALBERT SCHWEITZER GUNSBACH

suggests that these mothers may have been motivated by different reasons, which are difficult to discern from our sources.

Another example is from a letter written to Schweitzer by Dr. Wildikann in March 1936. Schweitzer did not reproduce the story in print, even though he enjoyed publishing such anecdotes of exotic and supposedly ignorant practices of locals. Wildikann reported the following:

> By the way, I recently experienced a delightful joke that I have to tell you in my 'obstetric practice'. A young Pahouin brings his pregnant wife (about 6–7 months) for examination. My stethoscope makes a big impression on both of them. After listening to the children's sounds, the man asks me: 'does my son already speak?' In my high spirits, I answer: 'yes, yes he starts to do so already', whereupon the good little negro shines so that his beautiful teeth become visible up to his ears and he asks me: 'What did he tell you?'[102]

---

102   Wildikann to Schweitzer, 25 March 1936, AMS.

Wildikann did not provide any further comment on this episode. As a result, we cannot tell if she thought that the husband was joking or ignorant. In any case, she did not simply dismiss the man's words as uninformed by correcting him or trying to impose her judgment. Instead, Wildikann responded in a humorous way, a reaction that at the same time acknowledged the man's point of view and denied its validity, which was one way to unknow local practices and perspectives.

In one 'African Story', a collection of which Schweitzer published in a booklet in 1939, he told of one of many women who believed that she was living under a 'taboo' that would kill her if her firstborn was a boy. When her first baby was delivered in her mother's village, it cried like a boy. After discovering that it was actually a girl, the new mother insisted that it had changed sex after delivery. A few days later, she was brought to the hospital 'severely emaciated' and could not be saved. Schweitzer believed that 'her illness was [...] of entirely psychological origin'.[103] Besides suggesting that locals perceived the hospital as a last resort in the case of certain afflictions, this example illustrates the inability of hospital staff to grasp issues that lay beyond the biomedical sphere.[104] Schweitzer did not deny that 'taboos' had real effects, but he referred to the woman's psyche and thus provided a rational interpretation. It is an illustration of how, when confronted with practices and attitudes that they considered primitive, staff unknew those by explaining them from a biomedical perspective or by making jokes. Instead of actively attempting to change local realities and practices, they were encouraged to find pragmatic solutions within the hospital.

Norwegian pediatrician Louise Jilek-Aall, who worked at the hospital in 1961, provides an account which suggests that Schweitzer was reasonably knowledgeable about local ideas on childbirth.[105] On one occasion, she accompanied the hospital's mechanic Siegfried Neukirch on a journey in a truck to collect plantains and other food. On their way, they were called into a hut, where an old woman lay seriously ill. To her own surprise, Jilek-Aall found the woman to be pregnant. At first, her husband reacted in a slightly offended manner: "'Why do you make a joke?" he asked, "we are prepared for bad news'". The doctor could not convince them of her diagnosis, but they readily agreed to visit the hospital to have Schweitzer solve the mystery. On confirming Jilek-Aall's verdict, Schweitzer commented to her pessimistically:

---

103   Schweitzer, *Afrikanische Geschichten*, 54.
104   See Chapter 5 for a discussion of this issue.
105   Jilek-Aall, *Working with Dr. Schweitzer*, 97–101.

What will the future hold for this child? To the African it is an unnatural event to bear a child at this mother's advanced age. Witchcraft will be suspected by the neighbors. Even the parents will be afraid of the child and probably let it succumb before long.

Schweitzer then confirmed the diagnosis to the disbelieving couple, adding:

I know it sounds impossible to you and you would rather not have another child at your age, but to us, this will be a special baby. We would like to make it a child of the hospital. Leave the child with us – if it is a boy, I shall give it my name; if a girl, we shall name it after la doctoresse. You need not tell anyone just stay at the hospital and look after your wife until she is well. When the child is born, we will keep it in our nursery. Should you wish to return at a later date to see your child, you will know which one is yours by its name.[106]

They were placed in quarters all by themselves, and the wife's condition improved. After a trouble-free delivery, 'the couple lingered on in the hospital much longer than we thought necessary. But we never saw them visit the nursery or display any interest in their child'.

A number of more general descriptions of non-hospital deliveries in Gabon emerge from the early 1960s. According to Jo Munz, a woman in labor would be watched over by a local birth attendant, usually an elderly woman. The former would lie on a banana leaf with her legs on the attendant's shoulders, her mother or another relative sitting behind her and holding her. According to Munz, the only course of action that a birth attendant could take if a delivery did not progress smoothly was to encourage the woman to push more forcefully; if unsuccessful, a failure of the cervix to open would often lead to the death of the mother or child.[107] When Dr. Müller explained local birth practices to a specialist medical readership, he also mentioned the older women who acted as birth attendants; however, he disagreed with Munz on the preferred position for delivery and claimed that 'as soon as the woman feels the urge to push, she goes into a squatting position and often only a few labor pains are enough to expel the infant'. Müller concluded that 'the majority of the deliveries runs smoothly', but shared Munz's general concern that 'a prolonged course, however, can lead to numerous complications: pushing when the cervix is often incompletely opened exhausts the woman and damages the

---

106   Ibid., 100.
107   Interview Munz and Munz.

child'.[108] Staff's preoccupation with the cervix reveals their biomedical training and its focus on anatomy. In their view, African ignorance in obstetrics was palpable and could prove to have fatal consequences in complicated cases.

According to some ethnographies, the sitting-on-banana-leaves birth position was customary throughout the study period,[109] but the birth position was not specified by the majority of the authors. They showed particular interest in the burying of the umbilical cord,[110] the placenta,[111] or both,[112] which they claimed to be of crucial importance for the new mother's family members. The exact details of this procedure, as well as the specific person responsible for its execution, remain vague. James Fernandez interprets the afterbirth as representing a kind of 'second person' or 'twin of the newborn who must die and be carefully buried lest animals or witches discover and devour it and bring harm to the newborn'.[113] Some colonial officials also recognized the deep significance of the practice. In 1934, for example, placentas were returned to the families of women who had given birth at the newly opened maternity ward in the Kong Hospital in Libreville.[114] In view of the great symbolic meaning attached to the afterbirth among the Fang, it is striking that this custom goes almost unmentioned in our sources relating to Schweitzer's hospital. The one exception was visitor Schoenfeld, who wrote that 'the grandmother disposed of the placenta (usually in the river)',[115] suggesting that it was a practice that frequently occurred.

Clear from the ethnographic writing is that childbirth was an exclusively feminine domain in Fang society. Men were not allowed in the same hut during the delivery. The ethnographic authors emphasized that the newborn baby's grandmother from the maternal side was normally present. According to Fernand Grébert, serving for the Paris Evangelical Mission in Gabon from 1913 to 1932, female birth attendants were fully competent and had long been powerful actors in Fang society.[116] Ethnographers who were not trained in medicine usually

---

108   Müller, '50 Jahre Albert-Schweitzer-Spital', 25–26.
109   Trilles, 'Les rites de la naissance chez les Fang', 407–9; Alexandre and Binet, *Le groupe dit Pahouin*, 91.
110   Trilles, 'Les rites de la naissance chez les Fang', 410; Alexandre and Binet, *Le groupe dit Pahouin*, 91.
111   Tessmann, *Die Pangwe*, 2:276; Gaulene, 'Coutumes des races gabonaises'. In: 'Rapport Annuel du Service de Santé de la Colonie du Gabon 1932', ZK 005-127. SHD.
112   Fernandez, *Bwiti*, 447.
113   Ibid.
114   'Rapport Annuel du Service de Santé de la Colonie du Gabon 1934', ZK 005-127, SHD.
115   Schoenfeld, 'A Summer at Dr. Schweitzer's Hospital (Draft)', AMS, 18.
116   Grébert, *Au Gabon*, 132. Tessmann is the only ethnographer who made no mention of birth attendants. See: Tessmann, *Die Pangwe*, 2:275.

did not judge their obstetrical ability, with the exception of Alexandre and Binet. According to them, 'the technique of midwives (*is*) extremely uneven: while some know how to perform artificial deliveries and even how to turn feti around, most of them are limited to massages and magical practices'.[117]

From the Albert Schweitzer Hospital, Dr. Wildikann claimed that it was the desire of African mothers-in-waiting to be attended to by a woman. She had 'the strong conviction that women have themselves examined with good confidence and less timidity by a female doctor'.[118] Schweitzer cited the same reason when he demanded the immigration permit for Wildikann during World War Two, insisting that 'indigenous women come more easily to a lady than a man'.[119] The argument that local women would only accept the care of female medical personnel, so overt elsewhere,[120] is less conspicuous in our case, but its maternity ward remained a largely female domain throughout the study period.[121]

Augustin Emane argues that giving birth at the Albert Schweitzer Hospital was considered a privilege by his informants, not only because Schweitzer himself provided protection from malign forces and submitted the birth certificate, but also because the baby was 'was surrounded by white women (known to be more competent and reliable) who will take care of him as well as dress him'.[122] According to this claim, it was not only European staff members at the hospital who considered Africans ignorant in matters of childbirth, but also African women themselves. This assertion, while difficult to evaluate, supports the argument that biomedicine diffused successfully in Gabon and changed perceptions of childbirth in the territory. As key to achieving the latter, Emane cites the free distribution of clothes for newborns, a practice that was also fondly recalled by my interviewees.[123] They

---

117   Alexandre and Binet, *Le groupe dit Pahouin*, 92. Italics mine.

118   Wildikann to Schweitzer, 18 June 1936, AMS.

119   He also underlined Wildikann's skills in dental care, a service from which many Europeans in the territory benefited; Schweitzer to Mandel, 26 January 1940, AMS.

120   Ndao, 'Colonisation et politique de santé maternelle et infantile au Sénégal'; Summers, 'Intimate Colonialism', 802f.

121   When the number of deliveries increased and the percentage of female doctors at the hospital decreased after 1960, female midwives continued to be hired for the purpose of routinely attending deliveries, as mentioned above. Throughout the study period, male doctors were occasionally present to perform episiotomies or sutures for perineal ruptures, as the protocols indicate.

122   Emane, *Docteur Schweitzer: une icône africaine*, 124. A more detailed discussion on the Albert Schweitzer Hospital as a place of safety will be provided in Chapter 5.

123   Group Interview Port-Gentil. This was also considered important by European personnel. See: Munz-Boddingius, 'Meine Chance und Freude, Hebamme in Lambarene gewesen zu sein', 68; Stocker, 'Diary 1961–63', 13.

also highlighted how valuable it was for mothers and babies to receive food.[124] These factors must not be underestimated when answering the question of why women chose to deliver their babies at Schweitzer's hospital. In other parts of the continent, including at the Berceau Gabonais in Libreville, the distribution of extra-medical items such as clothes or soap was seen as key to luring pregnant women to hospitals.[125]

5   Ignoring Context: Maternity Care as a Medical Service

Schweitzer and his staff ignored colonial discourses on depopulation and domesticity, but also rarely reflected on what would motivate a Gabonese woman to choose to deliver her baby at a hospital or in her community. When staff members discussed maternity care, this was usually in connection with complicated cases. This suggests that they conceived of obstetrics as a purely medical service, one of many offered at the hospital. While abnormal cases were considered worthy of reporting, general developments, overall numbers of deliveries, or simple updates were rarely provided. The protocols, on the other hand, reveal that the majority of deliveries occurred without problems. Usually, between 80 and 85 percent of births per year were categorized as 'normal', as Table 2 illustrates. Staff had a broad understanding of what constituted 'normal' (see Illustration 23). This could include stillbirths, breech presentations, perineal ruptures or episiotomies, deliveries in the hospital's living quarters or on the pirogues, and deliveries with the help of labor-inducing medication or by vacuum extractor. Categorizations varied over time and depended on the nurse; the classification in Table 2 thus cannot be provided with full certainty. Furthermore, as protocols for most years are missing, the available information is extremely fragmentary.

Technological artifacts were of some importance in obstetric practices at the Albert Schweitzer Hospital. Forceps had been in use since at least the early 1930s,[126] but by the early 1960s, staff made every effort to avoid using these. Jo Munz did so by turning the fetus over before the thirty-sixth week, a practice prohibited in Europe but that she had learned in Johannesburg as a way of preventing not only deliveries by forceps, but also cesareans and breech presentations. During her time at the hospital, a vacuum extractor was introduced, which quickly established itself as a key technology for easing deliveries.

---

124   Interview Marie-Joséphine Ndiaye-Boucah; Interview Daudette Azizet Mburu.
125   Headrick, *Colonialism, Health and Illness in French Equatorial Africa*, 271.
126   Bonnema to Schweitzer, 18 December 1932, AMS.

TABLE 2   Problematic deliveries

Year	Total number of deliveries	Not 'normal' deliveries (%)	By cesarean	By forceps	By vacuum extractor	Premature deliveries[a]	Other complications[b]
1938	82	14.6	2	2	0	0	8
1939	57	3.5	0	0	0	1	1
1940	55	16.4	0	0	0	3	6
1941	43	9.3	0	0	0	1	3
1953	70	24.3	5	7	0	3	2
1954	74	18.9	4	4	0	1	5
1959	176	18.8	18	6	0	4	5
1960	195	15.9	21	0	0	3	7
1961	320	13.8	23	2	0	6	13
1962	357	14.0	15	2	7	13	13
1963	350	20.6	11	1	45	7	8
1964	334	19.2	24	0	25	6	9

a   Premature deliveries were sometimes considered 'normal'. I have listed all premature deliveries referred to in the protocols in this column, even when these were categorized as normal.
b   This includes breech presentations, which were sometimes also categorized as normal', as well as other rare or unspecified complications.

Dr. Rolf Müller and Jo Munz tested it at the hospital on a few occasions as a potential replacement for forceps, after which Schweitzer was satisfied that it had demonstrated its superiority and lent his approval to its further use.[127] According to the birth protocols, it was used when the baby's heartbeat was irregular or when the mother had pushed for more than thirty minutes without result.[128]

The focus on irregular birth cases is especially noticeable in the sources from the 1930s onwards, when the new maternity ward was open and Schweitzer spent a considerable amount of time in Europe. In all her letters from 1936, Dr. Wildikann, who was at the time in charge of the maternity ward, reported irregular births to Schweitzer, but never discussed the general state of the

127   Interview Munz and Munz.
128   See, for example, the entries of April and July 1964.

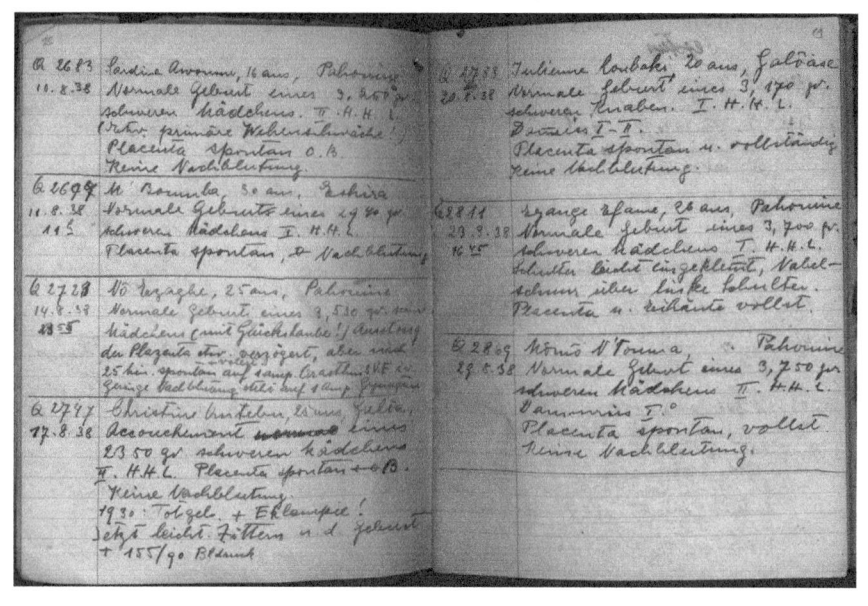

ILLUSTRATION 23   Delivery protocols of August and September 1938. All seven births were
'normal', despite a case of very tedious primary labor, a girl born with a
caul, two perineal ruptures, and a girl born with the umbilical cord over
her shoulder

© ARCHIVES CENTRALES ALBERT SCHWEITZER GUNSBACH

ward.[129] Some irregular cases were stillbirths, explained with reference to the
young age of the mothers and their narrow pelvises, a recurring concern to
which I will return below.[130] Other cases that Wildikann reported were those
that she considered strange. For example, a pregnant woman had shown mild
symptoms of smallpox one evening, upon which she was isolated. 'At the early
consultation the next morning I found the woman in hard labor, the baby's
head already visible', Wildikann wrote, continuning that 'as soon as I turned
around to gather the most necessary things for delivery, the child was already
there'.[131] In another instance, she considered the limits of their diagnostic possibilities. When the uterus of a dysentery patient became swollen, the doctors
suspected a tumor. One day, 'the woman felt a still desire' and went into the
bushes near the river, where she delivered 'a tiny child of seven months'.[132]

---

129   The same is true for her aide, the Swiss nurse Emmy Röthlisberger, who provided considerably less detail.
130   Wildikann to Schweitzer, 15 August 1936, AMS.
131   Wildikann to Schweitzer, 8 April 1936, AMS.
132   Ibid.

Such accounts contain a considerable degree of sensationalism, which is also a feature of Schweitzer's published writings. However, he preferred to print reports on huge cases of elephantiasis or on injuries suffered in animal attacks than on irregular deliveries. Presumably, he did not want to shock his supporters with stories of the deaths of innocent infants, but this publication strategy also reflects the marginal status of maternity care at the hospital. On another level, these accounts illustrate the agency of patients, as well as the limits of European doctors' knowledge and abilities.

Besides deliveries that were considered exotic or strange, medical personnel also deemed complicated ones worthy of reporting. A number of practices to extract babies were intrusive and potentially disturbing, as illustrated in a letter written in December 1934 by Dr. Ladislav Goldschmid, Wildikann's predecessor in the maternity ward.[133] A woman was brought to the hospital after she had been in labor for four days – '(supposedly!)', as Goldschmid remarked. He diagnosed a second-grade pelvis constriction and dismissed the option of performing a cesarean, because 'the woman was too dirty'.[134] Instead, he considered 'turning to the foot, high forceps, pulvotomy (sic) with Gigli saw, or craniotomy'. He chose to observe her condition for some time before making a decision, which he would base primarily on the 'further state of the woman', adding that 'of course I would also like to save the infant life'.[135] In the letters that followed, Goldschmid did not clarify which option he had chosen, but similar cases can be traced in other sources from throughout the study period.

The most invasive and disturbing practice was the skull perforation, also known as craniotomy. The practice was still being performed as late as 1953 and 1954, even if rarely.[136] A well-documented case occurred in 1936, when a pregnant woman arrived with seizures that the doctors identified as severe eclampsia. Dr. Wildikann wrote to Schweitzer that they carried out the perforation only 'after everything else had failed'. Dr. Heinz Barasch had to perform the procedure, 'because I lacked courage to do so'. Without further comment, she added that 'until now, the woman recovers fairly well'.[137] In his report, Barasch claimed that the unborn child had already been dead, a fact to which Wildikann did not mention at all. He underlined that it had been too late to perform a cesarean, ultimately justifying this serious intrusion with the need

133   Goldschmid to Schweitzer, 26 December 1934, AMS.

134   It is difficult to discern what Goldschmid meant to say with this statement, but it illustrates his concern about asepsis.

135   Goldschmid to Schweitzer, 26 December 1934, AMS.

136   Protocols reveal one case in each of these years, as well as one in 1938. See: L – P – A1, L – P – A3 AMS.

137   Wildikann to Schweitzer, 18 June 1936, AMS.

to end the birth process in order to save the mother's life. In a similar but slightly more optimistic manner to Wildikann, Barasch ended his account by assuring Schweitzer that 'the woman is well'.[138] In the Belgian Congo, medical personnel frequently employed craniotomy crotchets because Africans were said to believe that a cesarean would kill the mother. It was thus feared that attempting to perform one would damage the reputation of a hospital.[139] Gabonese were also reluctant to undergo cesareans, as we will see below, but craniotomies did not occur frequently enough at the Albert Schweitzer Hospital to argue that they served as a substitute for the former.

Like elsewhere in Africa, cesareans were rare at the Albert Schweitzer Hospital during the interwar period, as indicated in Table 2; from 1925 to 1941, only three instances were reported.[140] Indeed, this intervention was rarely performed anywhere in AEF. For 1935, for example, AEF records list only 3 cesareans in a total of 1,031 deliveries. In 1944, colonial authorities recorded 19 cesareans in a total of almost 7,500 births recorded in maternity wards throughout AEF.[141] This is somewhat surprising, since the procedure was performed frequently in predominantly Catholic metropolitan France, where medical tradition prioritized the life and baptism of the child. In Britain, on the other hand, priority was given to protecting the life of the mother and thus Cesareans were executed less frequently.[142]

There was no clearly stated policy on cesareans at the Albert Schweitzer Hospital. It was not specified if, in the case of severe complications, safeguarding the life of the mother or that of the child should be prioritized. Despite its staff members' diverse backgrounds and training – they were educated in a number of different countries and were of Protestant, Catholic, or Jewish faith – they tended to act first to save the mother. In December 1934, Dr. Goldschmid reported to Schweitzer what might have been the hospital's first cesarean, although his sober tone does not suggest a premiere had taken place. A woman who had been in labor in her village for two days was brought to the hospital. Goldschmid decided in favor of a cesarean, because 'otherwise I had to sacrifice the life of the child'. A 'fearful' period followed, during which the doctors suspected that the mother had caught a puerperal infection. Goldschmid blamed

---

138   Barasch to Schweitzer, 3 June 1936, AMS.

139   Hunt, *A Colonial Lexicon*, 223, 229, 235.

140   For the years prior to 1938, when the birth protocols become available, the annual 'Statistiques de l'Hôpital' only recorded one cesarean, which was performed in 1934. See: L – A – S2, AMS.

141   See the annual reports of the Service de Santé for AEF, ZK 005–121 (1933–36), ZK 005–160 (1939–44), SHD.

142   Moscucci, *The Science of Woman*, 141–43.

African ignorance for the possibility of this affliction to occur in this case. 'Only God knows what they had done to the woman in the village', he wrote. After two days, however, he was happy to report that 'now the mother is in an excellent condition'.[143]

Later in the decade, Wildikann and other staff members occasionally referred to the possibility of performing a cesarean. Yet, they never conducted one, in part because patients resisted. In 1936, the nurse Emmy Röthlisberger described a potentially complicated delivery, for which the husband accompanied his wife to the hospital. 'When we suggested to the husband to perform a cesarean, he left with her at night sauvé', she wrote.[144] 'Parti sauvé' was the expression used at the hospital to describe patients, cured or not, leaving for good without notice – a frequent occurrence not only at the maternity ward. The expression can be translated as 'departed to rescue oneself', which would concede that patients might feel better elsewhere and acknowledge their judgement on the chances of cure. The expression can be also understood as an emphasis of patients' lack of compliance; they 'departed and escaped'. Either translation becomes rather cynical in this particular case.

Two days later, Röthlisberger heard 'a tamtam from far and on the subsequent morning I learned that this poor woman had died, and that this was the reason for that tamtam', before concluding her account of the episode with the comment that 'it is a poor people'.[145] Wildikann described the same incident in more dramatic detail:

> We – all three physicians – then talked at the relatives for hours (in the true sense of the term) in order to receive permission for doing surgery, but in vain! The reply of the husband was: 'I prefer that my wife dies in the village without operation.[146]

Wildikann emphasized that this was the village where 'palm wine poisoning frequently occurred'. She ended the story writing that 'one day later, people told us that the woman died in great pain'. Wildikann then asked Schweitzer if he believed that 'in such cases, one had to force people. In Europe there are enough cases in which social welfare has to intervene and in which even

---

143 Goldschmid to Schweitzer, 21 December 1934, AMS. The woman died in February 1935. She had been well for weeks, but then her overall condition deteriorated, and she repeatedly vomited roundworms. See: Goldschmid to Schweitzer, 12 February 1935, AMS.

144 Röthlisberger to Schweitzer, 25 November 1936, AMS.

145 Ibid.

146 Wildikann to Schweitzer, 25 November 1936, AMS.

parents were put under tutelage if they resist better knowledge and judgement and we also have a welfare mission here'.[147]

Röthlisberger focused her account on the 'Tamtam', a recurrent trope in the
writings of hospital staff that seemed to provide them with particular fascination. Along with 'palavres', this drumming was depicted as typically local. Wildikann, in contrast, framed her version of the story around her medical duties:
obtaining relatives' permission for the operation, mentioning in a somewhat
derogatory manner the frequent episodes of poisoning in the village to emphasize the supposed backwardness of the woman's community, and ultimately
reflecting on the ethical responsibility that she believed would even justify co-
ercion. Above all, both of these medical practitioners portrayed African men
as uninformed decision-makers – without denying that these also existed in
Europe – and Gabonese women as passive victims.

In 1962, Dr. Müller claimed that, 4.2 percent of all deliveries at the hospital were cesareans. According to him, this number was distorted because
the neighboring government hospital, which recorded a similar number of
births, would not perform the intervention and sent all complicated cases
to Schweitzer's hospital. Müller argued that most of the cesareans were performed due to pelvis constriction. To clarify this, he had the pelvises of 288
women measured, with the result that 22 displayed 'extreme values'. Three of
them had to undergo a cesarean, which amounts to 13 percent. Thus, this very
small sample shows that the likelihood of women diagnosed with pelvis constriction to deliver their babies by cesareans was indeed considerably higher
than for those without.[148] In this study, Müller did not blame local maternal
ignorance for the high rate of cesareans, but cited the natural cause of pelvis
constriction.

Table 3 illustrates that the ratio of cesareans to normal deliveries at the hospital was often significantly higher than during Müller's time; our admittedly
small set of evidence suggests that it could reach over 10 percent. There are no
numbers for Gabon for the years after independence. Detailed records for the
Albert Schweitzer Hospital for the 1950s are also missing. This has resulted in a
data overlap of only two years, during which the total number of births at maternity wards was still very low and figures might not be representative for later
years. This extremely small sample suggests that cesareans were performed at
the Albert Schweitzer Hospital much more frequently than at government
hospitals.

Accounts of complicated deliveries, including those that involved craniotomies and cesareans, are only to be found in private letters. Schweitzer and his

---

147   Ibid.
148   Müller, '50 Jahre Albert-Schweitzer-Spital', 27.

TABLE 3 Cesareans as a percentage of total deliveries (number of cesareans)[a]

Year	AEF	Gabon	Albert Schweitzer Hospital
1953	0.9% (147)	0.6% (7)	7.1% (5)
1954	1.5% (277)	2.0% (32)	5.4% (4)
1955	1.9% (272)	2.8% (57)	
1956	2.0% (388)	2.7% (59)	
1957		1.9% (55)	
1958			
1959			10.2% (18)
1960			10.8% (21)
1961			7.2% (23)
1962			4.2% (15)
1963			3.1% (11)
1964			7.2% (24)

a The numbers for AEF and Gabon are taken from the annual reports of the Service de Santé for AEF, ZK 005–93 (1952–53), ZK 005–16 (1954–55), and ZK 005–95 (1955–56), SHD. For 1957, I used the annual report for Gabon, ZK005–005, SHD. The figures for the Albert Schweitzer Hospital are taken from the birth protocols. See: L – P – A1–8, AMS.

personnel unknew these practices and avoided discussing them in publications, which parallels their silence on the high prevalence of venereal disease in Gabon. They instead focused on the ignorance of Africans in matters of maternity care, thus underlining the hospital's self-proclaimed savior role.

The accumulation of accounts on complicated deliveries and the lack of updates on or interest in delivery numbers illustrate that personnel at the hospital perceived obstetrics as one of many medical services on offer. They did not connect it with a wish to increase the pool of African labor or domesticating African women to bring about their conversion to Christianity and adherence to the customs and values of 'European civilization'. In this manner, Schweitzer and his staff displayed a remarkable ignorance of influential colonial discourses behind maternity care. Unknowing this important part of their own medical culture, staff members constructed maternity care as a simple and purely medical service. A key question arising from these considerations is whether Africans also perceived giving birth at the Albert Schweitzer Hospital in this manner.

It is doubtful that there was an equivalent to the notion of a 'simple and purely medical service' in local conceptions of healthcare, as I have outlined in the Introduction. Indeed, this might be especially true for childbirth practices, in which so much cultural knowledge and meaning were embedded. Colonial government and missionary programs frequently targeted intimate spheres of African life in their zeal to reform diet, hygiene, or sexual practices while fighting the spread of sexually transmitted diseases.[149] At Schweitzer's hospital, on the other hand, personnel participated in no community outreach programs and had only a limited pedagogical mandate. This meant that only women who wanted to give birth in a hospital made use of the obstetrical services that Schweitzer and his staff offered; nevertheless, these were still as much in demand as those of the government hospital across the river.

Even though, as I have demonstrated, hospital births were in some ways compatible with local practices, their numbers rose slowly until they eventually became more accepted due to external push factors, such as the requirement to obtain an official birth certificate or the fact that families received a payment when mothers gave birth in hospitals. Murray Last has argued that 'people's disinterest in medicine is an important medical phenomenon'; patients normally do not care how a medical system works. According to his observations in Hausaland, patients did not 'switch codes' when going from one healer or doctor to another; instead, they 'simply switch(ed) off'.[150] When it came to childbirth, Gabonese women were not willing or able to do either. They did not switch codes by coming to the hospital, presumably because they did not switch off and *did* care about the meanings and customs attached to deliver a baby.

These observations suggest that childbirth was not easily medicalized in Gabon. Elsewhere on the continent, the medicalization of maternity care occurred during the interwar period.[151] Where this was the case, for instance in South Africa, it usually occurred due to the willingness of and demand from local mothers.[152] African midwives played a crucial role in fostering this acceptance, because they were able to merge different kinds of knowledge in a culturally meaningful manner.[153] Generally, only certain segments of the population sought medical assistance during and after childbirth, often the

---

149   Bruchhausen, 'Practising Hygiene and Fighting the Natives' Diseases', 100; Hunt, 'Le Bebe en Brousse', 431; Summers, 'Intimate Colonialism'.

150   Last, 'The Importance of Knowing about Not Knowing', 403.

151   Hugon, 'L'historiographie de la maternité en Afrique subsaharienne', 5; Schler, 'Writing African Women's History with Male Sources'.

152   Klausen, *Race, Maternity, and the Politics of Birth Control*, 111.

153   Barthélémy, 'Sages-femmes africaines diplômées en AOF'; Van Tol, 'Mothers, Babies, and the Colonial State', 119.

Christianized elite.[154] In this regard, given the numerous mission stations located in the vicinity of Lambaréné, it remains unclear whether the maternity ward at the Albert Schweitzer Hospital answered to or created a demand for its services.

6   Key Areas of Ignorance: Medication and Feeding

As we have seen, Schweitzer and his staff presented maternity care as a strictly medical service. However, they shared many of the same assumptions on African maternal ignorance that were integral to the wider colonial discourses on depopulation and domesticity. Occasionally, these assumptions revealed themselves in an overt manner. In 1934, for example, Schweitzer wrote:

> The presence of women with their newborns gives Miss Koch, who is in charge of this unit, an opportunity to work against the improper care of mothers and infants, which is causing such great suffering here. For example, the bathing of babies is misused. If they are ill, it can happen that they to endure long washings in the river, even in the morning and evening coolness, through which they of course loses more and more of their strength.[155]

Schweitzer blamed Africans for not possessing this knowledge, accusing them of simple not-knowing. Thirty years later, Dr. Müller expressed the same sentiment in slightly less harsh-sounding words. He explained that

> the raising of the many premature infants places a heavy burden on the nurses: for weeks the nurses have to take these children into their rooms at night, as the mothers are often too unreliable to allow them to take care of them on their own.[156]

Despite his softer tone, Müller now accused the mothers not of not-knowing, but of willful neglect, of not wanting to know. In contrast, other members of staff still placed more emphasis on their supposed ignorance as a case of not-knowing. Stocker noted in her diary how one mother was caring very well for

---

154   Kanogo, 'The Medicalization of Maternity in Colonial Kenya', 79; Hunt, *A Colonial Lexicon*, 226.
155   Schweitzer, 'Briefe aus dem Lambarene Spital Februar 1934', 4.
156   Müller, '50 Jahre Albert-Schweitzer-Spital', 29.

her newborn, who had been born prematurely, and wished that 'all of them would comprehend it so well'.[157]

Nurses frequently resorted to sheltering premature infants in their bedrooms at night to monitor them closely (see Illustration 24 and 25). Not only did this place an additional strain on the nurses, but, more importantly, illustrated their belief in the mothers' ignorance. Jo Munz abandoned the practice after she had to keep five babies at the same time in her room. When she handed this task back to the mothers, she nevertheless emphasized that she would continue to maintain 'supervision'.[158] Important to underline here again is that this distrust of maternal abilities was not a uniquely colonial attitude.

From the point of view of the European personnel at the hospital, one of the main signs of African ignorance in matters of childbirth was mothers' frequent application of what became known as 'médicament indigène'. Substances, mostly herbal, found in arriving pregnant women's genital areas were a recurring concern for staff in the maternity ward. In 1936 for example, Röthlisberger wrote to Schweitzer after a series of difficult deliveries, wondering what they could do 'against the terrible superstition of the blacks and against the Médicament Indigènes?'[159] Thereby she connected the use of such substances with the African worldview, which the European nurse considered backward and ignorant of proper medical practice.

One of the main worries that doctors and nurses had about *médicament indigène* was medical, namely that they would cause infection. In 1932, the wife of a catechist came to deliver her baby at the hospital. According to the nurse Lies Bonnema, Dr. Barend Bonnema's wife, the pregnant woman had had an opening of six centimeters for two days. When, on a ward round, they discovered her with 'much Medicament indigène in the vagina, my husband did not want to wait longer, as he feared an infection'. A biomedical solution followed: 'in lumbar anaesthesia he then applied the forceps and the baby came well and happy and cried immediately. Without having had a fever, the woman happily left with her boy on Sunday', Bonnema wrote.[160] Thirty years later, Jo Munz also voiced surprise that there had not been more infections due to *médicament indigène*.[161] As we have seen, this absence of infections on African bodies is a recurring trope in hospital sources, for example in relation to patients with a surgical wound.

---

157   Stocker, 'Diary 1961–63', 35–38.
158   Munz-Boddingius, 'Meine Chance und Freude, Hebamme in Lambarene gewesen zu sein', 66–68.
159   Röthlisberger to Schweitzer, 15 August 1936, AMS.
160   Bonnema to Schweitzer, 18 December 1932, AMS.
161   Interview Munz and Munz.

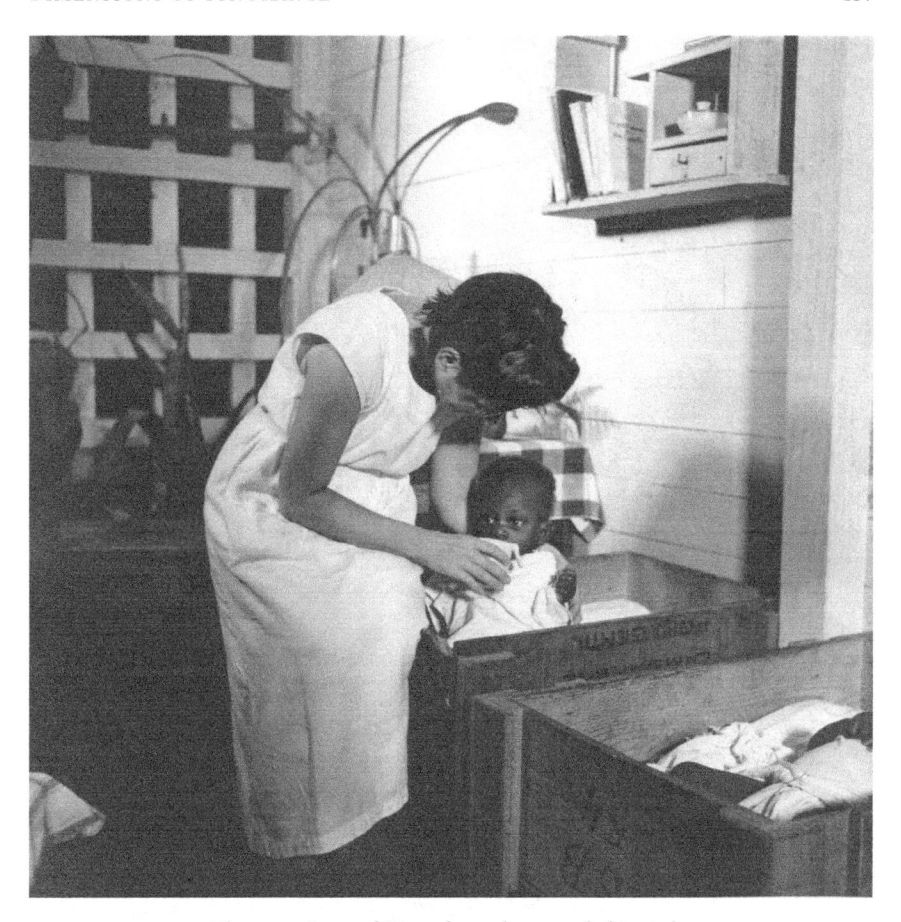

ILLUSTRATION 24   The nurse Irmgard Zinser has at least two babies in her room, ca 1951
            © ARCHIVES CENTRALES ALBERT SCHWEITZER GUNSBACH

Another medical problem associated with *médicament indigène* was the difficulties it posed to diagnosis. One of the few very detailed cases recorded in the
birth protocols illustrates this. In July 1941, the midwife noted:

> It is not possible to determine whether there is eclampsia or drug poison-
> ing (médicament indigène). In fact, the woman's relatives, since she has
> been in labor for 2–3 days, fed her with strong indigenous medicines until
> she passed out.[162]

162   This account is from the first volume of birth protocols that has survived. It covers the
      period from May 1937 to December 1941. The cited delivery took place on 25 July 1941. The
      nurse Maria Lagendijk and Dr. Anna Wildikann were working in the maternity ward at

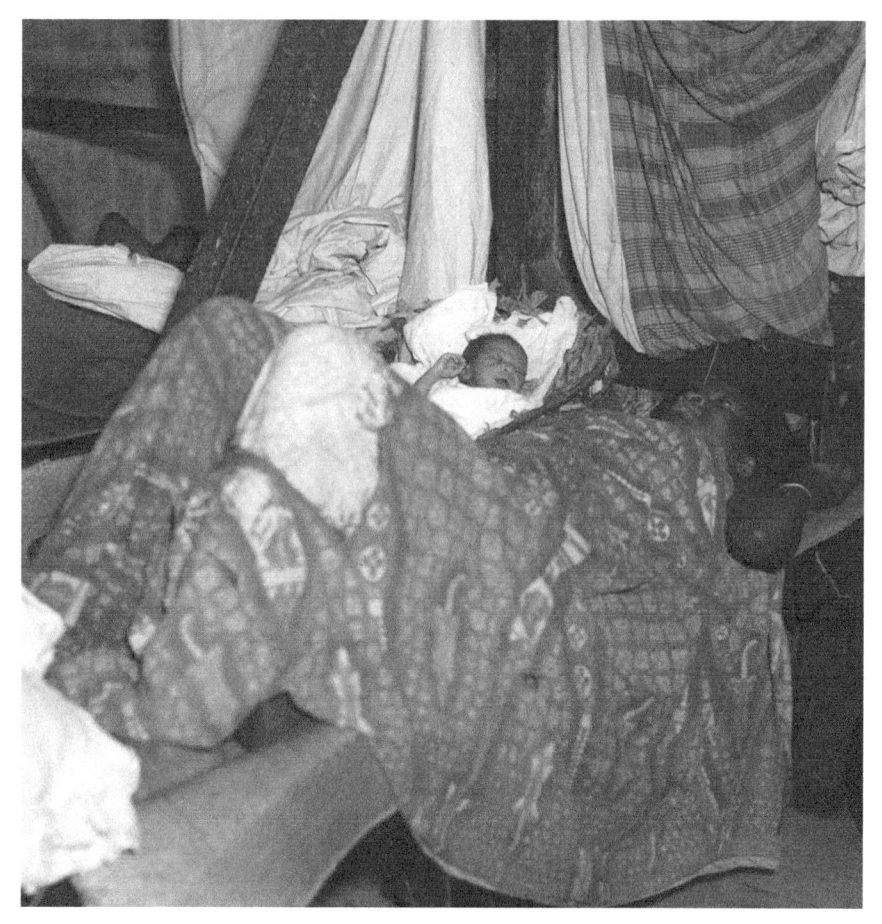

ILLUSTRATION 25   A mother with her baby in the bed, undated
© ARCHIVES CENTRALES ALBERT SCHWEITZER GUNSBACH

They were about to proceed with a cesarean, when suddenly the infant's head appeared. After a difficult yet successful delivery in which reanimating measures had to be applied, the baby died two hours later due to severe bleeding. In this case, *médicament indigène* had been swallowed rather than applied locally. The detailed description suggests that the nurse sought to blame the *médicament indigène*, and with it ultimately the ignorance of the mother's relatives, for the death of the baby. Just as in the previous example cited above, the mother herself is depicted as a rather helpless victim.

———————

the time. From the handwriting, it appears that Lagendijk recorded the above description. See: L – P – A1, AMS.

Sometimes staffs were more forthright in attributing deaths to the application of *médicament indigène*. In 1936, Dr. Wildikann wrote of a pregnant woman who had died a few hours after arriving at the hospital. Wildikann added that the woman had been 'too badly treated with Medicaments indigens, e.g. the eyes, into which a mixture of lemon juice, piman, and salt had been put, were like burned out'.[163] It is worthwhile pursuing how Schweitzer reported Wildikann's account in the leaflets that he sent to supporters in Europe. In October 1936, he wrote:

> Miss Dr. Wildikann tells me of several cases in which black women in childbed, brought to the hospital, had previously been treated with medicines of the natives and thus endangered their lives. One of them had been treated by putting acidic substances in her eyes so that the eyesockets looked like burned out. What suffering must she have endured before she finally arrived here?[164]

The rather common lemon juice, salt, and pepper mixture thus became an exotic and dangerous acidic substance. As observed earlier, Schweitzer did not explicitly mention the death of an individual woman, but wrote of a general danger to life, reluctant to overly shock his readers. The picture that Schweitzer conveys of his hospital here is that of a place of shelter, or even salvation, where women who had suffered terribly by being unnecessarily treated with life-threatening substances by ignorant practitioners would find their sanctuary. Modern biomedical know-how would thus heal wounds that had been inflicted by what were considered primitive methods. However, Schweitzer offered his refuge only to those who sought it; he did not seek to counter supposed ignorance in a proactive way.

While the doctors considered the use of *médicament indigène* as proof of African ignorance, they remained largely ignorant about the components of these substances. Dr. Wildikann, for example, wrote to Schweitzer in July 1936, reporting that a delivery had been successful; 'even though this woman too had been treated with médicaments indigens (from vagina and anus I pulled out rags soaked in who knows what!)'.[165] Even the protocols did not offer more specific details. In July 1959, a midwife noted that a woman had been 'brought in from village with retained products'. These were then expelled under anesthesia, and

---

163   Wildikann to Schweitzer, 18 June 1936, AMS.
164   Schweitzer, 'Briefe aus dem Lambarene Spital Oktober 1936', 2.
165   Wildikann to Schweitzer, 19 July 1936, AMS.

the baby was delivered easily. In 1963, Dr. Müller described Gabonese deliveries to a specialist medical readership, writing of a 'spice':

> A strong spice is then administered per orally and locally against secondary contractions. The spice is given in high amounts and strong concentrations. The already existing edema of the cervix and vulva is intensified by vaginal application. Such unfortunate cases are occasionally brought to hospital, while numerous vesicovaginal fistulas are signs of the other cases.[166]

Besides Müller's indifference to the exact composition of local medication, his use of biomedical language and invocation of indirect evidence, the fistulas, to supposedly prove African ignorance are notable. This example demonstrates that the question of ignorance is also one of perspective. From the point of view of European physicians, the exact composition of *médicament indigène* was unimportant. Its effects on the body and its functioning were considered much more significant.

However, staff's ignorance on the composition of *médicament indigène* was not complete. Jo Munz believes it was 'chili powder'.[167] In the already mentioned case from the 1941 birth protocols, the term 'indigenous medicines' was marked with an asterisk and defined as 'Cambo-Cambo-leaves as infusion',[168] a deviation from its typical description as a vaginal application in hospital- and non-hospital-related sources. In as early as 1910, Tessmann described the childbirth process in Fang society, remarking that 'of course it does not go without medicine'. This involved the juice of specific plants being trickled into the vagina. The liquid being 'slippery, "smooth"' was thus to guarantee the 'smooth completion of the process'.[169]

European medical staff at the Albert Schweitzer Hospital was ignorant about the application of such plant liquids, usually reporting the use of a powder or,

---

166   Müller, '50 Jahre Albert-Schweitzer-Spital', 25–26.
167   Interview Munz and Munz.
168   Rapoonda-Walker and Sillans write that the tree *Xylopia brieyi* was referred to as Kambo-gambo in Mitsogo. This tree is closely related to the one that provides what is commonly known as 'Grains of Selim' or 'African Pepper', seeds that were used as a spice, but also as a stimulant. Once decocted, its leaves were used to treat rheumatisms and as an emetic. There were numerous other plants used for the same purpose. See: Raponda-Walker and Sillans, *Les plantes utiles du Gabon*, 72.
169   Tessmann, *Die Pangwe*, 2:275. Tessmann lists this juice as coming from the following plants: *Cephalonema polyandrum, Cucurbitaceae, Fleurya aestauans, Urticaceae*.

more rarely, a concoction to drink. In their 1961 book 'Les plantes utiles du Gabon', André Raponda-Walker and Roger Sillans list six plants that were regularly administered to women shortly after they gave birth.[170] Most of these natural remedies were taken orally; the authors do not mention any powders and recount only one vaginal application.[171] Three of these plants were also used to treat gonorrhea, which was of great concern and for which the application of medication as enemas was common.[172] Given the high prevalence of the disease, it is not unlikely that women who arrived at the Albert Schweitzer Hospital with *médicament indigène* in their vaginas had used this to treat gonorrhea. Raponda-Walker and Sillans also list sixteen plants that women took to relieve pain or nausea during pregnancy. These too were usually consumed orally, frequently together with peanuts,[173] a combination which suggests that the latter were considered a key element in a pregnancy diet.

The dietary habits of mothers and infants were taken by Europeans at Schweitzer's hospital as another sign of African ignorance in the area of childcare. In 1931, Schweitzer summarized his view on the issue as follows:

> It is well known that women of primitive peoples do not breast-feed the child of a deceased woman, because in their superstition they believe that they are thereby falling under the power of the evil spirit which has killed the other woman.[174]

---

170   The subtitle of the book is 'essai d'inventaire et de concordance des noms vernaculaires et scientifiques des plantes spontanées et introduites, description des espèces, propriétés, utilisations économiques, ethnographiques et artistiques'. It was first published at Lechevalier in Paris. I am using a facsimile, reprinted in 1995 by the Fondation Raponda-Walker in Libreville.

171   Raponda-Walker and Sillans, *Les plantes utiles du Gabon*. Concoctions could consist of the leaves of a plant (in the case of *Crotalaria glauca*, a shrub, 249), its latex (*Lecomtedoxa klaineana*, 392), or its 'hearts' (*Aframomum giganteum*, from the ginger family, 427). It could also be a mix, (see for instance *Homalium letestui* and *Piper guineense*, 383f). In addition, *Entada gigas* (monkey ladder) was used for therapeutic baths or as enemas (242).

172   These were *Entada gigas*, *Crotalaria glauca*, and *Piper guineense* (see above footnote). In total, the authors list thirty-two plants that have been used to treat gonorrhea.

173   The authors mention the following medicinal plants whose cooked leaves pregnant women ate together with peanuts: *Culcasia scandens* (a climbing plant, 95), *Acanthus montanus* (Bear's Breech, 39), *Barteria fistulosa* (also important in female initiation rites, 345), *Bertiera racemosa* (a flowering plant, 360), Fleurya podocarpa (also important in female initiation rites, 420), and *Lygodium microphyllum* (the ornamental climbing maidenhair fern, 439).

174   Schweitzer, 'Briefe aus dem Lambarene Spital Pfingsten 1931', 8.

Numerous contemporaries shared this understanding into the 1950s.[175] Most agreed that Gabonese mothers usually breastfed their children for about two years (see Illustration 26).[176]

According to biomedical personnel of the 1930s, breast milk was the ideal diet for babies. Such promotion occurred in other parts of Africa at the same time, while in Europe breast milk had been endorsed as the best way to feed babies since the beginning of the twentieth century.[177] Sporadically in the 1930s, staff at the Albert Schweitzer Hospital had managed to obtain breast milk from African mothers. Dr. Barasch wrote to Schweitzer about a European newborn, whom he had fed first with the milk of the wife of the auxiliary Dominique Bouka and then with milk from another African woman, gradually adding more and more manufactured milk until he omitted breast milk entirely after three weeks.[178] The nurse Alice Weber reported about half a year later that a European family had brought their eight-week-old baby to be treated for malaria. The doctors successfully treated the child with quinine infusions, blood transfusions, and the milk of African women, without specifying how it was obtained.[179] These instances illustrate the pragmatic approach adopted at the hospital and modify the picture of colonial maternity programs that were, in the words of Nancy Hunt, 'permeated with a racism intent on protecting European children from African hands'.[180]

For orphaned babies who were placed in the hospital's care, often brought by desperate fathers, nurses aimed to substitute mother's milk with goat's milk and imported condensed or powdered milk. In 1933, the hospital's goats provided a fifth of its total milk supply.[181] During World War Two, staff had to abstain from drinking goat's milk because Schweitzer wanted to reserve it for babies.[182] At that point, Joy and Arnold blamed an unspecified maternal ignorance for the frequent need for hospital staff to feed babies at the hospital. In the caption of a photograph in their book, they explain that the mother

---

175   Alexandre and Binet, *Le groupe dit Pahouin*, 92; Lavignotte, *L'évur: croyance des Fañ du Gabon*, 82.

176   They were also claimed to be sexually abstinent during this period. See: Joy, Arnold, and Schweitzer, *The Africa of Albert Schweitzer*, 39; Naegele, 'Rapport Medical sur l'HAS 1951', AMS; Tessmann, *Die Pangwe*, 2:276. Only Fernandez claimed that infants were weaned in their third or fourth years. See: Fernandez, *Bwiti*, 199.

177   Dreier, 'Europäisch gebären', 164; Marland, 'Childbirth and Maternity', 561; Wylie, 'The Ignorance of Mothers and the Health of Children in 20th Century Pondoland', 109.

178   Barasch to Schweitzer, 15 December 1935, AMS.

179   Weber to Schweitzer, 18 July 1936, AMS.

180   Hunt, 'Le Bebe en Brousse', 415.

181   Schweitzer, 'Briefe aus dem Lambarene Spital Juli 1933', 7.

182   Schweitzer to Hume, 23 December 1940, AMS.

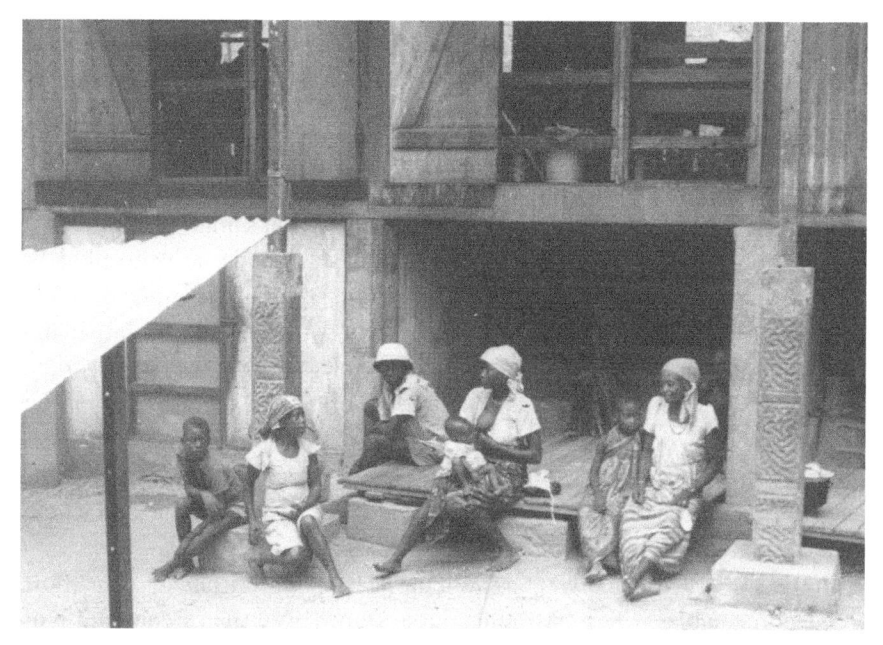

ILLUSTRATION 26   One of the very few pictures of a mother breast-feeding, undated
© ARCHIVES CENTRALES ALBERT SCHWEITZER GUNSBACH

depicted 'is unable to nurse her baby adequately, so she has brought her child to the Hospital for help'. Their solution was simple: 'The nurses prepare a special formula with powdered milk from the United States. Mother and child will stay in the Hospital until the baby is six months old and can take soft foods'.[183]

Some staff blamed the local environment, not African ignorance or super-stition, for fathers not being able to feed motherless babies. Writing about the 1930s, the nurse Marie Woytt-Secretan explained this perspective:

> In the past, if a mother died giving birth, the child was also condemned to death, because there is no milk in the whole country. Cows do not find food in the jungle and also succumb to sleeping sickness. [...] But since Dr. Schweitzer has been working in the country, the fathers have brought such babies to the hospital. Although they often arrive almost famished, we manage to save most of them and the canned milk from Europe does them good.[184]

183   Joy, Arnold, and Schweitzer, *The Africa of Albert Schweitzer*, 133.
184   Woytt-Secretan, *Albert Schweitzer baut Lambarene*, 102.

Once again, the trope of the hospital as a final refuge, a place of salvation, emerges. African children and their fathers are depicted as victims of the hostile vegetation and the tsetse fly. There is no pedagogical dimension in this account: like the mothers in the previous extract, widowers could solve the problem by bringing their children to the hospital, which possessed the necessary capacity and resources to obtain a substitute for mother's milk.

Occasionally, infants would be fed with more solid foods at the hospital. In 1936, Röthlisberger reported to Schweitzer that in addition to condensed milk, oatmeal gruel had been given to three-week-old babies, an approach that, according to her, had proven successful before.[185] In contrast, two years earlier, Schweitzer had emphasized the supposed ignorance of a mother, who had given birth in the morning by claiming that they 'found her busy feeding mush of rice to the world citizen who was only a few hours old.'[186] Feeding was thus an area of improvisation where babies received what was available and where staff could not uphold control.

In the late 1950s and early 1960s, staff at the hospital continued to put effort into feeding babies with breast milk, but acknowledged their frequent use of substitutes (see Illustration 27). Dr. Mai noted in his 1956 diary that a 'diet without breast milk is much more difficult with black babies than with white babies and almost never succeeds'.[187] Anderegg recalled that mothers would be kept at the hospital after a cesarean until it was certain that they could produce enough milk.[188] In 1962, Stocker tricked a group of mothers into providing additional breast milk to feed motherless infants, a request that they had previously refused. She told mothers of dysenteric children that 'the milk for the child is not good now, you have to empty everything'.[189] According to Stocker, the amount of milk that she obtained under this false pretense was still insufficient; she emphasized that many babies would have died without canned milk.[190]

Not only were infants' diets a concern for hospital staff, but even more so were those of expectant mothers. Numerous pregnant women arrived in a state considered undernourished, and doctors worried about the effects that this would have on their babies. Mothers-to-be were thus provided with calcium to supplement their diets for much of the 1930s, an approach that was

---

185   Röthlisberger to Schweitzer, 15 August 1936, AMS.
186   Schweitzer, 'Briefe aus dem Lambarene Spital Februar 1934', 4.
187   The diaries of Hermann Mai are held at AMS.
188   Interview Elisabeth Anderegg.
189   Stocker, 'Diary 1961–63', 55.
190   Interview Marianne Stocker.

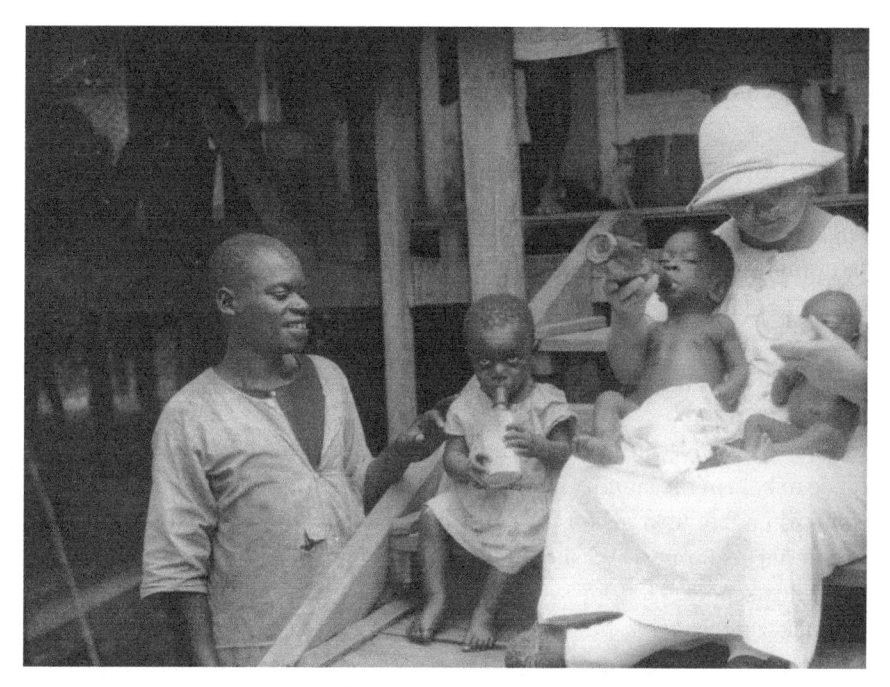

ILLUSTRATION 27   Gertrude Koch bottle-feeding, a father (?) watching, ca. 1950
© ARCHIVES CENTRALES ALBERT SCHWEITZER GUNSBACH

thought to make their babies stronger and more vigorous.[191] In 1936, Wildikann proudly reported to Schweitzer that 'our calcium-babies are splendid
specimens',[192] in the process invoking a somewhat dehumanizing image. In
1953, however, Schweitzer noted in one of his notebooks that calcium rendered
deliveries difficult, providing a short and rather unclear explanation in brackets: 'accumulation of calcium in the bones'.[193] The practice of providing calcium as a supplement had thus came to an end, but the diets of pregnant women
were still considered inadequate in the early 1960s. Here, however, the primary
concern for hospital staff was still that of the health of the infant: Jo Munz, for
example, claimed that expectant mothers' poor diets frequently led to premature deliveries. The solution, also noted in the birth protocols, resembled that

---

191   Schweitzer, 'Briefe aus dem Lambarene Spital Mai 1937', 3–4.
192   Wildikann to Schweitzer, 18 June 1936, AMS.
193   See the notebook '1953 Medizinische Notizen Lambarene', AMS.

of the 1930s. Instead of a regular dose of calcium, pregnant women received iron and vitamins every morning at eight o'clock.[194]

One way to counter perceived ignorance was to educate women, especially concerning diet. However, unlike at other colonial hospitals and especially at missionary ones,[195] neither Schweitzer nor any of his staff placed any great emphasis or attention on educating female patients in domestic responsibilities or 'proper' maternal practices during much of the study period. Instead, the focus of Schweitzer's 'civilizing mission' lay on manual and agricultural labor. It was thus left to Stocker to introduce what she claimed was the first 'maternity counseling' at the hospital, although she did note that some pedagogical measures had been implemented before her time. These included pregnant women who arrived at the hospital before their expected date of delivery being made to help in the laundry. According to Stocker, they also 'learned all sorts of things they should know for the care of their child'. She claimed that 'all this is only in its beginnings and should be expanded further. I think of some sort of maternity school'.[196]

Stocker introduced such a program during her second stay from May 1965. She organized this in loose cooperation with Dr. Munz; both wanted to leave Schweitzer out of its running because he was 'old and tired'. The lessons that it offered were mainly in 'diet and health', two areas in which Stocker and Munz had identified a supposed distinct lack of knowledge among local women. Pregnant women and those who had recently given birth at the hospital were thus taught, for example, to provide their children with more protein, such as eggs, milk, and fish.[197] As with the vacuum extractor, this is another example of staff introducing a new practice without informing Schweitzer; in this case, a preventive one, contrary to the hospital's usual focus on curative medicine. The measures taken by Stocker and Munz in this regard resemble those discussed at the Geneva conference on the African child more than thirty years earlier, which ignored the political, social, and economic circumstances of mothers in the region.[198]

Stocker's efforts were not without precedent at the hospital. Erika Taap, an evangelical sister from the Berlin Mission who visited in August 1960, claimed

194   Munz-Boddingius, 'Meine Chance und Freude, Hebamme in Lambarene gewesen zu sein', 66.

195   Addae, *The Evolution of Modern Medicine in a Developing Country*, 230; Coghe, 'Inter-Imperial Learning', 150; Hugon, 'La redéfinition de la maternité en Gold Coast', 157–58; Jennings, 'A Matter of Vital Importance', 246.

196   Stocker, 'Diary 1961–63', 7.

197   Interview Marianne Stocker.

198   Allman, 'Making Mothers', 1994.

that an important practice in the maternity ward was the counseling of pregnant women. Depicting a more idealized process than that outlined above, she described how staff asked women to arrive 'some time before the delivery to get used to the hospital organization' and to stay 'after the delivery in order to learn under the eyes of the nurses and doctors how to properly care for their child'.[199] More than ten years earlier, Joy and Arnold also referred to an educational aspect of maternity care:

> Mother and child will stay in the Hospital until the baby is six months old and can take soft foods. Meanwhile the staff will teach the mother how to make soup from bananas, and how to prepare rice, papaya and other foods for infant consumption.[200]

Given that at this time the number of deliveries at the hospital was rather low, it is unclear to what degree this was common practice. The quote certainly underlines the importance of dietary considerations in a more specific manner.

Staff members in the 1930s did not mention pedagogic measures. They were, however, convinced that Africans were ignorant in matters of childbirth and childcare and sought ways to mitigate this supposed ignorance. For example, Lies Bonnema wrote in December that she kept 'to this principle: from the moment the contractions begin, I do not leave a woman alone for even a moment!'[201] This was a command from Schweitzer himself. From Europe, he had written one of the very rare letters in which he voiced concern about the hospital's maternity services. To the physicians he explained how he wanted childbirth procedures to occur:

> I don't know if, tired at the time of departure as I was, I ordered clearly enough that a nurse who watches over an expectant mother should not leave her (even if the delivery is not anticipated for several hours) without another nurse replacing her, even if it is only for the quarter of an hour for lunch or dinner! If you please inculcate this instruction to the nurse, in each case anew! It is that the expectant mother should not have the slightest uneasiness. I have told you on my departure that I want the doctor in charge of the delivery to stay within easy reach of the woman during the last hours and to sleep in the room next to her at night, in

---

199 Taap, *Lambarener Tagebuch*, 58.
200 Joy, Arnold, and Schweitzer, *The Africa of Albert Schweitzer*, 133.
201 Bonnema to Schweitzer, 18 December 1932, AMS.

reference to a case that occurred years ago, when the doctor was not reachable for a birth.[202]

Schweitzer ultimately refers to a situation that had gone wrong years earlier to justify this command for upholding good medical practice and to prevent negligence from the side of his staff. Although he does not explicitly mention the ignorance of Africans and worries about their well-being, a clear mistrust in the abilities and knowledge of local mothers' shines through an order that strikingly resembles his instructions for control in the operating theater. In 1960 still, Schoenfeld reported that 'when labor was prolonged I would sleep on a table near the patient while Suzanne and the grandmother spread their mats on the floor'.[203] Similar doubts about mother's abilities persisted until after the delivery of the baby, as we have seen in the case of nurses keeping premature infants in their rooms.

7   Conclusion

In 1936, Dr. Wildikann recorded a vivid account of an anecdote from the maternity ward that illustrates many of the issues raised in this chapter. In a letter to Schweitzer, she wrote of a pregnant woman who had accompanied her husband, who had come to the hospital to have his hernia repaired. The night after the man's operation, his wife had gone into labor. She then retreated into the 'bush, because she did not want any help from whites for her delivery'. Wildikann informed the auxiliary Ambroise Nyama, a 'fellow tribe member', of the incident, who managed to persuade the woman to return to the hospital. Wildikann described the subsequent delivery procedure as follows:

> With tricks and cunning I managed to get the woman on the delivery table and to keep her on it during the whole process. If you did not hold her hands tightly, she tore herself away again and again, penetrated with monkey-like speed with one hand into the vagina and pulled at her uterus (no animal is so crazy!) in such a way that a severe bleeding was the result.[204]

---

202   Schweitzer to Bonnema and van der Elst, 1 August 1932, AMS.
203   Schoenfeld, 'A Summer at Dr. Schweitzer's Hospital (Draft)', AMS, 17–18.
204   Wildikann to Schweitzer, 8 April 1936, AMS. According to Wildikann, the baby was perfectly healthy, but it took two days to control the bleeding.

The coercive element of this intervention was exceptional for obstetrical practice at the Albert Schweitzer Hospital. Typically, procedures were not forced upon patients, as has been demonstrated in the cases of proposed cesareans that did not meet with patient consent. Wildikann's language is unusually harsh in this passage. She also takes the accusation of ignorance to the highest level: an animal would have acted more reasonably than the woman portrayed in the anecdote.

Wildikann's privately communicated account contrasts with the description that Barthélemy published thirty years later and quoted at the beginning of this chapter. He depicts cesareans as a routine procedure that occurred rather regularly, usually with a successful end result. He also acknowledges how strange the situation is for the woman, who nevertheless seems to quietly accept everything that is happening around her. Characteristically for a published account, mother and child are not pictured in an overly negative light or as suffering and vulnerable victims in a critical state. In private letters, however, the doctors often portrayed mothers, expectant and not, and her kin as primitive and ignorant.

Obstetrical services at the hospital were based on this premise that Africans were ignorant of proper biomedical childbirth and infant care practices. Doctors articulated supposed African ignorance in a more medicalized language, but nurses also expressed their frustration on the same topic. Infant and maternal diets, as well as the use of non-biomedical medicines during pregnancy, were taken as the main evidence of this ignorance. In most cases that were reported in detail, usually those that involved a difficult delivery or the discovery of the use of *médicament indigène*, it was not the mother who was blamed for her ignorance, but her relatives. Personnel were frequently confronted with practices that they considered ignorant, yet they did not choose to actively counter these; they unknew them. A strict staff recruitment and selection process, focused on personality traits rather than medical training, ensured this restraint, which was in accordance with the hospital's overall mission and vision.

Focusing on the many dimensions of (perceived) ignorance, this chapter has argued that the typical colonial explanatory frameworks for maternity services – depopulation and domesticity – were of little concern at the Albert Schweitzer Hospital. By ignoring these political, social, and economic justifications, staff constructed obstetrics as a simple medical service. They depicted the hospital as a place of universal refuge to which locals could flee to be saved from dangerous and unhealthy local practices. In the process, obstetrical personnel ignored details about how the delivery of babies occurred in the villages, while they took into account some of the preferences of African women on how to give birth. Nurses, midwives and doctors thus improvised during each delivery, for instance in regards to the presence of relatives or a woman's pre- and postnatal mobility. They reacted spontaneously to the practical challenges they faced, which varied from questions on how to feed women and infants to finding the most suitable way for resolving complicated cases.

CHAPTER 4

Trial and Error: Drugs and the Treatment of Infectious Diseases

'Idiot: he should try, not talk!'[1] In a rather unusual outburst of emotion, Schweitzer added these words in red pencil on a letter written to him by Dr. Heinz Barasch in Lambaréné in November 1936. The German physician had described his experiences with a novel combination of drugs that Schweitzer had proposed for the treatment of dysentery. Schweitzer apparently was unsatisfied with Barasch's initial reluctance to perform the new therapy, the way that he had eventually carried it out, and the results that it had generated.

This anecdote illustrates the pressure felt by doctors at the Albert Schweitzer Hospital to continually test new medication for the treatment of infectious diseases. Many examples of this 'trial and error' approach, as I will henceforth term it, are to be found in the sources. The regular execution of such testing suggests that Schweitzer and his doctors often doubted the usefulness of standard medicines and contradicts the optimism they displayed in public and private communications about many of these drugs.

The pharmaceutical treatment of dysentery, which has received very little attention from historians, and leprosy, which is very well researched, illustrate a central part of the daily clinical work in an institution that was primarily curative.[2] Doctors were constantly confronted with the question which one of the numerous drugs at their disposal they should give to a patient. They thus tested their suitability concerning efficacy, side effects, and dosage form and hence embraced an experimental approach to medicine. Historians have often used the metaphor of the laboratory or the experiment to describe such processes for a range of large-scale scientific and medical projects in Africa and beyond. My findings about daily practices in a small-scale and curative institution demonstrate that medicine works in a similar manner on a much more basic level.

---

1   Barasch to Schweitzer, 24 November 1936, AMS.
2   I have selected illnesses whose treatments can be easily traced throughout the study period. Syphilis and gonorrhea were also widespread, but sources are more silent on these diseases, as is true for malaria. Patients suffering from sleeping sickness were sent to government facilities from the mid-1930s. Tuberculosis became a major concern only after the hospital acquired X-ray equipment in 1954. Ulcers are discussed in: Mabika Ognandzi, Steinke, and Zumthurm, *Schweitzer's Lambaréné: A Hospital in Colonial Africa*.

1   Experiments in a Laboratory? the Treatment of Leprosy in
         Colonial Africa

Specialists at the first world leprosy conference in 1897 in Berlin concluded that complete isolation would represent the best form of treatment for patients with the disease. Colonial governments often ignored this recommendation for financial reasons.[3] In German territories, officials did not compel leprosy sufferers to isolate themselves. In most German-run leproseries, which were established in the period around 1910, patients were expected to perform agricultural work to guarantee the self-sufficiency of these facilities.[4] The most frequented German institutions lay in East Africa. These camps, which operated in partnership with missions, accommodated patients' non-affected family members.[5]

British colonial authorities established a number of leprosy settlements of their own in the late 1920s and early 1930s, such as in Uganda or Nigeria.[6] These were usually segregated, for example according to ethnicity, marital status, or stage of illness. Patients were also made to perform agricultural labor. Many of these settlements were conceived as 'native villages', not only architectonically, but also in terms of their hierarchical social structures.[7] For Megan Vaughan, the 'practices of twentieth-century sanitoria (*for TB*) in Britain make some of the African leper colonies look like holiday camps', since the enforcement of rules was not particularly strict in the latter.[8]

In French West Africa, conditions in early-twentieth-century leproseries were reported to be unsanitary, resembling 'more a prison for life than a health center'.[9] According to Eric Silla, colonial officials came to realize during the 1920s that 'treating patients more or less as criminals frightened them away from medical treatment'.[10] The open leprosery in Bamako, which provided food, accommodation, and agricultural land, was established in 1932. In the

---

3   Bado, *Médecine coloniale et grandes endémies en Afrique*, 141–42; Watts, *Epidemics and History*, 68.

4   Eckart, *Medizin und Kolonialimperialismus*. Camps in Togo and Cameroon had very limited success in terms of treatment; see 152–60, 210–14.

5   Ibid., 32–33. Members of the British Universities' Mission to Central Africa (UMCA) who took over the running of the settlement on the shores of Lake Malawi were horrified at the conditions they found there. See: Good, *The Steamer Parish*, 338.

6   Manton, 'Mission, Clinic, and Laboratory', 319; Vongsathorn, 'First and Foremost the Evangelist?', 552.

7   Vaughan, *Curing Their Ills*, 89–92.

8   Ibid., 96. Italics mine.

9   Bado, *Médecine coloniale et grandes endémies en Afrique*, 143.

10   Silla, *People Are Not the Same*, 101.

colony's new leprosy settlement system, which was designed to 'facilitate regular and prolonged treatment' instead of 'segregat(ing) the sick from the rest of the population', patient cooperation was crucial.[11]

Missions played a leading role in establishing many of these settlements. John Manton posits that 'leprosy served the relations between missionary and donor community far more than it informed evangelical strategies in Africa'.[12] In the process, colonial discourses were reframed. Benedictines depicted Africans suffering from leprosy as hard-working, grateful, and willing to suffer and submit to missionaries and their God. Their unafflicted counterparts, on the other hand, were presented as lazy, unappreciative, dull, and insubordinate.[13]

From a medical perspective, most leprosy programs had a limited reach and scope, especially during the interwar period. Any improvement in the health of leprosy patients during this period was most likely due to improved diets, sanitation, and nursing.[14] Missions and governments established leprosy settlements not only out of strictly medical considerations. The camps in Uganda, for example, represented a particular 'vision for the future of Uganda as a "civilised" and Christian country'.[15] In many parts of the continent, colonial governments aimed to establish closer cooperation with missions after World War Two, when the increasing availability of much more efficacious sulfone drugs allowed more and more leprosy sufferers to seek outpatient treatment.[16]

When Schweitzer first arrived in Lambaréné in 1913, biomedical practitioners routinely used substances extracted from the seeds of the Chaulmoogra tree to treat leprosy. Often, this was injected in the form of oil, with the shots being painful and the effects limited.[17] Medical professionals in the interwar period disagreed on how best to treat the disease, with chaulmoogra oil losing and regaining favor among doctors repeatedly.[18] Before 1945, from when the newly developed sulfone drugs promised to provide a more efficacious treatment, physicians throughout Africa experimented with different preparations from this plant,[19] as well as with a range of compounds varying from olive oil to

---

11 Ibid., 104.
12 Manton, 'Mission, Clinic, and Laboratory', 333.
13 Hölzl, 'Lepra als entangled disease', 111.
14 Vaughan, *Curing Their Ills*, 84. See also: Brydan, 'Mikomeseng', 637.
15 Vongsathorn, 'First and Foremost the Evangelist?', 544.
16 Manton, 'Mission, Clinic, and Laboratory', 327; Vaughan, *Curing Their Ills*, 90–92.
17 Digby, *Diversity and Division in Medicine*, 175–76; Eckart, *Medizin und Kolonialimperialismus*, 217; Good, *The Steamer Parish*, 339. The plant's latin binomial is *Hydnocarpus wightignus*. It is native to Southeast Asia.
18 Worboys, 'The Colonial World as Mission and Mandate'.
19 Addae, *The Evolution of Modern Medicine in a Developing Country*, 238; Good, *The Steamer Parish*, 341.

iodoform, trichloroacetic acid, and potassium iodide.[20] In the case of colonial Vietnam, Laurence Monnais argues that similar experiments and the perpetual replenishment of leprosy drugs by pharmaceutical companies transformed colonial health professionals' previously overriding therapeutic skepticism into a more optimistic attitude towards their ability to treat the disease.[21] For his part, Schweitzer had always displayed such therapeutic optimism, not only in relation to the treatment of leprosy.

The history of the distribution of sulfones in Africa is not yet fully understood. In Bamako, first experiments with these drugs were undertaken in 1948, but chaulmoogra was still widely used in French West Africa a decade later.[22] The Universities' Mission to Central Africa first made use of sulfone drugs in 1951 and soon realized that 'many new cases continued to emerge'.[23] Manton has revealed how in this context of therapeutic hope, small-scale experiments with a variety of drugs were central in research conducted at the leprosy hospital in Uzuakoli, Nigeria that led to the development of clofazimine, a medication still used today. He characterizes the scientific process of drug research at Uzuakoli as 'decentralized' and 'disarticulated',[24] insisting that 'the less than ideal physical and geographical circumstances of most leprosy research, the impossibility of cultivating leprosy outside a living human host, and the persistent privileging of local clinical knowledge' forces us to think of experimental research situations that simultaneously formed part of a treatment regime as 'characteristic rather than anomalous'.[25]

The situation in AEF was similar. A government report from 1955, when sulfones already constituted the standard treatment, claimed that 'like everywhere else in the French territories and elsewhere, many drugs have been tried'. The author concluded that, 'unfortunately, after slight improvements, not always very significant, it had to be agreed that there was no definite cure'.[26] Two years before, the director of the Service Général d'Hygiène Mobile et de Prophylaxie had distributed a guideline for leprosy treatment to all chief physicians in each sector of the colony. He recommended the exclusive use of sulfone-mère, a drug that is surprisingly never mentioned in sources relating to the Albert Schweitzer Hospital. Dapsone, as it was also known, was cheaper and, coming in the form of a pill, easier to administer than Promin and Diasone,

20   Eckart, *Medizin und Kolonialimperialismus*, 214–17, 337–39; Good, *The Steamer Parish*, 341.
21   Monnais, *Médicaments coloniaux*, 89–91.
22   Silla, *People Are Not the Same*, 107–10.
23   Good, *The Steamer Parish*, 344.
24   Manton, 'Trialing Drugs, Creating Publics', 87.
25   Ibid., 94–95.
26   Cheneveau, 'La lutte contre la lèpre en A.E.F', 1955, PR(H), 1 H 254.1. ANG, 1.

which had been the preferred drugs of doctors in AEF from 1941 to 1948.[27] Even though these government specialists attempted to unify and standardize treatment, they conceded that there were a great variety of possible medications, the potential efficacy of which depended on the local context as well as the condition and preferences of the patient and the views of the doctor.[28]

The 'laboratory' seems to be a useful metaphor for describing such experimental processes in science at large,[29] especially those in colonial contexts, drawing our attention 'to the prominence of scientific, notably, medical, research in imaginaries of Africa and, at the same time, to the tentative, exploratory nature, and often failure' of many research programs.[30] However, as a mere metaphor, indeed one that was invoked by colonialists themselves,[31] this analogy is not without its weaknesses, as Guillaume Lachenal highlights: 'the colonial opportunity gave rise to extraordinarily ambitious health policies, whose brutality and racism had absolutely nothing metaphorical about them'.[32] The other argument against using this comparison is that, unlike in a laboratory, conditions in the colonies were usually beyond the control of experimenters and, as such, not artificially created for the purposes of their experiments.[33]

Social and historical scholars of science have also frequently evoked metaphors around the term 'experiment' to examine scientific processes in laboratories and beyond.[34] Studies by Christoph Bonneuil and Helen Tilley emphasize the interdisciplinary and cooperative nature of the experiments that took place in the colonial 'laboratory' of Africa.[35] Furthermore, their work demonstrates how difficult it is to differentiate between the two metaphors of the laboratory and the experiment; these are often presented as interchangeable concepts in historical writing.

---

27   Richet, 'Lèpre. – Instructions, dépistages, traitements, pensions, statistiques', 1953, PR(H), 1 H 254.4. ANG, 2.
28   Cheneveau, 'La lutte contre la lèpre en A.E.F', 1955, PR(H), 1 H 254.1. ANG, 7–8; Richet, 'Lèpre. – Instructions, dépistages, traitements, pensions, statistiques', 1953, PR(H), 1 H 254.4. ANG, 6.
29   Knorr-Cetina, *Wissenskulturen*, 45.
30   Geissler, 'Public Secrets in Public Health', 13–14.
31   Bonneuil, 'Development as Experiment', 259; Tilley, *Africa as a Living Laboratory*, 5.
32   Lachenal, 'Le médecin qui voulut être roi', 128. Following Foucault, Lachenal suggests viewing the colonies as both real and imagined 'counter-emplacements' of the metropole.
33   Stoler and Cooper, 'Between Metropole and Colony', 5.
34   Knorr-Cetina, *Wissenskulturen*, 45. Dirk van Laak for instance proposes the term 'Experminetierfeld'. Van Laak, 'Kolonien als "Laboratorien der Moderne?"', 258–59. A recent example: Moore-Sheeley, 'The Products of Experiment'.
35   Tilley, *Africa as a Living Laboratory*, 27; Bonneuil, 'Development as Experiment', 264.

Recent studies on medical research in Africa focus on the experimental dimension in the testing of pharmaceutical and non-pharmaceutical therapies alike. They reach the conclusion that participants in research trials believed that they were part of a large-scale treatment program.[36] In fact, therapy and experiment were often conducted simultaneously, not only for leprosy. Both Lachenal and Wolfgang Eckart, the latter invoking the laboratory metaphor, have demonstrated for different periods and contexts how trial-and-error methods were used not only to determine a drug's efficacy in humans, but also as a means of treating the patients who participated in these very trials.[37]

Given that the first international guidelines on medical research on humans were loosely formulated in the Nuremberg Code of 1947 and more precisely in the Declaration of Helsinki in 1964, it is unsurprising, but nevertheless important to highlight, that the occurrence of such 'therapeutic experiments' was not limited to the colonies,[38] nor were they restricted to the pharmaceutical domain. 'Learning from mistakes' was the preferred approach adopted by early-twentieth-century surgeons to improve their skills.[39] A broad survey of the practices of German-speaking doctors in the nineteenth century has also revealed how highly this cohort valued personal experience and empirical knowledge over laboratory results and information derived from textbooks.[40]

While the central role played by hospital doctors in conducting pharmaceutical tests in colonial Southeast Asia, notably for dysentery drugs, is undisputed,[41] this issue has not been explored in detail for Africa. Medical research facilities on the continent were often attached to hospitals,[42] but it is not clear what role the latter played in experiments. Similarly, the function of experiments in hospitals that conducted their own research,[43] or in the

36   Graboyes, *The Experiment Must Continue*, 45; Malloy, 'Research Material and Necromancy', 435.

37   Eckart, 'The Colony as Laboratory', 202; Lachenal, *Le médicament qui devait sauver l'Afrique*.

38   Hess, Hottenrott, and Steinkamp, *Testen im Osten*; Marks, *The Progress of Experiment*, 159–62; Meier et al., *Testfall Münsterlingen*.

39   Wilde and Hirst, 'Learning from Mistakes'.

40   Kinzelbach, Neuner, and Nolte, 'Medicine in Practice: Knowledge, Diagnosis and Therapy'.

41   Gouda, 'Mimicry and Projection in the Colonial Encounter'; Monnais, *Médicaments coloniaux*, 124–30.

42   This was the case for the Wellcome Tropical Research Laboratories in Khartoum, founded in 1903, or the Pasteur Institute, opened in Yaoundé in 1959. See: Bell, *Frontiers of Medicine*, 88f; Lachenal, 'Franco-African Familiarities', 422.

43   This was the case, for instance, in Makere and Nairobi. See: Iliffe, *East African Doctors*, 174f.

numerous mission hospitals that were, like the Albert Schweitzer Hospital, run mainly as curative institutions, is also not evident.

Isgard Ohls has already observed how well Schweitzer's hospital, and especially its leprosy settlement, might reflect these experimental patterns. She writes of a twofold 'experimental field', one for the experimental development of new therapies and the second for 'practical training into the ethics of reverence for life in the clinical everyday life of the leprosy village'.[44] Ruth Harris terms the hospital a 'colony within a colony',[45] which would thereby render the leprosy settlement a colony within a colony within a colony. These images are useful when conceiving of the hospital, the leprosy village, or both as a laboratory for Schweitzer's ethics, as suggested in the Introduction. They are less accurate when describing the hospital's pharmaceutical treatment of dysentery and leprosy patients. For these small-scale tests, the results of which were intended only for internal use as guidelines for present and future physicians, I prefer the term 'trial and error'.

2   Leprosy in Lambaréné

According to Rita Headrick, leprosy was 'virtually ignored' in AEF, which is surprising in view of the significant efforts to combat the disease in other French colonies.[46] Still, the colonial government ran at least eight 'leprosy villages or agricultural settlements' in Gabon during the interwar period,[47] including a comparatively large settlement in Lambaréné. In 1936, Dr. Ladislav Goldschmid expressed doubt that conditions in this camp were adequate. He had heard that 'no fewer than 100 of [...] 140 lepers fled the camp. That says a lot, if it is true'.[48] Later that year, the government physician in Lambaréné and his superior from Brazzaville inspected Schweitzer's hospital and ordered that leprosy and sleeping sickness patients be sent to government facilities. Although 'quite a few' leprosy patients continued to seek treatment and shelter at the Albert Schweitzer Hospital after this inspection, Goldschmid sent them to the government's institution. This was not only 'because of formality', but also because he feared that in their increasing numbers leprosy patients would take up too much space.[49] Reports of the suffering of leprosy patients at the government

---

44   Ohls, *Der Arzt Albert Schweitzer*, 165.
45   Harris, 'Schweitzer and Africa', 1127.
46   Headrick, *Colonialism, Health and Illness in French Equatorial Africa*, 163.
47   Mabika, 'Médicalisation de l'Afrique centrale', 321.
48   Goldschmid to Schweitzer, 16 July 1936, AMS.
49   Goldschmid to Schweitzer, 24 October 1936, AMS.

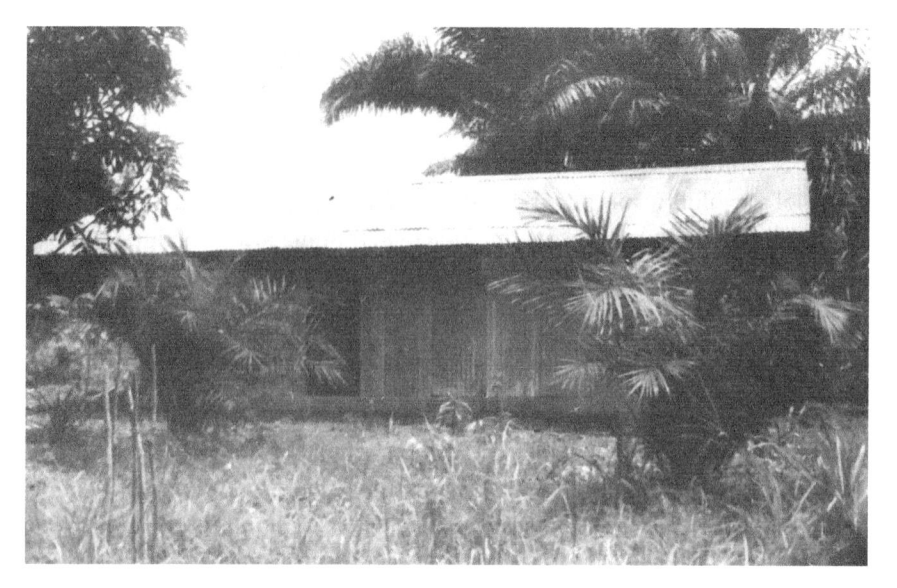

ILLUSTRATION 28   The hospital's isolation hut, away from the main buildings on a forest
                   clearing, early 1930s
                   © ARCHIVES CENTRALES ALBERT SCHWEITZER GUNSBACH

institution in Lambaréné, however, left him concerned. They 'tell us that they
are not treated, not bandaged, they hardly get anything to eat and moreover
they are maltreated with beatings'.[50]

It is difficult to verify these accusations; Goldschmid did hold a certain degree of resentment towards his colleague and rival from the nearby government facility, but his claims do reflect some of the findings of scholars who
have examined the history of African leprosy settlements in the early twentieth century. Despite these allegations of maltreatment, patients with leprosy
were sent to the sanitary formation of the government for the following two
years.[51] This arrangement remained in place for sleeping sickness patients for
the rest of the study period, but was to be revoked for those affected by leprosy
during World War Two.

The first steps towards establishing a leprosy settlement at the Albert
Schweitzer Hospital were taken in 1930, when an isolation ward was built (see
Illustration 28).[52] During the 1930s, an average of approximately forty leprosy
patients were treated at the hospital per year. In August 1936, when sixteen

---

50   Ibid.
51   See the 'Statistiques de l'Hôpital' for 1937 and 1938, L – A – S3, AMS.
52   Woytt-Secretan, *Albert Schweitzer baut Lambarene*, 78.

leprosy sufferers were present, two rooms had to be cleared in the ward desig-nated for tuberculosis patients.[53] The hospital staff's main motivation for seg-regating leprosy patients was to prevent the spread of the infection through the institution. It was also necessary to keep patients at the hospital to undergo long-term treatment with chaulmoogra drugs. Dr. Anna Wildikann, who was not sure how long they had to keep patients, raised doubts about this 'asylum policy' in 1935. The problem was that 'when they get bored, they just run away or – like some others do at the moment – they constantly revolt'.[54] As we will see below, patients did not like taking compounds from chaulmoogra, while doctors tried to find ways to make their application less unpleasant.

In the mid-1950s, the Service Général d'Hygiene Mobile et de Prophylaxie attempted to calculate the number of people affected by leprosy in AEF and to determine treatment for each patient.[55] By the end of the decade, almost 9,688 leprosy sufferers had been counted in Gabon.[56] This colonial effort was mod-elled on the successful campaigns against sleeping sickness orchestrated by Eugène Jamot in the early 1930s, in which mobile teams had distributed pills and administered injections. These programs were admired by colonial doc-tors because 'this "simple, efficacious" approach minimized the disturbances in the patient's life and permitted the complete avoidance of "segregation" and "detribalisation"'.[57]

The development of leprosy settlements in Gabon illustrates the shift away from isolation as the preferred means of treating the disease. In 1943, the colonial administration maintained ten leproseries in Gabon,[58] including one in Lambaréné with forty beds.[59] Ten years later, the eleven government 'leper colonies' provided a total of 930 beds.[60] French officials had envisaged es-tablishing villages 'like the others' that would enjoy maximal autonomy and self-sufficiency, but this plan was not realized due to financial restrictions

53   Goldschmid to Schweitzer, 11 August 1936, AMS.

54   Wildikann to Schweitzer, 15 December 1935, AMS.

55   Mabika lists the following possible treatments: 'oral, intravenous, at home, at the treat-ment centre, in the leprosy community, in hospital'. Mabika, 'Médicalisation de l'Afrique centrale', 219.

56   Ibid.

57   Silla, *People Are Not the Same*, 109–10. See also: Bado, *Médecine coloniale et grandes endé-mies en Afrique*, 359–60.

58   'Projet de Réorganisation du Service de l'A.M.I.', dated 15 January 1944 compiled by Médecin-Colonel Bizien, Inspecteur Général des Services Sanitaires et Médicaux de l'A.E.F., 117, ZK 005-127, SHD.

59   'Rapport Annuel du Service de Santé de la Colonie du Gabon 1945', ZK 005-005, SHD.

60   Mabika, 'Médicalisation de l'Afrique centrale', 322.

and because the 'displacement' of patients was not considered to be 'ideal'.[61]
In 1950, 1,185 leprosy patients lived in the government settlements of AEF,
while another 3,757 underwent outpatient treatment.[62] Schweitzer's hospital,
on the other hand, treated 204 leprosy patients, of which 146 were hospi-
talized.[63] In 1954, the Lambaréné government hospital recorded a total of
50 inpatients and 84 outpatients with leprosy,[64] whereas Schweitzer's newly
established 'village des lumières', as this settlement became known, then accommodated 250 patients.[65] In 1961, 857 individuals with the disease were
registered in Lambaréné District.[66] At this time, about one hundred patients
and approximately eighty of their family members lived in Schweitzer's leprosy settlement.[67]

In 1951, Dr. Jean-Pierre Naegele provided a detailed report on the state of
leprosy care at the Albert Schweitzer Hospital.[68] The number of leprosy patients had quadrupled between April 1950, when large quantities of sulfones
had first been provided to the hospital, and September 1951.[69] People seeking
leprosy treatment and their relatives had built four small settlements around
the isolation ward (see Illustration 29). They were segregated according to ethnic groups and housed a total of more than 300 patients. Naegele commented
that 'apparently, this is the kind of accommodation preferred by our patients.
They feel at ease and send for their sick relatives from far away to join them'.[70]
In agreement with other specialists as well as his predecessor, Dr. Wildikann,
Naegele emphasized that forced isolation was not a viable approach and that

---

61   Cheneveau, 'La lutte contre la lèpre en A.E.F', PR(H), 1 H 254.1. ANG, 10–13.
62   'Rapport Annuel du Service de Santé de l'Afrique Equtoriale Française 1950', ZK 005-91,
      SHD.
63   Naegele, 'Traitement des malades lépreux à l'Hôpital du Docteur Albert Schweitzer à
      Lambaréné au cours de l'année 1950', AMS, 8.
64   'Rapport Annuel Des Services Sanitaires de Lambaréné 1954'. 2 DC(I) 44.11, ANG.
65   Schweitzer, 'Briefe aus dem Lambarenespital Oktober 1954'.
66   'Rapport Annuel du Centre Médical de Lambaréné 1961', 1 H 226.1, ANG.
67   Goldwyn, 'Diary 1960', AMS, 31.
68   Naegele, 'Streiflichter aus Lambarene. 1951 III. Um die Lepra', AMS.
69   The number of leprosy patients can be accurately discerned from the *appels mensuels*, see
      L – P – AM7, AMS.
70   Fang patients, who had built their own houses, named their settlement 'Bingoung', which
      Naegele translated as 'tin roof'. Adouma, Bagota, Shake and other groups from the interior
      called their settlement of approximately thirty houses 'Bise-bouko-libengo', translated as
      'we are near the hole' because of a nearby well, that had been recently dug. Bapounou,
      Eshira, and Mitsogo lived on a nearby hill and called their settlement 'Labilila', which ac-
      cording to Naegele meant either 'far view' or 'to wait'. Members of a few local minority
      groups had started to build a fourth settlement. See: Naegele, 'Streiflichter aus Lambarene.
      1951 III. Um die Lepra', AMS, 2.

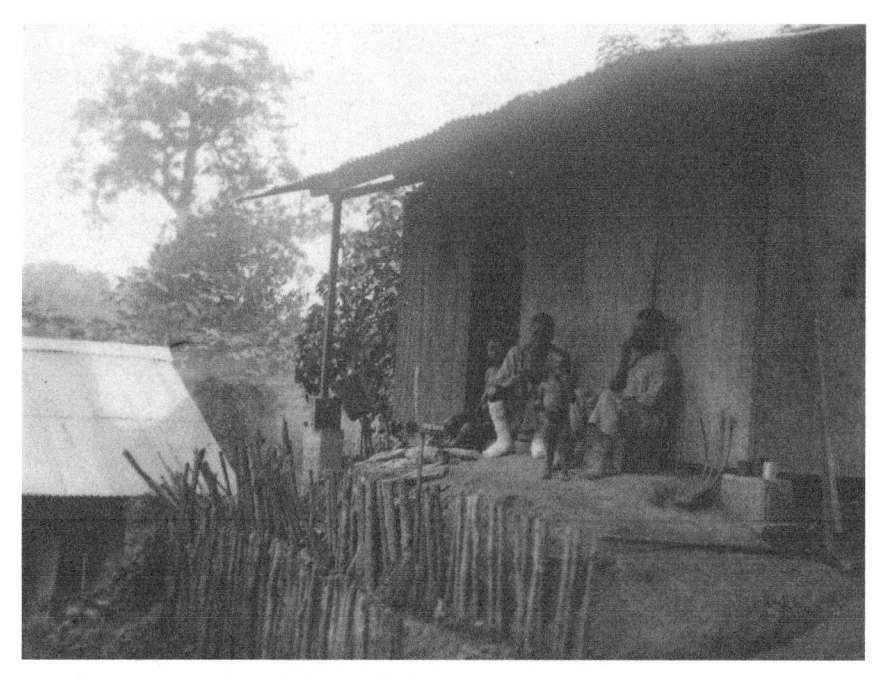

ILLUSTRATION 29   One of the huts in the first leprosy settlements, ca. 1950
© ARCHIVES CENTRALES ALBERT SCHWEITZER GUNSBACH

family members should be permitted to stay with their sick relatives in order to increase patients' willingness to remain at the hospital:

> It is needless to ask if one should send the healthy relatives of lepers back home or have them stay. If we send away the healthy wife, husband or daughter, we can be sure that the night after, the patient also disappears.[71]

In May 1952, Schweitzer proposed rebuilding the area where these settlements had developed,[72] plans that were realized one year later. The hill was flattened, and the bamboo cabins were replaced with buildings with concrete foundations, thereby creating what Schweitzer conceived of as a model village (see Illustration 30).[73] This went against the trend of decentralized out-patient treatment that was becoming standard in French colonies at the time and which was also the official approach of the colonial government in Gabon. In part, it also went against the recommendations of Schweitzer's

71   Ibid., 5.
72   Haussknecht to Royden, 1 May 1952, AMS.
73   Schweitzer, 'Briefe aus dem Lambarenespital Oktober 1954', 6–10.

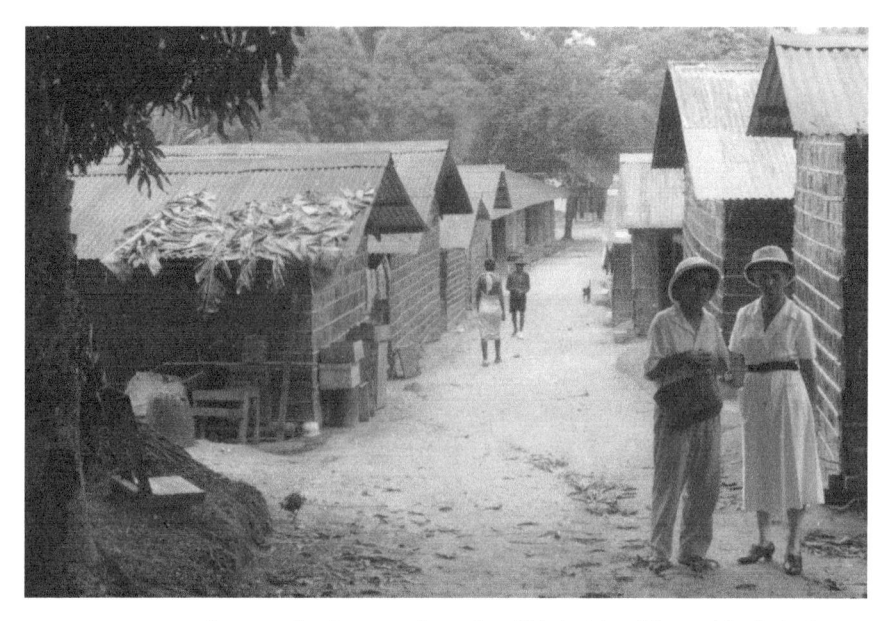

ILLUSTRATION 30   Long-serving Japanese doctor Isao Takahashi and Emmy Martin in the
                  hospital's new leprosy settlement, the 'village lumière', ca. 1960
                  © ARCHIVES CENTRALES ALBERT SCHWEITZER GUNSBACH

doctors and the preferences of Gabonese leprosy sufferers who sought care at
the hospital. Their numbers decreased by as many as 100 patients after the
opening of this new settlement for 250 people in early 1954.[74] By this time the
government had counted all leprosy cases in the colony during the course of
the above-mentioned campaign; Schweitzer's hospital had treated 649 leprosy patients since 1946. Only one-third of these patients came from the District
of Lambaréné,[75] which suggests that medication was not widely available
elsewhere. Despite the overwhelmingly positive reputation this part of the
hospital still enjoys in Europe,[76] we know very little about the patients who
were treated there.

   African societies confronted leprosy in different ways. In some locations,
affected individuals were isolated among themselves; in others, they were not

---

74   In September 1951, 350 leprosy patients were documented in the *appels mensuels*, L – P –
     AM1, AMS. One year later, Schweitzer even mentioned 400. See: Schweitzer and Mellon,
     Brothers in Spirit, 25–26. In the month in which construction of the 'village lumières' be-
     gan, Schweitzer still reported the presence of 300 leprosy patients. See: Schweitzer to
     Stoll, 18 May 1953, AMS.
75   'Hôpital Schweitzer – Lépreux recencés depuis 1947'. PR(H), 1 H 235.3, ANG.
76   Isgard Ohls quotes numerous contemporary sources and also assesses the leprosy village
     in a very positive manner. See: Ohls, *Der Arzt Albert Schweitzer*, 171–83.

stigmatized at all.[77] This wide range of responses to the disease – from complete isolation to partial marginalization with family visits allowed to no segregation at all – could be observed even within a relatively small territory.[78] It has been suggested that colonial segregation measures increased the general fear of the disease in societies where similar approaches had not been practiced before.[79]

In AEF in the mid-1950s, some colonial officials claimed that leprosy sufferers continued to work and were not considered a burden by their fellow villagers.[80] This view shaped the French preference for decentralized treatment. At the Albert Schweitzer Hospital, where a large leprosy settlement with an international reputation was about to be created, most staff believed that Gabonese leprosy sufferers were marginalized.[81] Augustin Emane's interviewees claim that leprosy patients would not only come to the hospital to be cured, but also for a place to stay after being ostracized from their villages.[82] Schweitzer, however, does not appear to have made this claim himself. Dr. Naegele, who was the first doctor at the hospital to make large-scale use of sulfones, agreed with government officials in favoring ambulant treatment in the short term. He claimed that 'the lepers of the Gabon are not rejected at all by their families and are therefore not forced to seek refuge in leper settlements and stay there if they do not like it'.[83] Similar discrepancies between public claims and personal correspondence have been observed in the previous chapter in the case of obstetrical emergencies. Since the treatment of leprosy was important for maintaining potentially lucrative relationships with the donor community, as argued by Manton above, Schweitzer was probably motivated to establish the settlement more by reasons other than strict medical imperatives.

Leprosy was a considerable concern among Gabonese communities. In their 1961 book on useful plants in Gabon, Raponda-Walker and Sillans list seven local plants used to treat the disease. For some of these plants, leprosy is the only indication listed, but specific details on how they were used to treat

---

77   Notably, the latter approach was considered less 'civilised' by European observers in the interwar period. See: Vaughan, *Curing Their Ills*, 80.

78   Bado, *Médecine coloniale et grandes endémies en Afrique*, 146; Eckart, *Medizin und Kolonialimperialismus*, 321.

79   Manton, 'Mission, Clinic, and Laboratory', 323.

80   Cheneveau, 'La lutte contre la lèpre en A.E.F.', 1955, PR(H), 1 H 254.1. ANG, 8–9.

81   Ohls, *Der Arzt Albert Schweitzer*, 173.

82   Emane, *Docteur Schweitzer: une icône africaine*, 2013, 203–4.

83   Naegele, 'Streiflichter aus Lambarene. 1951 III. Um die Lepra', AMS, 2.

the illness are not provided.[84] Most, however, were also recommended for a variety of other dermatological afflictions. The leaves and bark of the cashew tree were used for general skin care; its nuts provided oil for external application on ulcers and leprosy wounds.[85] Various plants were also used to cicatrize wounds.[86] It remains unclear how many of those plants were actually in widespread use; even less certain is how many relevant medicinal plants the authors did not list at all. They also included applications known from other contexts. In relation to *Caloncoba welwitschii*, for example, they wrote that 'the grains are very rich in chaulmoogric oils, highly praised for curing leprosy. But this property is not known to Blacks in Gabon'.[87] The local preference for using externally applied substances to treat skin afflictions found its equivalent at the Albert Schweitzer Hospital in the treatment of ulcers, including those caused by leprosy, with ointments. Sometimes made in the hospital's little pharmacy by nurses, these were used throughout the study period.[88]

Medical practitioners at the Albert Schweitzer Hospital had to respond to this local context when treating leprosy. They reacted to the complexity of the infection, the lack of efficacious treatments, and the sudden influx of patients by testing drugs using a trial-and-error approach. At the same time, these drugs also helped to shape this very context. Their availability enabled new types of leprosy settlements to be established, new therapeutic hope to flourish, more patients to seek treatment, and more difficult cases to be discovered. In turn, these developments shaped doctors' attitudes towards leprosy drugs and the disease itself.

---

84   This is the case for *Culcasia*, ('the leaves act against leprosy', 95) or *Drymaria cordatia* ('this herb is used to cure leprosy', 120) Raponda-Walker and Sillans, *Les plantes utiles du Gabon*.

85   Latin binomial: *Anacardium occidentale*. Ibid., 57.

86   For example, Gabonese Mint (*Ocimum viride*), ibid. 312; Leadwort (*Plumbago Zeylanica*), ibid. 349.

87   Raponda-Walker and Sillans, *Les plantes utiles du Gabon*, 181. The The Kew Species Profiles, describe the plant as follows: 'Uses: *Caloncoba welwitschii* has a wide range of traditional medicinal uses in Central Africa. For example, the leaves and bark are used for treating rheumatism, and are made into poultices for applying to abscesses. The leaf-sap is used to treat headaches, and the plant itself is prescribed as a means of killing body-lice. The fruit pulp is eaten in Gabon. It has been reported that the seed oil is used to treat leprosy in the Democratic Republic of Congo'. http://powo.science.kew.org/taxon/urn:lsid:ipni.org:names:365023-1#source-KSP (2 June 2020).

88   In 1937, Schweitzer explained to a former nurse that honey and cod liver oil were now used at the hospital for producing the ointments. See: Schweitzer to Stalder, 7 April 1937, AMS; Goldwyn mentioned 'liver paste, zinc oxide, Mercurochrome, and methylene blue'. Goldwyn, 'Diary 1960', AMS, 56.

3   Dysentery in Africa and Lambaréné

Dysentery in Africa has received much less historiographical attention than leprosy. It is linked with labor migration and unsanitary conditions,[89] frequently occurring at railway construction sites, on plantations, or along trade routes. Unlike leprosy, it often affected Europeans,[90] who typically blamed Africans for its spread by being ignorant of or unable to adapt to hygienic practices, such as using latrines.[91] Today, the main advice for avoiding contracting dysentery, which is considered highly contagious, remains to habitually wash hands and foodstuffs. Both its bacillary and its amoebic form, the latter being the main focus of this chapter, are believed to pass through fecal matter or contaminated food and water.[92]

Rita Headrick has described government measures taken during a series of dysentery epidemics in the early 1920s along construction sites of the Congo-Ocean Railway, where an estimated 20 percent of the population died of the disease. Colonial officials threatened local chiefs with imprisonment or fines if they failed to report cases. Infected individuals were quarantined, while canoes were confiscated and roadblocks erected to hinder the spread of the disease. Three of the eight doctors in AEF were called to the region. Headrick argues that these 'measures added up to an energetic and expensive response to the epidemic, rather uncharacteristic of the administration',[93] a sign of the priority given to the rapid construction of the railway.

Some French colonial medical officials believed that dysentery was unavoidable – an act of God, essentially – while others claimed that laborers could somehow acquire partial immunity. Colonial employers tried to avoid recruiting workers from distant areas where the disease was not endemic. They believed that these individuals would be more susceptible to the illness, having been weakened by a long journey and not being accustomed to the food served on construction sites. As dysentery came in two forms, difficulties in diagnosis added to the confusion as other intestinal parasites could provoke similar symptoms or cause simultaneous infections.[94]

---

89   Doyle, *Before HIV*, 97–98.

90   Good, *The Steamer Parish*, 333; Eckart, *Medizin und Kolonialimperialismus*, 232–33.

91   Eckart, *Medizin und Kolonialimperialismus*, 352–53; Headrick, *Colonialism, Health and Illness in French Equatorial Africa*, 167.

92   Marie and Petri Jr., 'Amoebic Dysentery'. See also: https://www.nhs.uk/conditions/dysentery/ (2 June 2020).

93   Headrick, *Colonialism, Health and Illness in French Equatorial Africa*, 165–67.

94   Ibid., 185–86.

The few historical studies that comment on the amoebic form of the disease mention emetine hydrochloride, made from the ipecacuanha root native to Central and South America, as the treatment that was preferred by colonial doctors in the period from 1920 to 1950. Accidents due to the compound's toxicity occurred repeatedly, but alternatives, such as Stovarsol, were not without their own problems.[95] It was hence recommended administering emetine via intravenous injections, which promised to be less painful than intramuscular ones, but underlined the need to closely monitor patients for potential side effects.[96]

It is no surprise that the crowded lumber camps in the region surrounding Lambaréné, that placed little emphasis on sanitation or balanced diets, provided an environment prone to the spread of dysentery. Indeed, Raponda-Walker and Sillans list no fewer than seventeen different local plants for treating the illness in their book. Once again, it remains unclear to what extent the authors incorporated their own knowledge about these plants into their descriptions. On water cabbage leaves, for example, they wrote that 'mixed with rice and coconut milk, they can be used against dysentery, but in Gabon these uses are ignored'.[97] According to Raponda-Walker and Sillans, different parts of a single plant often offered different medicinal uses. After being cooked before it ripened, soursop fruit was dried and then powdered to serve as a medication for dysentery; other parts of the tree were used to treat coughs and fever or as a tranquilizer or emetic.[98] Various parts of the African coralwood were said to treat toothache, yaws, gonorrhea, scabies, and wounds respectively, while 'the blacks use the boiled bark with that of Saccoglottis Gabonensis in enemas to fight dysentery'.[99] A range of crops were said to counter dysentery, including rice, through rice water 'as drink or enema',[100] and green bananas, 'grilled in ashes and into which bark rasps from wild mango or odika butter have been introduced'.[101] Notable in all of these examples is how the authors emphasized the combinations of various plants and their specific means of application in the treatment of different afflictions.

As a reaction to the dangers of emetine and the highly contagious nature of dysentery, a number of coercive therapeutic practices were followed at the

---

95   Ibid., 166; Good, *The Steamer Parish*, 233; Monnais, *Médicaments coloniaux*, 127.

96   Craig, *The Etiology, Diagnosis, and Treatment of Amebiasis*.

97   Latin binomial: *Pistia stratiotes*. Raponda-Walker and Sillans, *Les plantes utiles du Gabon*, 96.

98   *Annona muricata*. Ibid., 63.

99   *Pterocarpus soyauxii*. Ibid., 259.

100   Ibid., 191.

101   Ibid., 304.

Albert Schweitzer Hospital. When the hospital was located at its original site, dysentery patients were isolated in a building that was 'some sort of prison where we lock up the biggest banana thieves who loot Keller's beautiful plantations'.[102] Writing at the hospital's new location, Dr. Ilse Schnabel noted in her diary in 1929 that the 'the dysentery patients ask why they're kept locked up like prisoners'.[103] She also reported that they often escaped. The hospital's solution was to paint a blue sign onto each dysentery patient's forehead.[104] Two years later, dysentery patients were placed in an isolation ward that Schweitzer described as a 'spacious, airy barrack and a barred yard', which had formerly accommodated mentally ill patients.[105] Some patients attempted to hide their dysenteric symptoms in an effort to avoid being sent into isolation there.[106] This ward was still operational in 1948,[107] but was not mentioned in the sources thereafter. References to the disease are rarer after 1950, by which time emetine's negative side effects had been reduced and efficacious alternatives had become available.

On the one hand, coercive measures were justified with reference to the need to supervise patients' diets in order to minimize the negative side effects of treatment.[108] On the other hand, the fear of infection was deep-seated; forced isolation, so it was believed, would prevent the spread of dysentery through the hospital.[109] As with leprosy, the available drugs and the wider disease context shaped one another and the doctors' response to the illness. Trial-and-error testing of new drugs was the obvious reaction to a desire to avoid isolating patients or exposing them to unpleasant side effects. Unlike other doctors in the colonies, including some of his own, Schweitzer was more concerned about what he regarded as emetine's doubtful efficacy than its negative side effects, as will be discussed below.

Another strategy to stop the spread of the disease saw repeated measures being taken to improve the hospital's water supply in order to minimize

---

102   Nessmann, *Avec Albert Schweitzer de 1924 à 1926*, 192. Keller was a missionary at the neighboring Protestant station.
103   Schnabel, 'Von ärztlichen Verrichtungen', 57.
104   Ibid., 60.
105   Schweitzer, 'Briefe aus dem Lambarene Spital Pfingsten 1931', 2.
106   Schweitzer, 'Briefe aus dem Lambarene Spital März 1938', 5.
107   Schweitzer, *Das Spital im Urwald: Aufnahmen von Anna Wildikann*, 14, 20.
108   This was even more important for patients being treated for intestinal worms. See: Schweitzer, 'Neues von Albert Schweitzer Februar 1925', 5; Schweitzer, 'Briefe aus dem Lambarene Spital Februar 1939', 3–4.
109   Schweitzer, 'Mitteilungen aus Lambarene. Zweites Heft, 1924–1925', 140–41; Lauterburg-Bonjour, *Lambarene: Erlebnisse einer Bernerin im afrikanischen Urwald*, 16; Schweitzer, 'Briefe aus dem Lambarene Spital März 1938', 5.

contact with the amoeba-contaminated river water. For two days in 1927, for example, Schweitzer searched the local area for a longer pipe to serve the hospital's ever-deepening well, acquiring one 'by flattering and begging'.[110] The institution's pump was regularly out of order, during which time patients had no choice but to drink the contaminated river water from nearer to its bank. For this reason, a rainwater reservoir and a deeper well with its own pump were built during the dry season in 1931.[111] By the end of the decade, water supply had become insufficient once again. This forced patients to drink river water once more, in response to which another well was dug.[112] The pumps had to be replaced on a regular basis (see Illustrations 31 and 32). Fear of dysentery among patients in case of neglect was a main argument therefor. 'Because when the patients drink river water we constantly have dysentery', Schweitzer explained to Emmy Martin in June 1950.[113] Nurses who worked at the hospital in the 1960s recalled a still precarious water supply and claim that all water was boiled before consumption.[114]

The significant attention paid to dysentery at the Albert Schweitzer Hospital, and the isolation of African patients in particular, carried with it a racial dimension. Dysentery posed a threat to Europeans at the hospital and in its wider vicinity. Various hospital employees contracted the disease,[115] and it was among the three top reasons why Europeans were admitted to the institution, alongside malaria and gonorrhea.[116] Europeans were also accused by the staff of underestimating the disease and of being ignorant of its dangers and transmission paths. Mathilde Kottman deputized as hospital director during Schweitzer's absence in 1928, the year after a severe dysentery epidemic. She wrote to Emily Rieder bemoaning this lack of knowledge. 'Fortunately, this year dysentery is not so widespread among the natives', she wrote. It was, however, more prevalent among Europeans, 'who often face this disease in a harmless and optimistic manner. They often hardly know that dysentery is contagious and transmissible!'[117]

---

110   Schweitzer to Martin, 11 March 1927, AMS.
111   Schweitzer, 'Briefe aus dem Lambarene Spital Pfingsten 1931', 2; Schweitzer, 'Briefe aus dem Lambarene Spital Februar 1934', 6.
112   Schweitzer, 'Briefe aus dem Lambarene Spital März 1938', 6.
113   Schweitzer to Martin, 27 June 1950, AMS.
114   Interview Elisabeth Anderegg; Stark-Bernhard, 'Waschfrauen, Büglerinnen, Schneider und Matratzenmacher', 28.
115   Dr. Victor Nessmann was infected with dysentery several times in 1926. See: Schweitzer to Martin, 12 March 1926, AMS. Another case was the nurse Erna Frischknecht in 1938. She was sent home soon. See: Schweitzer to Martin, 6 September 1938, AMS.
116   These numbers are taken from the 'Statistiques de l'Hôpital', L – A – S1–3, AMS.
117   Kottmann to Rieder, 27 November 1928, AWHS.

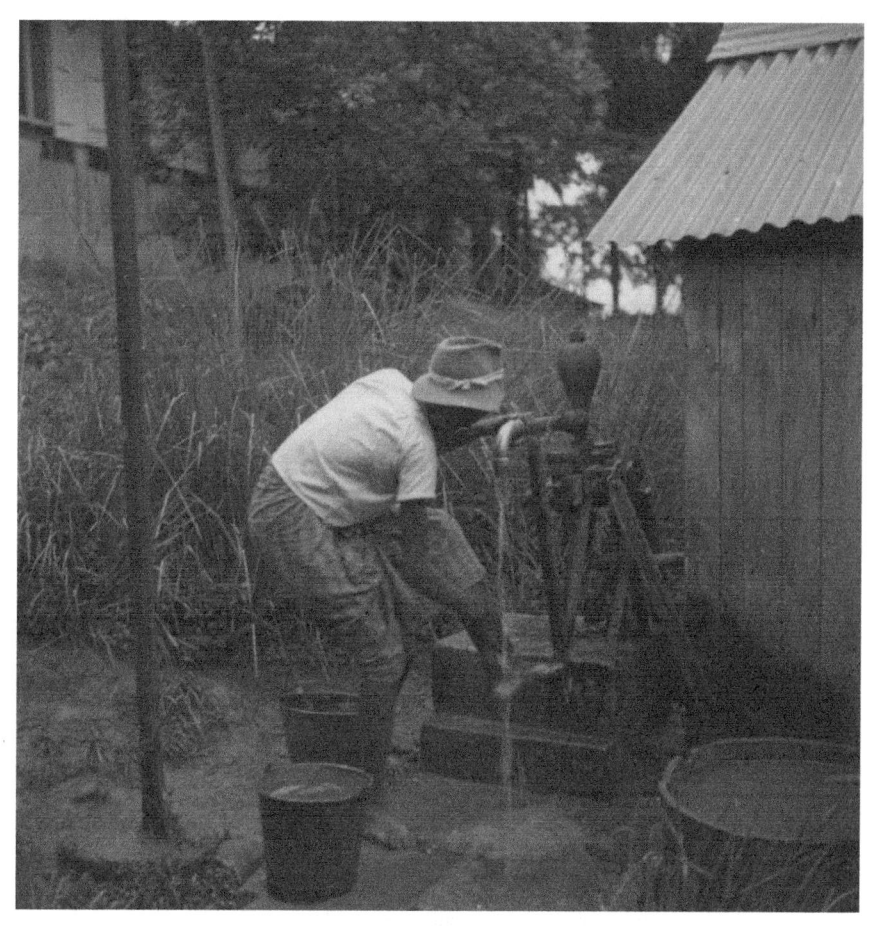

ILLUSTRATION 31   A pump at the hospital, undated
© ARCHIVES CENTRALES ALBERT SCHWEITZER GUNSBACH

At first glance, Figures 11 and 12 suggests that dysentery epidemics among Europeans did not necessarily coincide with outbreaks among Africans.[118] Europeans were affected by serious epidemics in 1933 and, to a lesser extent, 1934. In contrast, dysentery cases among Africans were not significantly higher in those years than in others, neither in absolute terms nor relative to total patient admissions. However, 1933 is one of the few years for which detailed statistics from the government clinic in Lambaréné are available. These show that it recorded 136 dysentery cases, 108 of which were among outpatients. In the previous year, a total of 63 cases among Africans were recorded, 71 percent of whom

---

118   The numbers for both figures are taken from the 'Statistiques de l'Hôpital', L – A – S1–3 AMS.

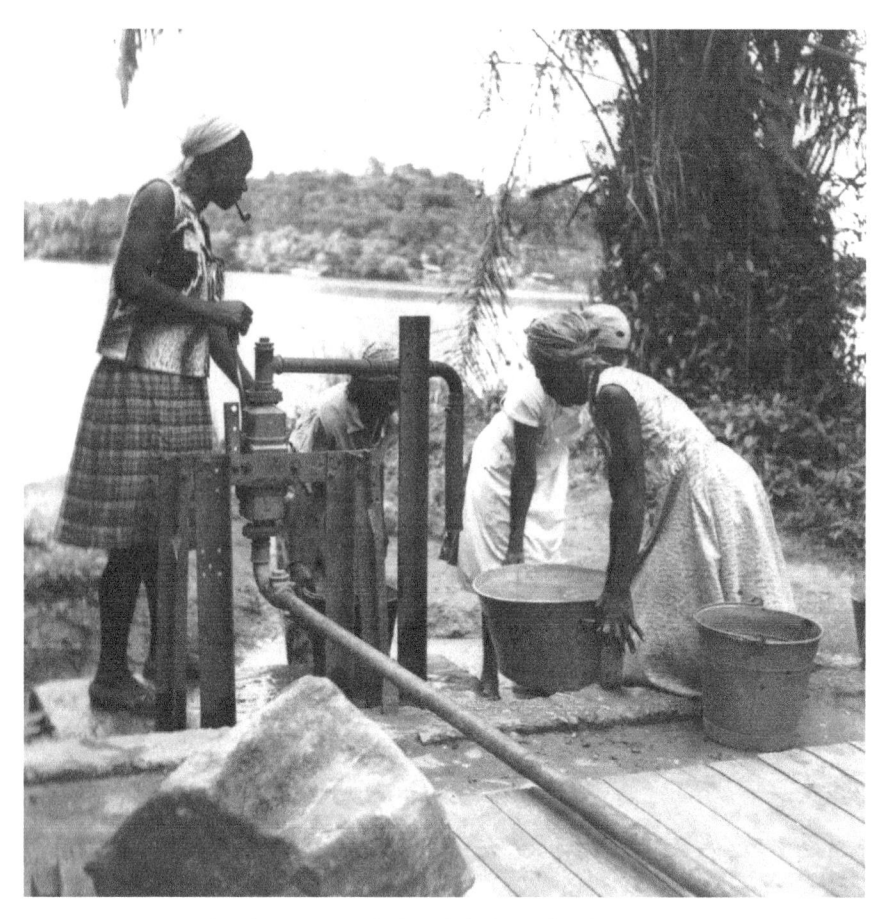

ILLUSTRATION 32   Another pump at the hospital, also undated
© ARCHIVES CENTRALES ALBERT SCHWEITZER GUNSBACH

were treated on an ambulant basis.[119] This small sample of evidence suggests that Africans were affected by the same dysentery epidemics as Europeans. This seems even more plausible when considering the fact that statistics from the Albert Schweitzer Hospital reveal that the total number of outpatients in both years was more than three times lower than the corresponding figures for the government facility, which Gabonese appear to have favored for ambulant treatment.[120]

---

119   See the Rapports Annuels du Service de Santé de la Colonie du Gabon for 1932 and 1933, ZK 005-127, SHD. The hospital did not provide statistics for 1934, while the Service de Santé's annual reports for 1935 to 1945 are missing in Toulon.
120   In 1933, for example, Schweitzer's hospital reported 1,829 ambulant cases, whereas the government clinic recorded at least 6,250, a figure that, considering unclear record-keeping, might have been as high as 8,866. In 1932, the government facility recorded 5,545

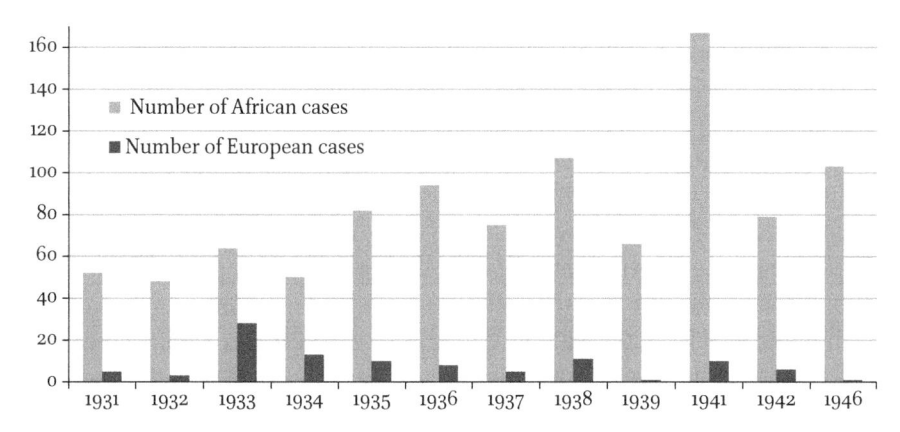

FIGURE 11   Patients diagnosed with dysentery

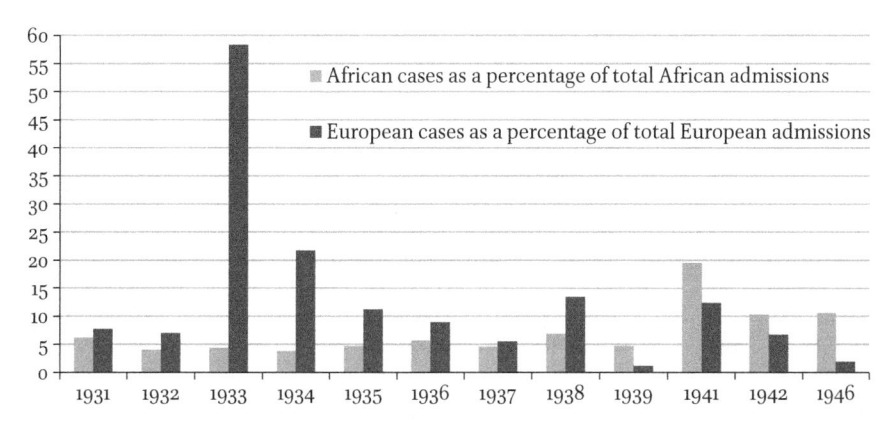

FIGURE 12   Dysentery cases related to total entries

The number of African dysentery patients at the hospital was particularly high during World War Two (see Figure 11), especially when considered in relation to total admissions during this period (see Figure 12). This implies that the disease was considered to be a serious concern, both by the patients, who actively sought treatment, and by the hospital staff, who admitted them while rejecting persons with other afflictions. It might further suggest local food scarcities, increased population densities in the area, burgeoning local lumber exploitation, and/or a closure of the government hospital. A more detailed analysis of these issues is beyond the scope of this chapter.

outpatients, as opposed to 1,445 at the Albert Schweitzer Hospital. For the source of these statistics, see the previous two footnotes.

4   Trials and Errors: the Use of Pharmaceuticals at the Albert
         Schweitzer Hospital

In the treatment of dysentery and leprosy patients with pharmaceuticals a
pattern can be discerned. Towards public and private sponsors, Schweitzer
would praise a globally known standard drug, which was routinely administered to patients (see Illustrations 33, 34, and 35).[121] In daily practice, however,
doctors' in Lambaréné had to confront the fact that every drug came with its
own flaws, which could relate to the form in which it was administered, its
efficacy, and/or its side effects. In an attempt to mitigate these faults, the doctors tested alternative or additional options via a trial-and-error approach. In
this subchapter, I analyze efforts to find more patient-friendly dosage forms,
improve efficacy, or reduce side effects respectively by way of three examples:
chaulmoogra, emetine, and sulfones. These drugs, or their trialed alternatives,
were most frequently discussed in the sources in relation to the issues raised

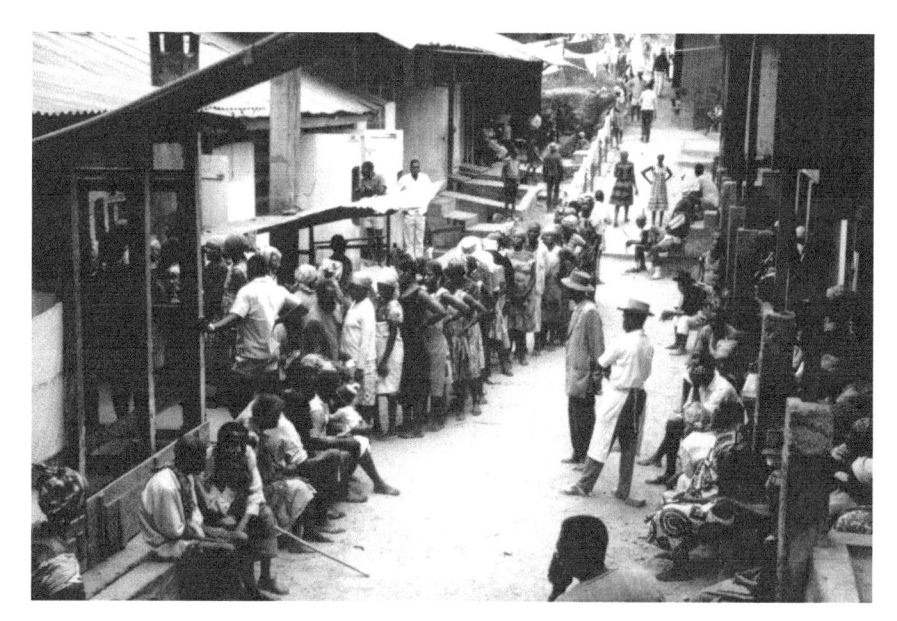

ILLUSTRATION 33   Patients queuing in front of the 'Grande Pharmacie', possibly for drugs,
                   mid-1950s
                   © ARCHIVES CENTRALES ALBERT SCHWEITZER GUNSBACH

---

121   See Chapter 1 for a description of how the distribution and administration of drugs
       occurred at the hospital.

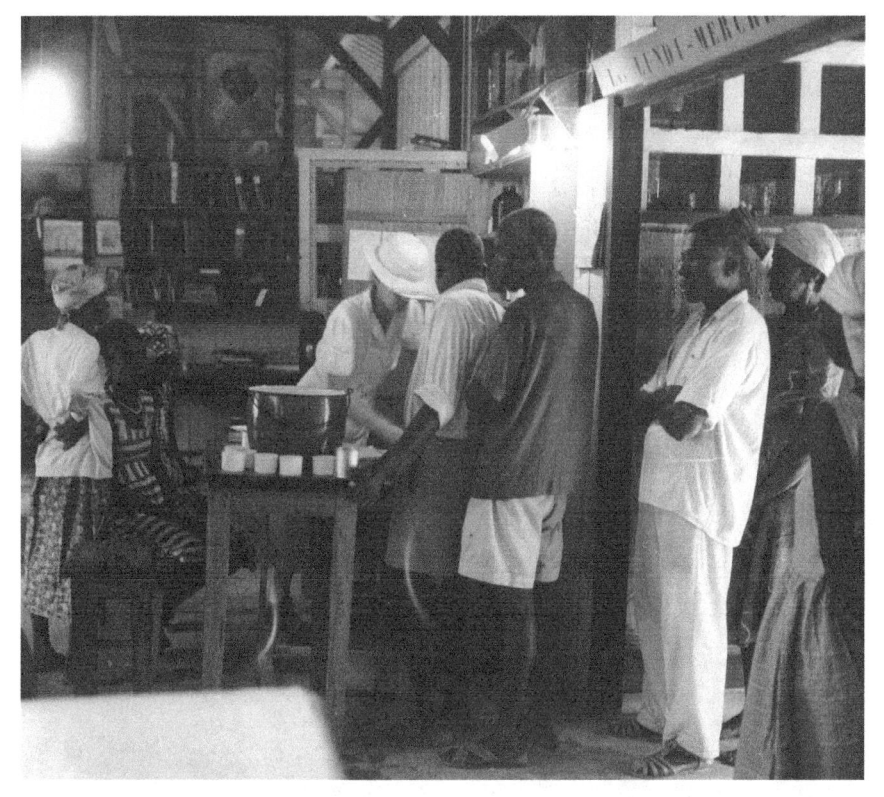

ILLUSTRATION 34   Inside the 'Grande Pharmacie' during the distribution of medication,
mid-1950s
© ARCHIVES CENTRALES ALBERT SCHWEITZER GUNSBACH

in the respective examples, which is not to imply that these concerns were not
expressed in relation to other drugs.

I argue that the treatment of leprosy and dysentery was rather representative of drug use at the Albert Schweitzer Hospital, and presumably beyond it.
Certainly, some common infectious diseases, such as yaws and syphilis, could
be treated with relatively efficacious drugs. Others, such as malaria or tuberculosis, would need a more detailed analysis to make more informed claims. The
frequent parasitic diseases habitually demanded a combination of various
pharmaceuticals; a trial-and-error approach for determining the most appropriate arrangement would be no surprise. My observations from the surgical
and obstetrical wards have shown that staff administered drugs in a liberal
manner. The same is true for the psychiatric unit, where the process of decid-
ing which medication to administer to a patient followed a pattern that was
similar to the one being described now. Ulcers could likewise be targeted with

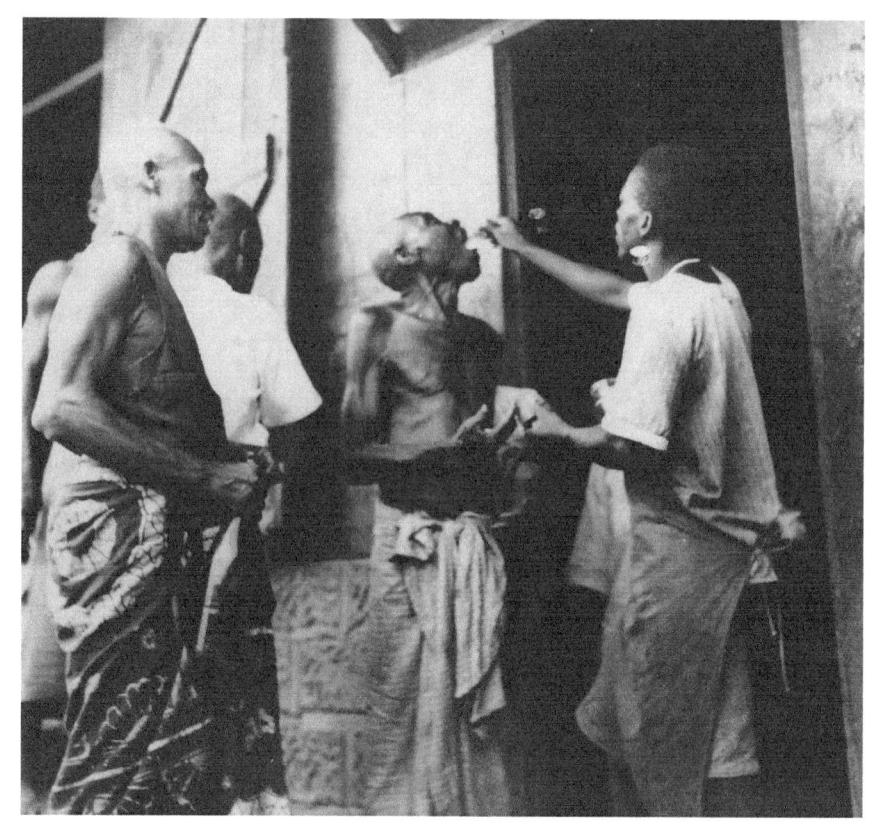

ILLUSTRATION 35   Patients receiving their medication under the supervision of medical
personnel, mid-1930s
© ARCHIVES CENTRALES ALBERT SCHWEITZER GUNSBACH

a range of pharmaceutical options. Staff's methods to find the most effective
approach and substance clearly resembled those observed in this chapter.[122]

Schweitzer, like many other colonial doctors in the 1920s and 1930s, had a
reputation for conducting trials. Some pharmaceutical companies shipped
their new drugs directly to Lambaréné without prior arrangement, expecting
reports on the results obtained in tests on patients.[123] Others, such as the French
company Poulenc Frères, delivered Schweitzer's orders with the request that

122   Mabika Ognandzi, Steinke, and Zumthurm, *Schweitzer's Lambaréné: A Hospital in Colo-
      nial Africa.*
123   The Chemisch-Pharmazeutische Aktiengesellschaft Bad Homburg sent four cases of vari-
      ous medications, as its director informed Schweitzer in an accompanying letter. See:
      Abelmann to Schweitzer, 28 August 1929, AMS.

he would communicate 'the results of (*the*) experimentation', as was the case for a consignment of emetine in 1929.[124] One year later, Schweitzer agreed to test Simaran, another dysentery drug, for the German firm Degen and Kuhn.[125] In 1931, the German corporation Bayer contacted Schweitzer, locating him in 'La Mbarene, Belgisch Congo'. The company sent a 'trial amount' of its new arsenic 4005, for which encouraging reports had emerged from dysentery treatment trials in Spanish Guinea. The Bayer representative, aware that various drugs were trialed at Schweitzer's hospital, added that his employer would be 'be very grateful if you could also include this preparation in the frame of your experiments'.[126] None of these companies specified what kind of comments or results it required or expected; instead, they were simply interested in the information that could be derived from Schweitzer's 'experiences' in testing a drug's effects on actual patients.

4.1   *Chaulmoogra and Dosage Form*

Disregarding the pain of the injections and their doubtful impact on the disease, Schweitzer described the treatment of leprosy with chaulmoogra oil in his first newsletter from Lambaréné as being very successful. 'You don't really achieve real cure. But at best you get results that are so perceptible and durable that it almost equals cure', he wrote.[127] After his return to Europe, he reviewed these circulars and published them in his popular memoir *On the Edge of the Primeval Forest* in 1921. In his revisions, Schweitzer was even more optimistic about the therapeutic potential of chaulmoogra, claiming that 'in any case, one can observe improvement and long lasting arrestment of the disease, which sometimes almost equals cure'.[128]

It has been well documented how Schweitzer aspired to contribute to the advancement of chaulmoogra oil therapy in the 1920s.[129] His efforts focused on making its associated injections less painful in order to increase patients' willingness to undergo the treatment. He aimed to find a diluter that would allow injections to be administered using the less painful subcutaneous method. He was thus willing to pay Professor Gustav Giemsa of the Bernhard Nocht Institute of Tropical Medicine in Hamburg for advice. Giemsa had conducted a series of tests on dogs, ultimately recommending peanut oil as a diluter. In his trials, this had allowed chaulmoogra oil to be injected subcutaneously,

---

124   This letter is catalogued as: De Pulligny to Schweitzer, 30 April 1929, AMS. Italics mine.
125   Degen & Kuhn to Schweitzer, 28 August 1930, AMS.
126   Bayer to Schweitzer, 7 August 1931, AMS.
127   Schweitzer, 'Notes et Nouvelles de la part du prof. Albert Schweitzer Lambaréné', 11.
128   Schweitzer, *Zwischen Wasser und Urwald*, 87.
129   Ohls, *Der Arzt Albert Schweitzer*, 199–205.

presumably without complications,[130] which would nevertheless develop when the method was later applied to patients in Lambaréné.

Aware of the limited efficacy of chaulmoogra, Schweitzer conducted trials with an arsenic compound in 1931 at Giemsa's request. Although the latter had tested this successfully on dogs, Schweitzer reported negative results after he had administered it to some of his patients, as did other doctors in various parts of Africa. He did, however, report some promising test results for fighting leprosy with Trypaflavin, a well-known medication already used to treat sleeping sickness. Giemsa was enthused by these and encouraged Schweitzer to continue the trials:

> I would be extremely interested to hear from you about your further experiences with trypaflavin, on whose results it will depend, whether it seems necessary to further expand the chemotherapy of leprosy with acridine derivatives. What an unexpectedly beautiful surprise it would be if it would finally be possible to free humanity from this probably worst of all scourges![131]

In a typically optimistic and exaggerated tone, Giemsa assigned a key role to Schweitzer in the fight against leprosy. However, no correspondence between the two doctors from after January 1933 is held in Gunsbach, suggesting that their cooperation ended abruptly.[132]

During their Trypaflavin trials, doctors at the Albert Schweitzer Hospital still preferred to treat leprosy with Bayer's chaulmoogra compound, Antileprol.[133] This was a widely-used drug that was administered using the painful intramuscular method.[134] In April 1934, however, Dr. Goldschmid began injecting it intravenously and was pleased with the outcome, which promised better results and less frequent side effects. He also emphasized that patients preferred this method and were willing to submit to it more readily, aspects not typically

---

130   Giemsa to Schweitzer, 6 September 1924, AMS.

131   Giemsa to Schweitzer, 14 January 1932, AMS. The digitized file is wrongly dated 13 November 1932.

132   Isgard Ohls, who has consulted the archives of the Bernhard Nocht Institute in Hamburg, also does not refer to any documents relating to Giemsa from after 1933, but she does not reflect on this sudden rupture in his relationship with Schweitzer. See: Ohls, *Der Arzt Albert Schweitzer*, 223–24. Support for Hitler shown by Giemsa, the institute's founder, Nocht, and its director, Peter Mühlens, might be one explanation for this cessation of correspondence. See their entries in: Klee, *Das Personenlexikon Zum Dritten Reich*.

133   Schweitzer, 'Briefe aus dem Lambarene Spital Pfingsten 1931', 7.

134   Klingmüller and Grön, *Die Lepra*, 697.

considered by doctors at Lambaréné. Respecting Schweitzer's desire to cast a controlling eye over his hospital, Goldschmid sent the following favorable synopsis of his trials:

> Also, the results of intravenous injections are much better than those of intramuscular ones. With intramuscular injections I also observed too many abscesses (almost every week I had to cut open an abscess). Since we have been injecting intravenously, patients have been much more willing to undergo Antileprol injections. I am waiting for further instructions from you in this regard. I can say that I can take responsibility for the efficacy of the intravenous method.[135]

However, doctors at the Albert Schweitzer Hospital were not fully satisfied with the intravenous Antileprol method and continued to look for alternatives throughout the 1930s. In October 1934, Goldschmid tested methylene blue injections in the hope that they would complement the Antileprol treatment and render it more efficacious, reporting to Schweitzer that the 'results justify the continuation of the tests'.[136] Methylene blue was used extensively in the hospital throughout the study period as a disinfectant for ulcers and other skin lesions,[137] but it would never become a viable alternative for the treatment of leprosy as such.

During World War Two, diphtheria toxin was used to treat leprosy. Once more, Schweitzer was optimistic about its efficacy, writing to Edward Hume that 'with this drug you really see successes'.[138] In his first circular after the war, Schweitzer revealed that the compound would be combined with chaulmoogra, arsenics, Trypaflavin, and methylene blue in an injection. The efficacy of this cocktail is doubtful, the shots were painful and their side effects severe. In Schweitzer's view, however, the main obstacle to a cure for leprosy was African patients' inability to comply with doctor's orders. 'Today, as in the past, the poor sick lack the necessary patience', he reasoned. He further declared that there was new hope for fighting the disease more effectively in the future due to promising trials conducted by French doctors in Madagascar with a drug

---

135   Goldschmid to Schweitzer, 12 June 1934, AMS.
136   Goldschmid to Schweitzer, 31 October 1934, AMS.
137   Schweitzer, 'Mitteilungen aus Lambarene. Erstes Heft, 1924', 44; Goldwyn, 'Diary 1960', AMS, 56. Elsewhere in the tropics, it was also used to treat malaria. See: Prins, 'But What Was the Disease?', 160.
138   Schweitzer to Hume, 6 April 1943, AMS.

derived from the plant *Hydrocotylus asiatica*, while American trials with Promin had yielded similarly encouraging results.[139]

4.2   *Emetine and Efficacy*

The treatment of dysentery at the Albert Schweitzer Hospital followed a plot that resembled the one of leprosy until the end of the 1940s. The standard drug, equivalent to chaulmoogra for leprosy, was emetine. Schweitzer had praised emetine's efficacy since his first stay in Lambaréné. In *On the Edge of the Primeval Forest*, he wrote about its miraculous effects: 'If you inject it for several days in a row into the skin, improvement, and usually lasting cure, can soon be observed. Successes resemble a miracle'.[140] In 1931, Dr. Bonnema reported more soberly that 'emetine provides good benefits, usually people don't need more than 40 mg per day'.[141] In addition, Yatren, a sulfonic acid combined with iodine and manufactured by Behring, was administered on a regular basis, especially for chronic cases.[142] In 1936, Goldschmid assessed the treatment of dysentery, concluding that 'the combined emetin and yatrène treatment still proves to be the best therapy'.[143] Side effects, for which emetine was frequently known and which often led to forced isolation of patients, were not mentioned. This positive, straightforward evaluation notwithstanding, the sources reveal that a variety of trial-and-error tests on patients were undertaken with further drugs.

Patient records provide only a limited insight into dysentery treatment patterns. However, there is an eleven-month period from July 1928 to May 1929 when the records of European and African patients overlap, as illustrated in Figure 13.[144] During this time, dysentery cases were relatively frequent among both groups. Emetine constituted the major treatment for both groups, with 88 percent of African patients and 81 percent of European patients receiving it. Approximately one-third of patients in each group were treated exclusively with emetine. When additional drugs were administered, these often included medications to treat other afflictions, such as heart conditions, intestinal parasites, or to improve their general state of health. The limited data overlap suggests that Yatren was more frequently prescribed to Europeans (in 35 percent

---

139   Schweitzer, 'Briefe aus dem Lambarene Spital März 1946', 12–13. Possibly, Schweitzer meant *Hydrocotyle asiatica*.

140   Schweitzer, *Zwischen Wasser und Urwald*, 88.

141   Bonnema to Schweitzer, 2 March 1932, AMS.

142   Schweitzer, 'Mitteilungen aus Lambarene. Zweites Heft, 1924–1925', 140–41.

143   Goldschmid to Schweitzer, 16 July 1936, AMS.

144   European patient records commence in this period, just as African patient records come to an end. See: L – P – C1–16, L – P – E1, AMS.

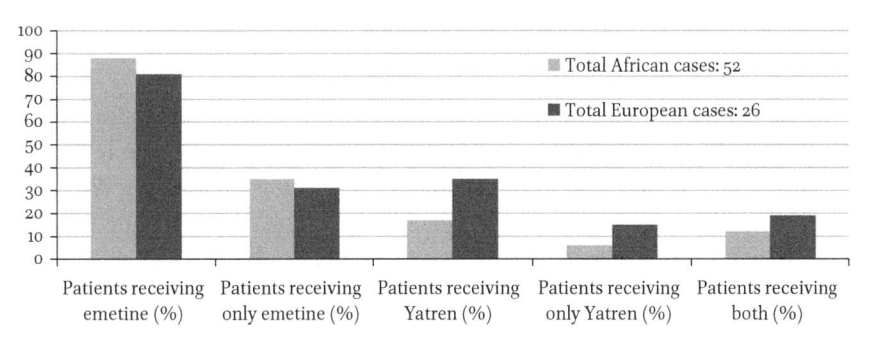

FIGURE 13   Dysentery treatment, July 1928 to May 1929

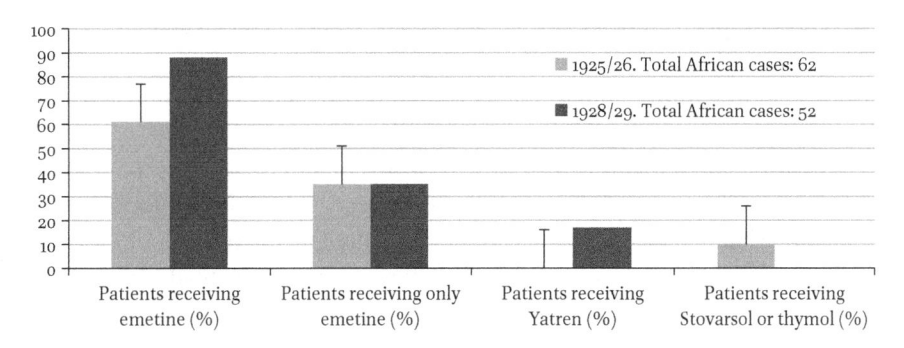

FIGURE 14   Developments of dysentery treatment

of cases) than to Africans (in 17 percent of cases). This tendency was based on medical observations: European cases were more often diagnosed as chronic, and cysts were more regularly detected among Europeans, both indications for the use of Yatren. However, the time period for the comparison is too narrow and the number of cases too low to draw broader conclusions from these observations.

A slight change can be observed when comparing the treatment of Africans in 1928/29 to that at the corresponding time of three years earlier, as Figure 14 illustrates.[145] As Schweitzer described in a newsletter, the summer of 1925 was marked by a dysentery outbreak. 'The contamination of the hospital with dysentery is progressing', he wrote, specifying that 'almost every day a new patient

---

145   The records from 1925/26 list a further ten dysentery patients without specifying the treatment that they underwent. As a result, it is not known whether they received any medication, and, if they did, whether this was emetine, the most likely prescription. In Figure 14, this uncertainty is represented by the vertical black lines in each category.

who has contracted the disease is discovered. And dysentery patients continue to be brought in'.[146]

Yatren is mentioned for the first time in the same publication, with Schweitzer claiming that it worked better for chronic cases than emetine.[147] The latter was already the most commonly used drug for treating Africans at the time, albeit to a lesser degree than in 1928. The percentage of African patients who only received emetine was identical in both periods. Despite Schweitzer's praise for Yatren, it was not administered to Africans in 1925. Instead, Africans were treated with thymol and Stovarsol, among other drugs, but both of these medications do not appear in the records three years later. This limited set of data suggests that some drugs, such as Yatren, were prioritized for Europeans, a practice justified with reference to medical imperatives. Given that Africans did receive Yatren in 1928, it could indicate that promising drugs were first tested on Europeans, but there are no remarks in the sources to support such a reading.

As with chaulmoogra in relation to leprosy, emetine's leading role in the fight against dysentery was frequently challenged. While dosage form represented a primary concern in the case of chaulmoogra, the main doubt arising from trials with emetine was the drug's efficacy, and not, as might have been expected, its side effects. A variety of compounds were trialed as alternatives, as the quotation at the beginning of this chapter suggests. Schweitzer's comment cited there was his response to the following paragraph written by Dr. Barasch in November 1936 and illustrates the doctors' hope to find a more efficacious drug against dysentery:

> According to your wish I treat some cases of dysentery with iodalgin-emetine instead of yatrine-emetine. Maybe – but I don't believe it – it will be possible to do without the yatrine in the future; you certainly won't be able to do without the emetine because so far it is the only reliable remedy against the amoebae themselves. Iodine preparations only have an effect on the kysts.[148]

Throughout 1936, Schweitzer had regularly inquired about the effects of Jodalgin, a compound distributed by his friend Paul Gloess, who had a pharmaceutical laboratory in Paris, as a substitute not only for Yatren, but also emetine. In

---

146   Schweitzer, 'Mitteilungen aus Lambarene. Zweites Heft, 1924–1925', 156–57.
147   Ibid., 140.
148   Barasch to Schweitzer, 24 November 1936, AMS.

August, there were not enough dysentery cases at the hospital to allow meaningful conclusions about Jodalgin's efficacy to be drawn.[149] Two weeks before Barasch's above-cited letter, Goldschmid also expressed his doubts about the drug, explaining to Schweitzer that 'it is very difficult to indicate the value of Gloess' iodine preparations for dysentery, as it would be too risky to use them without emetine'.[150] Goldschmid thereby invoked his clinical experience to reject Schweitzer's request to have the new drug tested, arguing that the existing treatment was sufficiently efficacious. As we will see below, Schweitzer employed similar reasoning himself on a number of occasions.

In the case of Jodalgin, it was Schweitzer who requested the testing of the new drug, rather than any doctors at the hospital out of their daily practices and observations. The trials were not successful, if indeed any were ever held. Less than a year after the above exchanges with his doctors, Schweitzer wrote in his notebook that the 'Gloess preparation is not so effective against dysentery itself, but it increases the effect of emetin and reduces its side effects'.[151] While Schweitzer did refer to side effects here, he claimed that Jodalgin had been rejected because its efficacy was lower than that of emetine. Jodalgin does not appear again in the sources; other drugs once considered failed could regain favor at a later stage.

The arsenic Stovarsol, which was manufactured by Poulenc and was a well-known treatment for syphilis, was used at the Albert Schweitzer Hospital to combat dysentery in the mid-1920s.[152] In the first week of May 1925, Schweitzer was called to a lumber camp where 31 out of 107 workers had contracted dysentery in mid-April, 16 of whom passed away within the following two weeks. Schweitzer reported to the district administrator that the sanitary conditions were nevertheless 'perfectly satisfying' and treated all affected persons with three shots of emetine. Patients who continued to excrete blood were taken to the hospital, while the rest were left in isolation at the camp, where they received Stovarsol.[153] At the hospital, Stovarsol was prescribed alongside emetine, but was also considered sufficiently efficacious to be administered on its own, as Figure 14 indicates. After 1928, the drug was no longer prescribed for dysentery. In contrast, Dr. Ilse Schnabel, who served at the hospital from 1928 to 1930, expressed her doubts about its efficacy in a medical journal article,

---

149   Goldschmid to Schweitzer, 16 August 1936, AMS.
150   Goldschmid to Schweitzer, 10 November 1936, AMS.
151   See of the notebook '1930 Therapeutische Notizen', 111, AMS. Schweitzer used the book until 1940. It is not possible to discern the exact date of each passage, since Schweitzer only occasionally entered dates in these notebooks.
152   Trensz, 'Le médecin', 214.
153   Schweitzer to Garnier, 5 May 1925, AMS.

claiming that Stovarsol would not deliver 'encouraging successes'.[154] The drug does make another appearance on Schweitzer's personal list of seven different dysentery treatments in 1934 (see Illustration 36).[155] In the 1940s, it was routinely applied in combination with emetine and coffee charcoal to treat chronic cases.[156]

A similar case was that of Enterovioform, an antifungal and antiprotozoal drug produced by the Swiss company Ciba. Schweitzer wrote in his notebook that he had recorded positive results with the drug in February 1939 and had thus requested 'larger trial quantities to test the drug on the (good old) emetine'.[157] Enterovioform was frequently prescribed at the hospital by the end of the 1950s, but details on how exactly and rapidly doctors at Schweitzer's reached a positive conclusion about its usefulness cannot be discerned from the sources.[158] Common to the Enterovioform, Stovarsol, Jodalgin, and Yatren trials was that they were not conducted with the primary aim of finding a dysentery treatment with fewer side effects.[159] Instead, these drugs were trialed because it was hoped that they might prove to have greater efficacy than emetine or be able to maximize its effects.

In a letter to Eugen Bernoulli, a leading Swiss pharmacist, Schweitzer maintained that emetine, when injected subcutaneously, was both non-toxic to humans and highly efficacious against the amoebae that cause dysentery, but on the condition that one always uses 'freshly prepared solutions, not older than 24 hours and stored away from light, no ampullae'. Schweitzer justified his challenge of Bernoulli's pharmaceutical authority with reference to his own abundant experience. 'I who so often work with emetine, practically don't know of any malfunctions or toxic side-effects', he wrote.[160] Schweitzer emphasized

---

154   Schnabel provides a long list of compounds that were given to dysenteric patients, often alongside emetine: calomel, bismuth subnitrate, kaolinite, Elkosam, simaruba, as well as tea and rice gruel, and Yatren for chronic cases with cysts. See: Schnabel, 'Medizinisches aus Albert Schweitzers Urwaldspital', 3.

155   Schweitzer's six other treatment options were: two different mixtures containing Yatren, bismuth, and chalk; emetine; Novarsénobensol; Yatren; and Rivanol. See the notebook '1930 Therapeutische Notizen', 59, AMS.

156   Schweitzer, *Das Spital im Urwald: Aufnahmen von Anna Wildikann*, 13.

157   See the notebook '1930 Therapeutische Notizen', 133, AMS.

158   The hospital issued about 3,000 pills per month, approximately 1,000 of which were given to leprosy patients, to treat unspecified forms of diarrhea, or amoebic dysentery. See: Friedmann to Schweitzer, 6 November 1957, AMS.

159   Although no side effects were reported from the trials, it is unlikely that none occurred.

160   Schweitzer to Bernoulli, 20 April 1950, AMS. In this letter, Schweitzer thanked Bernoulli for having published the seventh edition of his pharmaceutical encyclopedia in 1949, which he considered to be the most practical handbook on the market. Bernoulli and his co-editor therein recommended emetine to be injected either intra-muscularly or intravenously. In the next edition of 1955, they do not mention the subcutaneous option

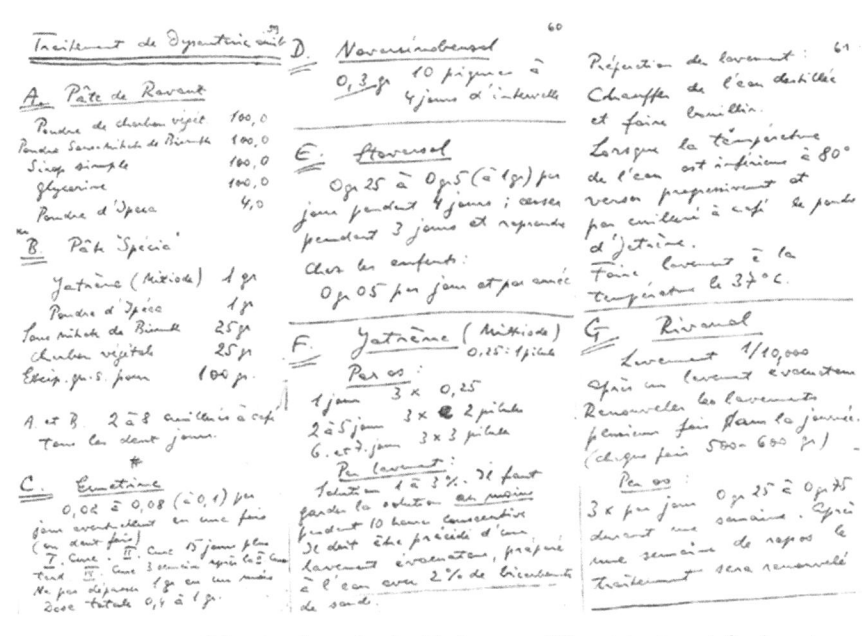

ILLUSTRATION 36   Schweitzer's notebook with the seven different treatments for dysentery, 1934
© ARCHIVES CENTRALES ALBERT SCHWEITZER GUNSBACH

his belief that, contrary to common perceptions, emetine had almost no side effects, but he also highlighted its high efficacy. Emetine trials were mostly concerned with efficacy, but it is likely that these trial-and-error tests also revealed a method to reduce its side effects. While not denying either of these benefits, specialists advised against injecting amoebic dysentery patients with emetine because this could render the disease-carrying amoebae resistant.[161]

Emetine was still in frequent use at the Albert Schweitzer Hospital after 1960.[162] A 1969 report by the WHO indicates that this was not unusual at the time. The drug's side effects remained the major concern, to mitigate against which the report recommended emetine's use in combination with antibiotics.[163] At

anymore. See: Lehmann and Bernoulli, *Übersicht der gebräuchlichen und neueren Arzneimittel*, 298.

161   In 1941, Philip Manson-Bahr, for example, recommended administering emetine bismuth iodide in capsules. See: Manson-Bahr, 'Amoebic Dysentery and Its Effective Treatment'. Philip Manson-Bahr was Patrick Manson's son-in-law and had adopted the family name after marriage. He edited the seventh to fifteenth editions of *Manson's Tropical Diseases*, a handbook first published by his father-in-law in 1898. The twenty-third edition was published in 2014.

162   Cousins, *Dr. Schweitzer of Lambaréné*, 209; Müller, '50 Jahre Albert-Schweitzer-Spital', 11.

163   Powell, 'Drug Therapy of Amoebiasis'.

Schweitzer's hospital, antibiotics were frequently prescribed in the post-surgery ward. Chloroquine was administered as a malaria prophylaxis, as was quinine for severe cases of the disease; penicillin injections were given to treat yaws; and gonorrhea and ulcers were treated with unspecified antibiotics.[164] In 1963, amoebic dysentery still represented a significant worry at the hospital, as Dr. Rolf Müller revealed in a medical journal article. In addition to emetine, he listed five further antiprotozoal drugs – but no antibiotics – as treatment options, of which Enterovioform is the only one discussed in this chapter.[165] These preparations were considered to have a higher degree of efficacy than emetine and doctors had learned how to offset its side effects, both factors that go a long way towards explaining why references to dysentery largely disappear from the sources after 1950. It is conspicuous, however, that neither Schweitzer nor any of his doctors praised these new compounds in the manner that they had done for emetine or for sulfones in the case of leprosy.

4.3   Sulfones and Side Effects

While emetine remained an important option in the fight against dysentery throughout the study period, chaulmoogra fell considerably out of favor in the treatment of leprosy as a result of the development of sulfone drugs during World War Two. In 1946, Schweitzer expressed his optimism about these new drugs, writing that 'in America, a substance related to the sulfanilamides, Promin, is also being successfully tested. How glad we doctors who deal with leprosy patients will be once we have a faster and better treatment'.[166] Two years later, he told Albert Einstein that the new drugs being used at the hospital, Promin and Diasone, 'really achieve what those used until today could not'.[167]

In 1946, there were 34 leprosy patients at the hospital.[168] This number rose to 150 in January 1951 and 350 in September of the same year,[169] with some patients coming from as far as 400 kilometers away. Schweitzer believed that this

---

164   Müller, '50 Jahre Albert-Schweitzer-Spital', 12–13. In this article, Müller analyzes the diagnoses of 2,500 patients, including, unusually, those of outpatients. Infectious diseases represented 13.9 percent of these diagnoses, rendering them the second most common disease category after parasitic diseases (14 percent). Without providing further details, Müller briefly refers to 'anthelmintic therapy and iron therapy' as treatments for parasitic diseases (10).

165   The others were Entobex, Intestopan, Bemarsal, and Atebrin. Ibid., 11.

166   Schweitzer, 'Briefe aus dem Lambarene Spital März 1946', 13.

167   This letter is published in: Bähr, *Albert Schweitzer: Leben, Werk und Denken*, 187.

168   'Statistiques de l'Hôpital 1946', L – A – S3, AMS.

169   See the *appels mensuels*, L – P – AM7, AMS.

influx of patients was due to the efficacy of the new sulfone drugs.[170] With numerous variants of the drugs available, many trial-and-error tests were conducted at the hospital. These did not, however, provide conclusive evidence of the drug with the fewest side effects.

Despite this usual optimism, Schweitzer initially had his doubts about the efficacy of sulfones. In January 1950, he wrote to Robert Weiss, his long-time pharmacist in Strasbourg, explaining that he still preferred using chaulmoogra oil as the basic drug to dissolve the wax layer of the leprosy bacilli. These could then be targeted with copper or Trypaflavin, 'with which I have always seen successes in association with chaulmoogra oil'.[171] At this point, Schweitzer believed that the new sulfone drugs should be administered in combination with these proven compounds.

Schweitzer's initial perception of sulfones as merely complementary changed radically in a short period of time. Just four months after writing to Weiss, he sent Emmy Martin the following decidedly enthusiastic assessment:

> I'm completely consumed by correspondence about new leprosy medications! A Parisian house 'Theraplix' has sent me a cheaper and at least as effective remedy to try, which is related to the American drugs but has the big advantage that it is taken through the mouth instead of intravenous injections. Yesterday I left everything, studied the question in the literature sent to me and placed my first order directly with the house, which I pay for from here. That leaves no time for anything else. But it is something wonderful, this simplification and price reduction of the whole fight against leprosy. All day long I staggered around like a donkey stunned by happiness (this time not by incense). The new remedy is called 'Disulone' with the scientific name 'Diamino-4-4Diphenylsulfone DDS. Sulfone 1350 F'. Please learn by heart...[172]

Ultimately, Disulone would not become the standard drug for the treatment of leprosy at the Albert Schweitzer Hospital. It is noteworthy, however, that Schweitzer underlined not only its lower cost and higher efficacy, but also its oral mode of application, which was favored by both patients and medical personnel. Diasone, which would become the most extensively used leprosy drug

---

170   He expressed this view in another letter to Einstein. See: Bähr, *Albert Schweitzer: Leben, Werk und Denken*, 209.

171   Schweitzer to Weiss, 9 January 1950, AMS.

172   Schweitzer to Martin, 16 May 1950, AMS.

at the hospital, was also ingested orally, an advantage referred to elsewhere,[173] but curiously rarely highlighted in the sources analyzed for this study.

Naegele, who arrived in February 1950 and served until May 1952, was the first doctor at the hospital to prescribe sulfone drugs on a regular basis. In 1950, he carried out a series of tests on which he reported in detail.[174] Diasone was given on its own to 167 out of a total of 265 leprosy in- and outpatients. Naegele then matched the length of treatment and the amount of Diasone that each patient received with his or her condition, which he defined as 'improved, stagnant, aggravated, cured, deceased'. He concluded that 'the effect obtained is more or less directly proportional to the amount of sulfones ingested', but acknowledged that the number of patients was too low to draw any confident conclusions. Naegele was also interested in the question of side effects, summarizing that 'in general we had no difficulty with our four-week treatment (on average 15 g of Diasone) cut by a fifteen-day rest period', albeit with the qualification that an aggravation of typical leprosy symptoms often occurred immediately after the first application of the drug.[175] Thirty of the remaining patients received Diasone as well as an additional drug – most frequently Trypaflavin. This trial also indicated encouraging results, but the hospital ran out of Trypaflavin during the course of the year. In a final trial, sixteen patients received either Disulone, which had excited Schweitzer so much, or its American prodrug equivalent, Promin, as a complementary treatment to Diasone. Naegele noted very promising results with Promin. It positively affected 'cases with general skin infiltration' and had 'a very noticeable influence on leprosy wounds'.[176]

Half a year after these trials, Naegele provided updated results. He now claimed that Promin was the 'most superior sulfone'[177] in terms of efficacy, but a closer examination of his explanation reveals that this observation was based on inconsistent evidence.[178] Naegele observed that different patients reacted

173   Faget, Pogge, and Johansen, 'Present Status of Diasone in the Treatment of Leprosy', 961. See also: Gould, *A Disease Apart*, 290.

174   Naegele, 'Traitement des malades lépreux à l'Hôpital du Docteur Albert Schweitzer à Lambaréné au cours de l'année 1950', AMS.

175   Ibid., 3.

176   Ibid., 4.

177   Naegele to Schweitzer, 4 June 1951, AMS.

178   A total of 21 patients received Promin, 106 received Diasone, and 32 received Disulone. In each trial, between 46 and 50 percent of the patients' conditions improved (10 with Promin, 49 with Diasone, 16 with Disulone). Between 38 and 46 percent of patients showed no change (8 with Promin, 49 with Diasone, 12 with Disulone). At 12 percent, Disulone provided the highest percentage of patients whose condition deteriorated. All three sulfones were administered for at least six months, 'because this seems to be the "time limit"

differently to different sulfones and concluded that 'probably those people are right who call for selecting the most effective and best tolerated sulfone for each patient anew'.[179] This approach differed from that of many doctors in Africa and Europe alike, who aimed to find a standard drug or establish a standardized treatment regime for leprosy. At the end of 1951, Naegele shifted his focus back onto side effects. In this regard, he named Diasone as the 'best tolerated sulfone', but acknowledged that more conclusive claims could not yet be made given the drug's estimated application period of two to three years.[180]

When Naegele left the hospital in 1952, Schweitzer recorded his doctor's recommendations and observations in his notebook. The conclusions of both men reveal that they weighted efficacy less heavily than side effects when evaluating a drug's potential. They declared Promin to be the most efficacious drug, but also the one with the most regular side effects, and recommended using it only when other drugs did not work. Both still considered Diasone to be the drug with the fewest side effects, even when taken in very high doses.[181] Schweitzer explained to Robert Weiss that 'Diasone has proved to be the most useful, albeit slow acting remedy because of its relative harmlessness'. However, Schweitzer was aware that there were less expensive alternatives and expressed his intention to conduct further trials.[182]

Cost was a constant concern for Schweitzer. Later in 1952, Dr. Emeric Percy, who took over from Naegele, updated Schweitzer on 'new ways in leprosy therapy'. Unlike Naegele, Percy trialed chaulmoogra again, while the other compounds remain unknown. Schweitzer did not reproduce these findings in detail, and Percy's letters have not survived, but the results Percy had summarized pleased the hospital director.[183] These promised a reduction in side effects and an end to the 'ghost of anemia', and would enable the doctors to return to using the 'cheaper Disulone', Schweitzer's initial preference. Percy's trials also confirmed Schweitzer's belief that 'chaulmoogra doesn't lose its significance next to the sulfones',[184] a conviction he had already professed in his letter to Weiss some three years earlier, before Naegele had started trialing sulfones.

In 1953, Schweitzer once again listed detailed guidelines on the treatment of leprosy in his notebook. These were a combination of Naegele's and Percy's

---

after which first effects occur on a regular basis, after "primary deteriorations", which also occur on a regular basis, have abated following the first or second course of treatment'.

179   Naegele to Schweitzer, 8 June 1951, AMS.
180   Naegele, 'Streiflichter aus Lambarene. 1951 III. Um die Lepra', AMS, 3–4.
181   See the notebook 'Medizinische Notizen, Albert Schweitzer Lambarene 1953', 41ff, AMS.
182   Schweitzer to Weiss, 8 January 1952, AMS.
183   Schweitzer to Percy, 14 August 1952, AMS.
184   Schweitzer to Percy, 13 November 1952, AMS.

findings, and incorporated the notable return of chaulmoogra. Under the heading 'treatment of the lepers: fundamentals', Schweitzer determined that each patient would receive a 'base therapy' with a sulfone drug, either Disulone, Diasone, or Promin. He did not stipulate how the specific drug was to be selected, but defined the subsequent procedure as follows:

> Keep up this treatment if permanent improvement is shown after controls every 6 weeks. If there is stagnation of various months, then add injections of Promin or Disulone Retard or both, and in any case chaulmoogra. If that doesn't help then change fundamentally.[185]

The many 'ifs', 'ors', 'whens' and 'thens' in this excerpt reveal the hospital's adoption of the case-to-case approach that Naegele had already recommended after his first trials and which would be implemented more frequently in the following years. In a jointly written document entitled 'medical work at the Hospital', Percy and Schweitzer insisted in 1955 that 'more and more we expand the principle that leprosy must be treated individually and not schematically. This means that not only the drug itself, but also the dosage has to be adapted individually'.[186] As a result of this policy, a large variety of sulfone drugs were used at the hospital.

In 1956, Schweitzer wrote to Bernoulli again, disclosing further information on the properties that a drug needed to possess in order to be prescribed at his hospital. The pharmacologist had claimed in the eighth edition of the pharmaceutical encyclopedia he co-edited, published in 1955, that Promin was no longer used. As in the case of emetine, Schweitzer invoked his experience to correct Bernoulli. 'But for those working with leprosy that verdict is not valid. For those, Promin remains one of the best, if not the best, remedy against leprosy!' he wrote.[187] According to Schweitzer, Promin's main disadvantage was that it had to be injected daily. This was practically impossible in most parts of the world in which leprosy was prevalent, where there were typically few medical practitioners as well as a trend towards the abandonment of the asylum model due to financial considerations. This letter is a rare instance in which Schweitzer or his staff discussed the preferences of their patients. He claimed that

---

185 See the notebook 'Medizinische Notizen, Albert Schweitzer Lambarene 1953', 33f, AMS.
186 As the following page of this document is missing, there are no further details on the treatment of leprosy to be found. It is unclear if the document was written for internal use or public discussion. It is kept among Emeric Percy's correspondence at the AMS.
187 Schweitzer to Bernoulli, 20 October 1956, AMS.

My patients keep asking me to treat them with Promin. The reason for this is that it is administered intravenously, meaning that there is no risk of abscesses, which often occur with even the best intramuscular techniques.[188]

Schweitzer did not disclose that the hospital's favored leprosy medication, Diasone, was administered orally, and not by injection, and that the doctors had found it to have the fewest side effects of all sulfone drugs. Instead, he focused on Promin's supposedly superior efficacy, but claimed, somewhat contradictorily, that patients preferred it because of its comparatively few side effects, while his doctors had concluded that the drug had many of them.

Such confident statements notwithstanding, trials with further leprosy drugs continued at the hospital. A trial-and-error approach was imposed on patients when their condition would not improve, as a report on Leprosan trials illustrates.[189] Starting in October 1956, twelve patients received this new Austrian sulfone brand. Eight of these patients had lived at the hospital for five years or more, during which time their condition had not improved despite having been given as many as seven different leprosy drugs during the course of their stay, not including those administered to treat secondary afflictions such as skin infections. It is not known whether these were the only patients whose conditions did not improve, which seems unlikely; neither is it possible to reconstruct the criteria by which they were selected to receive Leprosan. Besides one exception who suffered 'severe reactions', the other eleven patients showed promising signs after taking the drug for five months. Although this was admitted to be too limited a trial period to deliver meaningful results, Schweitzer ordered a large quantity of Leprosan, which he classed as 'excellent'.[190]

This document on the Leprosan trials also illustrates that even sulfones, which were regarded as fairly efficacious, were not without alternatives (see Illustration 37). Five of the twelve patients had received an antibiotic, Citocilline, to target the bacilli. A more illuminating case, on which further details are available, was Vitamin D. The document lists one patient as having also been treated with the vitamin at some point of his or her stay.

---

188 Ibid.. As if the authors followed Schweitzer's suggestion, unlike in the case of emetine, they changed the entry on Promin in the next (ninth) edition of 1959. They wrote that Promin 'must, because not well tolerated int., be administered i-ven., but is a very efficacious remedy if controlled well'. Lehmann and Bernoulli, *Übersicht der gebräuchlichen und neueren Arzneimittel*, 330.

189 This document is entitled 'Leprosan Patienten' and dated 14 February 1958; the author is unknown. It is kept in an unnamed box at the AMS.

190 Schweitzer to Kik, 6 June 1958, AMS. I could not obtain any further useful information on Leprosan.

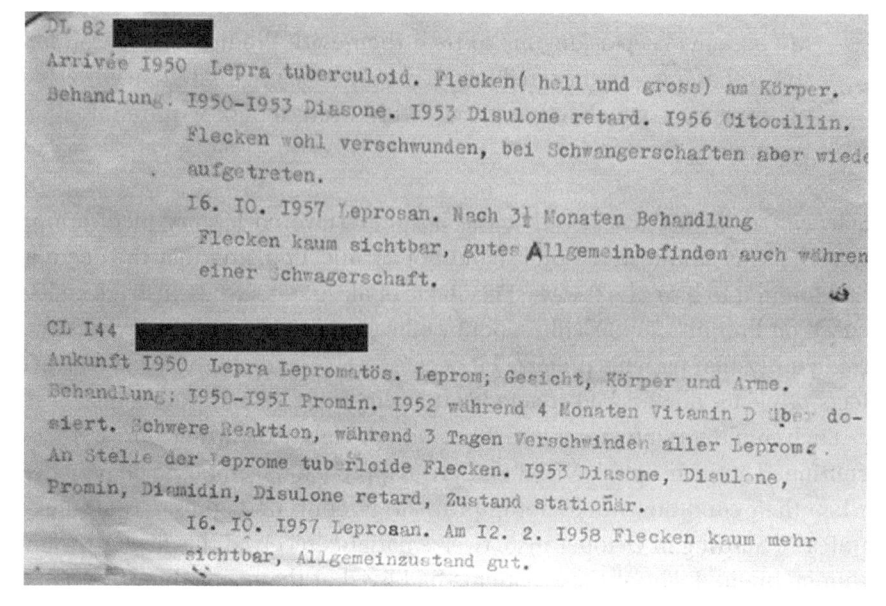

ILLUSTRATION 37   From the Leprosan trials; list of drugs that a patient had received, 1958
© ARCHIVES CENTRALES ALBERT SCHWEITZER GUNSBACH

Naegele had noted in his 1951 report that a 'very small' number of patients had received high dosages of Vitamin D and that the results were 'promising'.[191] The doctors soon realized, however, that the vitamin was highly problematic due to its side effects, and thus agreed to suspend testing. In 1953, Schweitzer recorded in his notebook that Vitamin D was 'too dangerous in greater quantities'; a woman who had been given ten grams per day for a period of six weeks was now in 'danger of life'. Schweitzer concluded that 'the efficacy is there, but you need to go almost to the toxic dose'.[192] Vitamin D and chaulmoogra – as well as Stovarsol and Jodalgin in the case of dysentery – were thus seriously considered to replace or complement an efficacious standard drug, emetine or Diasone, which had received such a reputation by a process that was by no means straightforward. In their daily practices, doctors were regularly confronted with the shortcomings of these new drugs, which they attempted to overcome via further trial-and-error tests.

The last file relating to leprosy among the archival sources, probably from 1958, is entitled 'leprosy medicaments' and was intended as a guideline for

191   Naegele, 'Streiflichter aus Lambarene. 1951 III. Um die Lepra', AMS, 3–4.
192   See the notebook 'Medizinische Notizen, Albert Schweitzer Lambarene 1953', 45f, AMS.

prospective personnel at the hospital.[193] The doctors now attempted to standardize treatment and provide an alternative for each option. As stated in the document, chaulmoogra was no longer used. Diasone had become the standard drug, with Promin prescribed to patients who did not react to Diasone, and Leprosan to those who did not respond to Promin. These sulfones were not to be given in combination with other drugs, except when a patient suffered from chronic rheumatic diseases or had a heart condition. Other diseases were always to be treated before administering sulfones. Antibiotics were considered useful in halting secondary infections and thus improving a patient's overall condition. Given the constant shifts in treatment detailed in this chapter, it is doubtful that this neatly structured treatment regime remained in place for long at the Albert Schweitzer Hospital.

5 Conclusion

Leaving aside the pharmaceutical treatment methods employed there, Schweitzer's leprosy settlement represented somewhat of an anachronism. In the 1950s, at a time when French colonies were directing their efforts towards outpatient treatment, Schweitzer's leprosery operated as an open-access space where patients could bring their families and stay for an extended period of time. Contrasting with the earlier harsh treatment of dysentery patients, who were regularly forced into isolation in a locked ward, this arrangement was not only a manifestation of Schweitzer's particular socio-medical ideology and his ethics, but was also dependent on the nature of the available pharmaceuticals.

Pharmaceutical treatment of infectious diseases followed the pattern sketched out in this chapter. A single drug – chaulmoogra, emetine, or Diasone – would be used as the standard treatment for a disease. However, this would often be rejected by patients, provide unsatisfactory results, or provoke adverse side effects. A range of other drugs would then be trialed as alternatives or additional treatment options. Pharmaceutical innovations promised more efficacious treatments, thereby attracting patients in greater numbers, the treatment of whom exposed the limitations of new drugs. Doctors were forced to react to this pattern by conducting trial-and-error tests with other drugs or drug combinations.

---

193   This document is not dated, but in all likelihood originates from 1958, when results of the Leprosan trials became known. It is kept with the file on the Leprosan trials in the same unnamed box at the AMS.

While the laboratory or experiment metaphor might be useful for understanding scientific practices in the colonies and even the metropole, it is less applicable to the Albert Schweitzer Hospital and presumably to other hospitals with a focus on curative services. Doctors at the hospital did not seek to participate in the wider circulation of scientific knowledge; their aim was not to test whether a drug could be universally applied, nor was it to draw universally applicable conclusions from the trials that they conducted. Instead, doctors aimed to find a treatment model that was easily adaptable to their daily practices. They tested a drug's suitability for their own patients, inquiring whether a particular individual could tolerate a specific drug. Such improvised trials could be performed easily at the Albert Schweitzer Hospital, where a constant supply of a large variety of medications was available.

Healing and 'Civilizing': Community and Safety in Psychiatric Care

In early 1927, Schweitzer informed his supporters in Europe about Njambi, a patient who had been brought to the Albert Schweitzer Hospital in chains a few months earlier:

> In mental derangement, he had killed a woman. In the cell he slowly calmed down. Now he has reached the point where he is allowed to move around freely under surveillance and to occupy himself. He sharpens axes and goes into the forest with Miss Russell and helps cutting down trees.[1]

Since this is not a horror thriller, I can assure you that the story continued well for Miss Russell.[2] Njambi's subsequent story would be marked by numerous ups and downs. While his cell would frequently become the source of security concerns – a scene of recurring violence and, in response, involuntary drugging – he and his fellow psychiatric patients were to be 'civilized' through occupational therapy.

An analysis of psychiatric care and the reasoning behind it allows reconstructing how the latter influenced the former. Like many of their colleagues all over the world, Schweitzer and some of his psychiatric personnel believed that the modernity imposed by colonialism represented a threat to the mental health of colonized persons, but at the same time suggested that the existing beliefs of their patients were to blame for their mental illnesses. While the number of psychiatric patients at the hospital was relatively low, it rose from six in the late 1920s to twenty-five in the 1960s, the many case studies in the sources allow for an analysis of how patients and their communities understood their own disorders.

---

1 Schweitzer, *Mitteilungen aus Lambarene. Drittes Heft, 1925–1927*, 53.
2 Lilian Russell returned repeatedly to Lambaréné to work in the plantations, a task that would later be performed by psychiatric patients. She also supported Schweitzer from abroad, for example by translating parts of his work. Russell was the first person to bring a video camera to the hospital. The short film 'Aus dem Urwaldspital von Dr. Albert Schweitzer in Lambarene (1935)' was made from her material.

1   Psychiatric Services and Ideology in Colonial Africa and at the
         Hospital

In colonial Africa, few hospitals offered beds to psychiatric patients, and the
number of asylums remained constantly low.[3] This indicates that the Foucauldian confinement of deviant individuals was not common during this period.[4]
Before asylums began to be established on a more regular basis in African colonies in the opening decades of the twentieth century, it was not unusual for
psychiatric patients, African and European, to be sent to facilities in the metropole.[5] Early African asylums did not differ significantly from those in Europe,
with mental institutions on both continents custodial in nature.[6] Numerous
observers compared the conditions in African asylums to those of prisons, often unfavorably.[7] A more therapeutic and less restrictive approach was only
adopted in African institutions after 1950.

   Until at least 1950, the so-called ethnopsychiatrists, colonial doctors and
medical researchers working at the interface of psychiatry and ethnography,
were important drivers of debates on African mental health. Their underlying
assumption was that the minds of Africans functioned differently to those of
Europeans. They began by explaining 'African inferiority […] in terms of physical endowment and brain structure', then with reference to 'cultural patterns
and child-rearing conventions'.[8] While these findings were challenged by a
number of peers, they were more often reinforced by contemporary scientific
methodologies.[9] Since the 'Other' was located within the colonial subject in
this construction, mentally ill Africans, unlike their European counterparts, became 'insufficiently "Other"', as Megan Vaughan terms it. They were individuals
'who spoke of being rich, of hearing voices through radio sets, of being powerful, who imitated the white man in dress and behaviour'.[10] Such discussions on

---

3   One of these was Mengo Hospital in Uganda. See: Pringle, 'Neurasthenia at Mengo Hospi-
     tal, Uganda'.
4   Keller, 'Madness and Colonization', 313; Vaughan, 'Psychiatry and Empire, Introduction', 2.
5   Ngalamulume, 'The Regulation of Madness in Sénégal, 1890–1914'; Scarfone, 'Italian Colo-
     nial Psychiatry', 397.
6   Porter, 'Madness and Its Institutions', 278.
7   In East Africa, asylums emerged out of the prison system, with patients usually forcibly
     committed. See: Mahone, 'East African Psychiatry and the Practical Problems of Empire',
     43. On the comparison with prisons, see: Vaughan, 'Psychiatry and Empire, Introduction', 2.
8   McCulloch, *Colonial Psychiatry and the African Mind*, 141.
9   Ibid., 75; Vaughan, *Curing Their Ills*, 109–15.
10   Vaughan, *Curing Their Ills*, 101. Lynette Jackson underlines how, given this discursive con-
     text, mentally ill African women, as the 'others' other', posed a particular challenge for
     colonial officials. See: Jackson, *Surfacing Up*, 102.

racial difference were at the core of a wider debate, 'namely whether the emphasis of the colonial regime should be on providing stability to the subject population or on undertaking grand projects of social transformation'.[11] Ethnopsychiatrists, and a broad variety of colonial interest groups who shared their views, favored the latter option because they assumed that Europeans, their minds, and their 'civilization' were superior to the societies of colonized peoples. This belief persisted well into the 1950s before coming under increasing challenge from anti-colonial movements across the world.[12]

In his early years in Gabon, Schweitzer subscribed to Darwinian ideas in this respect. He believed that different societies possessed essentially the same culture, but were at different stages in their evolutionary journey towards 'civilization'. Matthieu Arnold, who has analyzed the sermons that Schweitzer gave in Lambaréné until 1934, offers an intriguing analogy to describe this asymmetric relationship between societies: 'the one between the doctor, who rescues, and the patient, who is saved'.[13] The well-known analogy that Schweitzer proposed himself in 1921 is that of an older and a younger brother.[14]

In later years, Schweitzer stopped referring to evolutionary stages, choosing instead to emphasize inherent differences between cultures. In 1953, he wrote a letter to the French writer Marcel Thiébaud, asking him to treat it 'absolutely confidential'. Nowhere else did Schweitzer express his thoughts on the political and social state of France's African colonies in such an outspoken manner:

> The big question: Will the natives be capable of administering themselves? The answer of those who know their mentality: they are not capable and will never be. [...] Living with the least effort is his ideal. [...] This is his mentality. We'll never change it. [...] They live in a world that is a product of civilization. They live in this world, they inhabit it, but they do not belong to it spiritually.[15]

Besides the negative and static image of Africans that Schweitzer conveys here, it is noteworthy that he considered spirituality to be an important feature of his conception of 'civilization'. According to his theory, 'civilization', which was by definition Western, shaped and encompassed people's life all the way to Lambaréné. Africans, who defied the principles that underlay Schweitzer's

---

11   Heaton, *Black Skin, White Coats*, 32.
12   McCulloch, *Colonial Psychiatry and the African Mind*, 138.
13   Arnold, 'Vous les noirs, nous les blancs', 440.
14   Schweitzer, *Zwischen Wasser und Urwald*, 124.
15   Schweitzer to Thiébaud, 24 July 1953, AMS.

ideal, were not really part of it. This understanding influenced the way in which patients were treated at the hospital, as is especially obvious in the case of the mentally ill.

However, as discussed in the Introduction, Schweitzer also viewed Western 'civilization' in a negative light and wanted to protect Africans from its adverse influences. As argued in Chapters 2 and 3, he refrained from intruding into certain spheres of African life. Such an approach to healthcare in developing countries had become more widely accepted by the 1960s, by which time the notion of a European 'civilizing mission' no longer went unquestioned. In the words of Michael A. Woodbury, who was part of a team of psychiatrists who visited Lambaréné for two weeks in late 1963, Schweitzer

> shows no great desire to impose any part of a civilization that may have produced the most beautiful bathrooms in the world but has also developed the most efficient man-killing machines ever devised. And as psychiatrists we know, moreover, that cleanliness, anal training, and destructiveness may be closely related.[16]

The omnipresence of African labor at the hospital suggests that Schweitzer believed that the institution should serve as a vehicle to diffuse a particular version of the 'civilizing mission' rooted in manual labor and shaped by Christian ethics and spirituality. For Schweitzer, infrastructure development and schooling were not central aspects of this quest, as he stated in 1924. According to him, the key question was 'how will the blacks become hardworking people?' He offered a simple answer, namely that 'they become hardworking through religious and moral instruction and through workmanship'.[17] Thirty years later, he expressed his views on the topic in very similar words. 'One of the great tasks facing those who work with primitives and semi-primitives is to educate them in the right estimation of manual labor', he wrote.[18]

The central position assumed by labor in Schweitzer's conception of the 'civilizing mission' is especially evident in the case of psychiatric care. Manual

---

16   Woodbury et al., 'Psychiatric Care at the Albert Schweitzer Hospital', 149. Woodbury was the director of research and psychotherapy at the Prangins clinic in the Swiss canton of Vaud. He was accompanied to Lambaréné by Elizabeth S. Palacios, a psychiatrist based at Chestnut Lodge, a psychiatric institution in Maryland, and William Thomas, an auxiliary at Crownsville State Hospital, Maryland. They were sponsored by the Visiting International Psychiatric Teams, Inc. No further information on these individuals or this corporation could be found.

17   Schweitzer, 'Mitteilungen aus Lambarene. Zweites Heft, 1924–1925', 130.

18   Schweitzer, 'Briefe aus dem Lambarenespital Oktober 1954', 16.

labor had long been an everyday feature of life at institutions for the mentally ill in colonial and metropolitan settings alike. In the first half of the nineteenth century, inmates of European asylums were typically put to work, 'partly for reasons of economy, partly implementing an ideology of cure through labour'.[19] These two motives also drove practices in colonial asylums, except in the case of European patients, who were exempted from duties of manual labor.[20] Since most studies of psychiatric institutions in Africa do not focus on aspects of patients' day-to-day life, the role of work in African asylums remains unclear. Ingutsheni Mental Hospital in colonial Zimbabwe is one exception; there, 'work was such a central feature of the psychiatric hospital routine that many patients, when asked why they were at the hospital, replied that they had been sent there to work'.[21] In the mid-1920s, African patients at the institution were ordered to grow cotton.[22] When the superintendent attempted to compel European inmates to likewise participate in such work, he risked upsetting the colonial social order so deeply that he was dismissed from his post.[23]

For the most part, work in colonial asylums was intended as a means of keeping patients busy rather than healing them. Efforts to cure patients became more widespread only in the late 1930s, when new therapeutic technologies, such as lobotomies and electroconvulsive therapy, became available.[24] In the mid-1950s, psychoactive drugs, known today as antipsychotics or neuroleptics, renewed hopes of developing cures for mental illness.[25] A variety of drugs had hitherto been used to treat mental afflictions,[26] but the extent of drug use in psychiatric cases now rose to a new level. Doctors appreciated the ability of

---

19 Porter, 'Madness and Its Institutions', 296. In Germany, encouraging 'usefulness' among psychiatric patients was considered important in the early twentieth century, but occupational therapy never enjoyed a prominent status, unlike in Switzerland, for example, where it generated more interest. See: Schott and Tölle, *Geschichte der Psychiatrie*, 443.

20 In South-East Asian asylums, whereas local patients participated in harvesting crops, construction work, painting, and laundry tasks, European inmates enjoyed 'outdoor leisure activities'. Edington, *Beyond the Asylum*, 153.

21 Jackson, *Surfacing Up*, 161.

22 Ibid., 50–51.

23 Ibid., 150–55.

24 Psychiatrists in Algeria were at the forefront of testing and administering these therapies, achieving curative success rates far exceeding those in metropolitan France. See: Keller, 'Taking Science to the Colonies', 27–28. In relation to Nigeria in the 1930s, Sadowsky notes that 'although officials usually saw little ambiguity in the identification of African lunatics, the cure of these persons was seen beyond colonial competence'. Sadowsky, *Imperial Bedlam*, 37.

25 Keller, 'Taking Science to the Colonies', 34–35; Heaton, *Black Skin, White Coats*, 161.

26 Pringle, 'Neurasthenia at Mengo Hospital, Uganda', 255. The Albert Schweitzer Hospital is a further case in point, as we will see.

antipsychotics to suppress the major symptoms of a range of mental illnesses. Their apparent universality 'also helped to foster the reemergence of biological notions of the nature of the human mind'.[27] These drugs were popular among patients, or more precisely their therapy management group, too. Mentally ill individuals in colonial Zimbabwe, for example, were taken to psychiatric clinics to be pacified, but continued to consult local healers when seeking a diagnosis or a cure.[28]

Antipsychotics were considered crucial for the success of the new therapeutic approaches that emerged in the late 1950s, such as that exemplified in the Aro Village Scheme established and operated by a group of Nigerian psychiatrists. In line with contemporary global trends, participating doctors administered antipsychotics to stabilize patients in order to perform 'psychoanalysis, community therapy, or other forms of social psychiatry'.[29] They also cooperated with local traditional healers during therapy.[30] In Dakar, the Fann neuropsychological clinic introduced an open-door policy that permitted relatives to stay with patients. It also regularly organized a '*Penc*, a meeting of the hospital ward, modeled on a village palaver'.[31]

At the Albert Schweitzer Hospital, the wider community was granted no role in therapeutic practices. Instead, psychiatric patients were sought to be included into a community *within* the hospital. Occupational and pharmaceutical therapies were applied for this purpose from very early on. The ways in which labor, drugs, and community were intertwined in this process is a central focus of this chapter. Unlike other colonial doctors and consistent with the therapeutic optimism he displayed in the fight against leprosy and other infectious diseases, Schweitzer had already envisioned being able to cure mentally ill patients in the 1920s.[32] In 1931, he reported to the congregation at the Guildhouse in London, whose members were particularly supportive of his psychiatric endeavors, that 'several of our insane people were cured'.[33]

---

27   Heaton, *Black Skin, White Coats*, 26.

28   Jackson, *Surfacing Up*, 11.

29   Heaton, *Black Skin, White Coats*, 176. However, frustration at the use of these drugs soon grew in Nigeria. Psychiatrists felt that they were not able to execute proper psychotherapeutic work because antipsychotics were being used simply to reduce the number of staff working at psychiatric institutions.

30   This pushed Nigerian-born, Western-trained psychiatrists into a specialist role as gatekeepers who claimed to be uniquely capable of understanding issues arising in the fusion of traditional therapies with biomedical practices. See Chapter 5 of: Heaton, *Black Skin, White Coats*.

31   Collignon, 'Some Aspects of Mental Illness in French-Speaking West Africa', 172.

32   Schweitzer, 'Mitteilungen Aus Lambarene 1924–25', 157.

33   Schweitzer to Schweitzer Comittee, 2 July 1931, AWHS.

In the early 1960s, by which time it was more widely believed that the mentally ill could be cured of their afflictions, a number of visiting psychiatrists expressed their esteem of the therapeutic practices at the Albert Schweitzer Hospital. George R. Andrews, who visited the hospital from Wisconsin for one week in 1961, praised the institution's combined approach of pharmaceutical and occupational therapy as effective in 'helping the patient make a transition as quickly as possible back to the community'.[34] Three years later, Woodbury declared that Schweitzer's 'psychiatric service is a more therapeutic ward than the majority I have visited in the United States or in Europe'.[35] Dr. Louise Jilek-Aall, who would later become a professor of psychiatry at the University of British Columbia, claimed that 'many a psychiatric patient had recovered enough under the care of the hospital staff to return to his village', although 'some would come back looking for help again when they felt a relapse threatened their lives or that of other villagers'.[36] The confinement and isolation of psychiatric patients was thus presented as being in the best interests of their communities, while at the same time offering the best hope for a cure.

Despite such claims that emphasize the therapeutic nature of the hospital's approach, in practice staff was more concerned about enforcing confinement. Doctors at the hospital did regularly acknowledge failures to heal the mentally ill. Many admitted the limits of their understanding of local lifeworlds. Such instances furnish the historian with opportunities to study doctors' beliefs about what caused mental illness among Africans.

Schweitzer often attributed unsuccessful attempts to cure patients, including mentally ill, to his belief that they had been poisoned, an opinion that he and others maintained throughout the study period.[37] At the same time, he also speculated that poisoning was an overly invoked explanation for mysterious deaths or symptoms.[38] In one way or another, however, poison features in most of the examples presented in this chapter. Besides explaining diagnostic and therapeutic limits, doctors attributed poisoning to the worldview of their patients, which many perceived as fundamentally different from their own, backward and irrational. According to the doctors' argumentation, only such contexts would enable poisoning and only individuals adhering to such beliefs would suffer from fear of being poisoned. In 1936, for example, Dr. Heinz

---

34 Andrews, 'Psychiatric Facilities at the Albert Schweitzer Hospital', 526. No further information on Andrews could be found.

35 Woodbury et al., 'Psychiatric Care at the Albert Schweitzer Hospital', 149.

36 Jilek-Aall, *Working with Dr. Schweitzer*, 163.

37 For a summary of examples thereof, see: Ohls, *Improvisationen der Ehrfurcht vor allem Lebendigen*, 184–88.

38 Schweitzer, *Zwischen Wasser und Urwald*, 47.

Barasch reported that 'we house a new insane man; a schizophrenia with persecution ideas. (Supposedly, his family wants to poison him)'.[39] Here, Barasch considered the fear of poisoning to be a form of persecution mania. In this reasoning, the patient's adherence to his 'irrational' worldview made him sick, with his beliefs in the possibility of being poisoned to blame for his pathological fear.

Schweitzer likewise believed that their 'superstition' was not beneficial for his patients' mental health. He maintained that he and his staff were unable to fully understand those 'superstitions'. In 1939, he reflected in great detail on his inability to relate to his patients or their lifeworlds:

> The natives who come to us in our hospital and let us treat them often have thoughts of which we do not know anything. As a result of a taboo, a curse or a spell, their soul is in an emotional distress that remains hidden from us. [...] We always regret that our patients so rarely bring it about themselves to let us take a look at the emotional misery in which they find their soul. If they did, we could help in many a case in a very different manner. Psychotherapy as a supplement to purely medical treatment is sometimes much more necessary for the savages than for the whites.[40]

From this perspective, African patients' worldview was the cause of their pathological anxieties. 'Civilizing' their minds was thus a fundamental task for any colonial doctor. Schweitzer assigned psychotherapy a central role in this process. Not proposing a culturally adapted treatment, he aimed to use psychotherapy to bring about a radical change of mindset among African patients towards a worldview based on Western values and conceptions and, above all, devoid of 'superstition'. He justified this version of the 'civilizing mission' with reference to psychiatric imperatives:

> Anyone who has ever penetrated a bit into the primitive imagination and knows something about the states of anxiety in which people can find themselves, for whom taboos, unpreventable curses, and effective magic spells exist, is no longer in doubt that we have to attempt to cure them of these superstitions.[41]

---

39   Barasch to Schweitzer, 3 June 1936, AMS.
40   Schweitzer, *Afrikanische Geschichten*, 61–62.
41   Ibid., 62.

In practice, however, Schweitzer's 'civilizing mission' focused on disciplining African bodies through manual labor, rather than on civilizing the minds of his patients by indoctrinating them with Western ideas.

In East Africa in the 1930s, colonial doctors considered the 'clash of cultures' and 'detribalization' as the main causes of mental illness among Africans.[42] Since the early twentieth century, neurasthenia, for instance, had become 'part of a wider discussion about detribalisation, in which a person's social environment was as important as race'.[43] In Europe the condition was also associated with the stress of 'modernity', but its main trigger for Europeans in the tropics, besides climate, was thought to be separation from 'civilization' and urban life.[44] In contrast, urbanity represented a key risk factor for mental illness among Africans, as Lynette Jackson argues. Her explanation focuses on her assertion that the mental health of Africans was more likely to be scrutinized in urban environments.[45] The implication thereof was that men were more likely to be committed to mental institutions. They 'surfaced up', 'because of their formal incorporation into colonial institutional frameworks', while women were more likely to be committed for 'their lack of incorporation'.[46] For the case of Algeria, Nina Studer has coined the term 'hidden patients' for these mentally ill women who would usually not end up in colonial facilities.[47]

Arguing that colonialism produced mental illness and molded its symptoms,[48] Frantz Fanon warned of the severe effects of colonial rule and colonial psychiatry on colonized individuals.[49] The tensions that Fanon highlighted between colonial rule and the so-called 'civilizing mission' or between a supposed modernity and mental health had been key concerns for doctors before him and remain prevalent.[50] Conservative psychiatrists had documented

---

42 Mahone, 'East African Psychiatry and the Practical Problems of Empire', 47–48.

43 Pringle, 'Neurasthenia at Mengo Hospital, Uganda', 243, 253. Pringle hence links Neurasthenia with education and class, rather than race.

44 Crozier, 'What Was Tropical about Tropical Neurasthenia?'.

45 Jackson, *Surfacing Up*, 70–71.

46 Ibid., 103. At the root of this claim was the argument that 'African women were characterized as normally abnormal, even without the 'civilization' that was needed to unbalance the minds of native men', ibid., 107.

47 Studer, *The Hidden Patients*,.

48 For a discussion of these arguments, see: Sadowsky, *Imperial Bedlam*, 3.

49 Fanon argued that depicting the colonized as lazy, criminal, and violent made them resist colonialism in precisely these ways. For a deeper analysis of this argument, see: Studer, *The Hidden Patients*, 24–25. Frederick Cooper argues that such a simple transfer of 'issues of state sovereignty to personal autonomy' might neglect the 'multidimensional contexts in which personalities are actually shaped'. Cooper, 'Conflict and Connection', 1542–43.

50 For example, René Collignon writes: 'Current economic changes facing Africans and their devastating effects on the traditional family and other solidarity-enhancing groups have

how colonialism alienated individuals from their self and the surrounding environment, but concluded that the colonized were too slow to adapt, thus bringing mental instability upon themselves.[51] According to mainstream psychiatric thinking, "'the African" in the twentieth century, like the European woman in the nineteenth century, was simply not equipped to cope with "civilization"'.[52] Many colonial doctors, including Schweitzer, identified two apparent forms of madness among Africans: their innate irrationality and their inability to cope with 'modernity'. Education and economic change were seen as possible remedies for the former, but these came with the disadvantage of inducing the latter.[53]

There is evidence that Schweitzer's understanding of what caused mental illness among his African patients had altered by the 1960s, as had his ideas of how to cure them. In a purported conversation with Dr. Edgar Berman, he discussed how the inherent characteristics that he claimed to have identified among Africans affected their mental health. Schweitzer and Berman talked about a woman known as Mama Sans Nom, one of the most recognizable individuals with an apparent mental illness at the hospital. In many ways, Mama Sans Nom was an atypical patient or inmate, although neither of these designations is appropriate in her case. She was of unknown origin and name, spoke an unidentified language, slept outdoors between two buildings, smoked a pipe, ate worms, regularly sang and danced, walked around without clothes, and came and went as she pleased.[54] Berman was surprised that she had been diagnosed with dementia 'not, as is generally conceded, resulting from the modern family and the fast sophisticated living we endure, but derived from

---

forced the individual to face the challenges of competition, including the management of aggressiveness. The development of clinical material over the years seems to emphasize the progressive appearance of guilt in association with increasing modernity'. Collignon, 'Some Aspects of Mental Illness in French-Speaking West Africa', 172. Other authors place more emphasis on the enduring personal impact of emotional trauma suffered during conflict as well as on the effects of macroeconomic decline on the individual. See: Akyeampong, Hill, and Kleinman, 'A Historical Overview of Psychiatry in Africa', 5–10.

51   Vaughan, 'Psychiatry and Empire, Introduction', 1–2.

52   Vaughan, *Curing Their Ills*, 107.

53   This contradiction has been identified by: Chakrabarti, *Medicine and Empire*, 135. For a case study, see: Keller, 'Taking Science to the Colonies'. For psychiatrists in Algeria, 'primitivism' was 'a real social problem rather than an intellectual curiosity' (25). According to them, North Africans were inherently mad, a condition that manifested itself especially when faced with 'civilization' (27).

54   Breitenstein, 'Meine Arbeit mit den geistes- und gemütskranken Menschen in Lambarene', 72–73; Oswald, *Mein Onkel Bery*, 167–68; Stocker, 'Diary 1961–63', 13.

the most primitive milieu'.[55] Schweitzer struggled, meanwhile, to reach a definitive diagnosis:

> She's obviously not sane; yet she fits into no usual pattern of abnormal behaviour. Perhaps it was the influence of her primitive upbringing and the society she had always lived in that has ameliorated her actions and made her such an (sic) unique mental patient. She may have stranger habits than most of us, but maybe we have worse ones that we tightly control.[56]

Berman's reports are not to be taken at face value, but it was indeed common practice at the time to link tensions between a 'primitive upbringing' and the colonial encounter with mental illness. The quoted conversation illustrates how these discourses were linked with Schweitzer's static and somewhat romanticized picture of Africans and their culture.

In 1961, visitor Andrews was also drawn to the association between intercultural difference and mental health. Having learned from staff members that 'attitude and practice among the native population toward sexuality is [...] almost completely permissive, and without the neurotic guilt and anxiety characteristic of our own culture', Andrews proclaimed his regret that no anthropologist had yet worked in the local area. Referring to Freud, he implied that such permissive sexual attitudes and practices could be expected to lead to a lower rate of 'neurotic anxiety and related symptoms'. He concluded that the area around Lambaréné, which he described as 'still essentially unaffected by the moral concepts of Christianity', 'might yield data that would be of value to psychiatry in theory and application'.[57]

When Woodbury and his team of colleagues visited two years later, they maintained that the underlying cause of the professed rise in mental illness among Africans was fairly obvious. They saw the reason for 'the apparent increase in depression among Africans' in 'the internalization of a more individualized superego as detribalization proceeds'. This would result in 'feelings of low self-worth [...] as the native populations become more exposed to an alien but supposedly superior culture'.[58] In their view, members of the Gabonese upper class, such as teachers or church ministers, were especially prone to 'what one would call "transcultural anomie", missing the closeness of belonging to

---

55   Berman, *In Africa with Schweitzer*, 64.
56   Ibid., 65–66.
57   Andrews, 'Psychiatric Facilities at the Albert Schweitzer Hospital', 527.
58   Woodbury et al., 'Psychiatric Care at the Albert Schweitzer Hospital', 148.

the tightly knit inner tribal group, yet too Europeanized to accept its restrictions'.[59] The logical implication thereof was that 'local culture' constituted a positive influence on mental health. Woodbury and his co-authors were intrigued by the relatively high recovery rates for 'functional psychoses'. They ascribed these to 'permissive child-rearing practices', explaining that 'return from regression is facilitated by the lack of guilt about primary process thinking and activities associated with childhood', while 'in our culture, where punishment and disapproval are common in child rearing, chronicity may be related to guilt about regressed or childlike behavior and thinking'.[60]

Like Schweitzer and the ethnopsychiatrists, these visiting psychiatrists employed a vocabulary of difference, but at the same time conceded that Africans and Europeans found themselves on the same evolutionary path, albeit at different locations. They spoke of 'regression' or of Christianity having *not yet* penetrated African culture. In their view, Africans were childlike, their sexual morality retarded. The authors romanticized these societies, imagining an ideal state in which all individuals were at ease with themselves and their surroundings.

Psychiatric care at the Albert Schweitzer Hospital sought to recreate such circumstances. While these visitors insisted on the beneficial influence of 'permissiveness', staff members struggled to find a balance between leniency and control in all areas of hospital life, and especially in the care of the mentally ill. Unlike Schweitzer some twenty years earlier, who had aimed to eradicate African 'superstition', these early 1960s Western psychiatrists recommended preserving patients' cultures in order to maintain their mental health.

Dr. Richard Friedman was, while also having other duties, responsible for psychiatric patients at the Albert Schweitzer Hospital from 1956 to 1969 (see Illustration 38). He was of Hungarian origin and had gone to a Protestant school in Czechoslovakia, after which he converted from Judaism. Nevertheless, he was deported to Auschwitz and Dachau with his parents. After World War Two, he left for Israel where he worked for the army and in hospitals. In summer 1955, he saw a picture of Schweitzer and Dr. Emeric Percy in a newspaper. He recognized the latter from their studies, which encouraged him to reach out to the former, asking if he might serve in Lambaréné. Schweitzer agreed, as Friedman promised to be a long-term option. On several occasions, Schweitzer expressed that he was very satisfied with Friedman on a personal and professional level.[61]

---

59   Ibid., 150.
60   Ibid., 147.
61   See: Schweitzer to Martin, 6 July 1955, 21 October 1956, 25 November 1956, AMS. No information about Friedman's post-Lambaréné biography could be obtained.

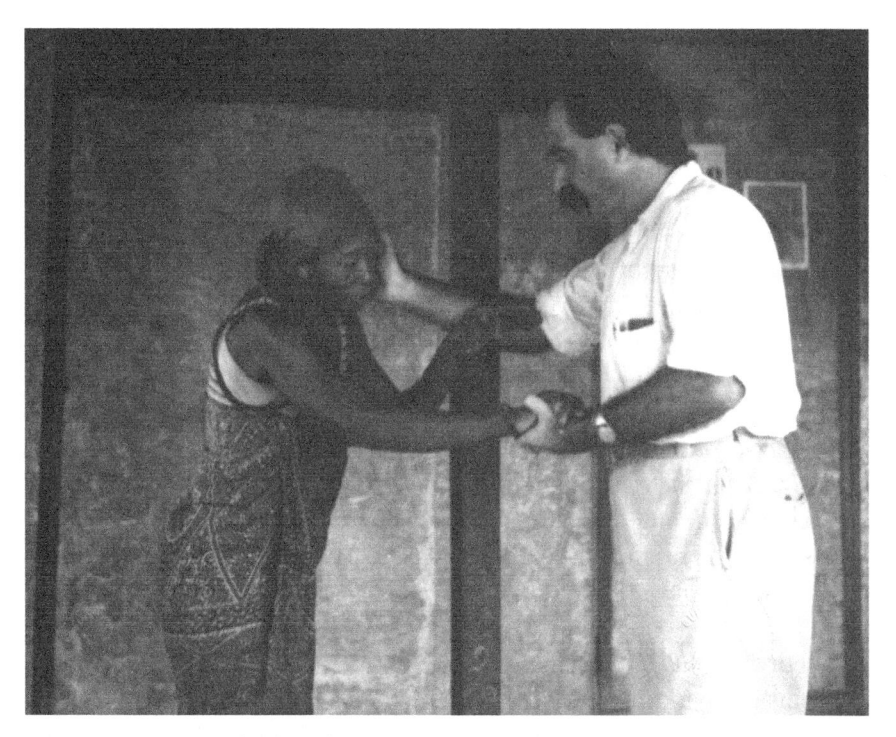

ILLUSTRATION 38   Richard Friedmann and a patient, late 1950s
© ARCHIVES CENTRALES ALBERT SCHWEITZER GUNSBACH

Even though Friedman co-authored Woodbury's paper, he was aware of the limits of his understanding of African lifeworlds and expressed thoughts that were similar to the views held by Schweitzer in the late 1930s. After Friedman had unsuccessfully attempted to ameliorate the condition of a psychiatric patient, Gerald Götting, a visiting official from the German Democratic Republic, summarized the doctor's reaction: 'He found the story distressing because he was unable to make progress with his conventional medicine. According to him, it is difficult to help here because it is about "powers", which can hardly be analysed'.[62] For Friedman, one of the most fundamental tasks for a psychiatric doctor was to free the patient from 'various deep-seated fears'. He found this aim extremely difficult to fulfil in Gabon due to what he described as 'the power of magic and the old imaginations of animism', which he thought to be 'overly powerful' in the region.[63] Successfully treating his patients thus often appeared to Friedman as an impossible challenge, which supposedly was the

62   Günther and Götting, *Was heisst Ehrfurcht vor dem Leben?*, 173.
63   Ibid., 189.

result of their radically different conception of a reality that he did not fully understand in the first place. 'They were talking about things that were much more important to them than any reality. Their entire world is often cruelly different from our own', he said.[64]

Friedman, who believed in intercultural difference and maintained that this had consequences for the treatment of the mentally ill, doubted the effectiveness of Western psychiatric treatment in the case of many of his patients. He thereby contradicted both Woodbury and Andrews, who were remarkably optimistic about their ability to overcome many of the limitations of transcultural psychiatry. Andrews was confident that he could reach a diagnosis by relying on

> criteria of the grosser but important sort, such as motor activity, facial expression, tone of voice, ability to relate to examiner and others, response to presumably delusional and hallucinatory material, and resemblance to categories of psychiatric illness encountered elsewhere.[65]

Woodbury and his co-authors went a step further, claiming that 'ordinarily, problems in diagnosing the patients were minimal'. Placing less emphasis on intercultural difference, they underlined that 'we were dealing with people who had already been classed as mentally ill in their own culture'.[66] The universality of their outlook becomes even more evident in their descriptions of common therapeutic practices at the psychiatric unit of the hospital. They were convinced that 'the dynamics were familiar, and our treatment concepts were resisted by the natives neither more nor less than at a psychiatric clinic in the United States'.[67] Many of these contradictions of colonial psychiatric care endure even when examining in more detail the practices that were employed to treat the mentally ill at the Albert Schweitzer Hospital.

2 The Mentally Ill in Colonial Gabon and at the Albert Schweitzer Hospital

Very little is known about colonial psychiatric services in Gabon, or even in AEF as a whole.[68] In 1923, Albert Sarraut, France's minister of the colonies,

---

64   Ibid., 169.
65   Andrews, 'Psychiatric Facilities at the Albert Schweitzer Hospital', 525.
66   Woodbury et al., 'Psychiatric Care at the Albert Schweitzer Hospital', 148.
67   Ibid., 149.
68   Neither Headrick nor Mabika provide any information on this topic.

proposed establishing an 'asylum for the insane' in Brazzaville, because doctors at the local hospital did not have anywhere to accommodate the 'poor excited or demented ones'.[69] By 1935, most dispensaries and hospitals in the colony of AEF had buildings to house the 'severe cases'. The *médecin général* was convinced, however, that 'alongside these severe cases, there are many chronically insane people who live on the fringes of the village and for whom it is essential to create asylums with a special psychiatric service'.[70] In 1950, there was still no 'psychiatry' in the whole colony, only a 'mediocre asylum' in Brazzaville. It was equipped with an electroshock device, which doctors reportedly did not use.[71]

In the early 1930s, Gabon's medical services were underfunded and primarily occupied with the fight against sleeping sickness. When the *chef du territoire* asked Schweitzer to accommodate psychiatric patients from Libreville, the latter refused because all of his hospital's cells for the mentally ill patients were occupied 'by insane persons who, according to our predictions, will be staying there for a long time to come'.[72] The government mission that inspected the territory's medical facilities in 1954 made no mention of any psychiatric institution. The hospital in Libreville hosted an unknown number of mentally ill patients, whose living conditions were, according to the mission report, 'certainly below those of ordinary prisoners'.[73]

Given this context, it is unsurprising that not only did the Gabonese colonial government request Schweitzer's assistance in providing psychiatric treatment, but relatives of mentally ill persons also sought to take advantage of these services. Schweitzer treated his first psychiatric patient shortly after his arrival in Lambaréné in 1913, healing her after fourteen days 'for some time at least', as he wrote.[74] When he recounted this story in his memoirs a decade later, he claimed that 'thereupon the rumour spread that the doctor was a great

---

69   Sarraut, *La mise en valeur des colonies françaises*, 437. At the time, the general hospital in Brazzaville had 44 beds for Africans and 16 for Europeans, ibid., 433.

70   'Rapport médical sur le fonctionnement durant l'année 1935 des services sanitaires et médicaux civils de l'Afrique Equatoriale Francaise'. ZK 005–121, SHD.

71   Baudoux, *La situation psychiatrique au Congo et au Ruanda-Urundi en 1950–1951*, 8.

72   Schweitzer to Monsieur le Gouverneur de FOM, Chef du Territoire du Gabon, undated, AMS. Schweitzer mentions in this letter that the hospital had a total of only five places for mentally ill patients. The letter must therefore have been written before 1934, when an additional building for psychiatric patients was built.

73   'Rapport fait par M. Petitjouan, Inspecteur de 3ème Cl. de la France d'outre-mer, concernant la vérification (du) Service de Santé Publique du Gabon à Libreville à l'époque du 3 Avril 1954', ZK 005-174, SHD. The hospital in Libreville received unsatisfactory assessments concerning its maintenance and the state of its equipment and financial resources.

74   Schweitzer, 'Notes et Nouvelles de la part du prof. Albert Schweitzer. Deuxième rapport', 19.

magician and could heal all the insane'.[75] This reputation has persisted into the present. Even André Audoynaud, one of Schweitzer's harshest critics, concedes that he was able to handle agitated cases that not even the police could.[76] Augustin Emane asserts that 'for my interlocutors, the fact that Schweitzer could calm down those they called the fools was particularly important and was part of the magic of this man'.[77] Emane's main informant, Janvier, underlined how 'Schweitzer was even able to be in command of them, while no one else could control them',[78] implying not only the police here, but also local healers.

Despite this widespread praise for Schweitzer's natural gift in dealing with mentally ill people, the number of psychiatric cases at the hospital remained relatively low. Prior to 1934, when an additional building was constructed to accommodate what they called 'loud' patients,[79] there were no more than six beds for psychiatric cases.[80] By 1950, there were two buildings with six well-ventilated compartments each.[81] A decade later, Dr. Jilek-Aall reported that the psychiatric compound consisted of 'three buildings constructed around an inner yard',[82] offering a total of eighteen rooms, which were all reportedly occupied in 1961.[83] Like the rest of the hospital, this unit grew rapidly over the following four years. Woodbury and his colleagues then provided the following overview:

> The psychiatric service, which is contiguous with the rest of the hospital, consists of four small zinc-roofed huts and one wooden building with heavy bolts that was built 30 years ago to accommodate very disturbed patients. One European nurse assisted by a native male aide runs the service. All patients receive a thorough physical examination and are treated in the general hospital for their numerous somatic ailments: malaria, amaebiasis, intestinal parasites, gonorrhea, and so on. At the time of our study, there were 25 psychiatric inpatients at the hospital – 15 men and 10 women.[84]

---

75   Schweitzer, *Zwischen Wasser und Urwald*, 48.

76   Audoynaud, *Le docteur Schweitzer et son hôpital à Lambaréné*, 152.

77   Emane, *Docteur Schweitzer: une icône africaine*, 159.

78   Ibid.

79   Schweitzer, 'Briefe aus dem Lambarene Februar 1934', 4.

80   Schweitzer, 'Briefe aus dem Lambarene Spital Pfingsten 1931', 8.

81   This detail is taken from the incomplete and muddled 'Statistiques de l'Hôpital' of 1950, L – A – S3, AMS.

82   Jilek-Aall, *Working with Dr. Schweitzer*, 163.

83   Andrews, 'Psychiatric Facilities at the Albert Schweitzer Hospital', 524.

84   Woodbury et al., 'Psychiatric Care at the Albert Schweitzer Hospital', 146.

The visiting psychiatrists then provided a statistical analysis of key details about these psychiatric patients. They emphasized that the majority had consulted a 'feticheur' before coming to the hospital, usually together with their family.[85] At least twenty of the inpatients had been 'admitted involuntarily'. The authors did not specify what exactly this meant, but examples of psychiatric patients being brought to the hospital by force will appear repeatedly in this chapter. Six people had already been treated at the hospital on a previous occasion. Ten patients had been there for between six months and two years, eleven for less than half a year, and four for more than two years. In addition to these inpatients, there were fifteen unspecified outpatients.[86] At 44 percent, the most common reason given for psychiatric treatment was that the patient presented 'a threat to the community' by being 'assaultive', 'destructive of property', or 'thought to be possessed by evil spirits [...] considered "contagious"'. Another 25 percent 'had become a burden to his family and community', while the remaining 31 percent were brought to the hospital due to their 'inability to communicate verbally'.[87] Woodbury and his co-authors did not further specify why they defined such obviously overlapping categories. Their classification highlights the role of the community in defining when a mentally ill patient required hospital care.

The idea that the hospital's psychiatric ward served primarily as a relief for local communities can be discerned from many of the detailed cases found in the sources. Staff and visitors at the Albert Schweitzer Hospital were very concerned about the fate of mentally ill persons who remained in their communities. There are numerous reports from the hospital's initial years that detail mentally ill individuals being chained, restrained with ropes, or even killed in their villages. Schweitzer claimed that the mentally ill could not be confined in a room or cage in their homes because they would always break the weak bamboo bars typically used for this purpose.[88] In 1925, however, he refused to accommodate more psychiatric cases, arguing that they would disturb other patients at the hospital. 'Hence I have to let them return to their village bonded, where they may be tortured to death, while in my care they may become healthy', he claimed.[89]

---

85   Ibid., 149.

86   Ibid., 147.

87   Ibid., 148.

88   Schweitzer, 'Notes et Nouvelles de la part du prof. Albert Schweitzer. Deuxième rapport', 19–20.

89   Schweitzer, 'Mitteilungen aus Lambarene. Zweites Heft, 1924–1925', 157.

The account of the nurse Emma Ott from December 1938 invokes similar images of ropes, chains, and a gloomy fate that would await the mentally ill in their villages:

> Shortly before lunch, a young, well-grown insane man was brought to us, his legs tied together, his hands tied, and a big chain around his body. In a whisper he spoke to us, with big gleaming eyes. His escorts didn't want to leave him here, they just wanted to get drugs. After a long discussion they left him here. In the village he would have had to be on the chain all the time, here at least he is free in his cell, and if he is calm and not too dangerous, he may sit outside for a few hours under surveillance.[90]

In this particular case, as was typical in other African contexts, the therapy management group did not bring the patient to the hospital for therapy or a cure in the strict sense, but to obtain drugs for temporary relief of symptoms.[91] From Ott's description, it is unclear whether his escorts agreed to leave the patient at the hospital in order to grant him more freedom of movement, because they started to believe that he would be cured there, and/or because they sought to relieve themselves of the responsibility of caring for him. Meanwhile, Schweitzer and his staff viewed themselves as saviors, believing that their methods of treatment were more humane than the supposedly ignorant approaches resorted to in local villages.

In the 1960s, it was not only the use of ropes and chains in local communities' treatment of the mentally ill that caught the attention of Europeans, but another supposedly common element of (mental) illness in Gabon, namely spirits. By then, psychiatric staff and visitors at the hospital had become eager to obtain a better understanding of patients' mindsets as well as local manifestations of mental illness. Woodbury explained that 'in this region of the world, the mentally ill person is thought to be invaded by spirits', reporting that 'if exorcism, which often includes physical beatings, does not cure the patient, he is abandoned in the jungle to starve or be devoured by wild animals'.[92]

The German psychiatrist Christoph Staewen visited Lambaréné in early 1964 in the course of an educational journey through Africa, which marked the beginning of his interest in the continent. In the following years, he would practice as a general physician in Niger, Congo, and Chad. He would also publish memoirs and handbooks, for example on the 'cultural and psychological

---

90   Ott, 'Natur, Mensch und Tier', 138–39.

91   Jackson, *Surfacing Up*, 11.

92   Woodbury et al., 'Psychiatric Care at the Albert Schweitzer Hospital', 145.

conditions' of 'cooperation with Africans'.[93] In a text on his stay in Lambaréné, he equated, like Woodbury and his colleagues, Gabonese therapies for mentally ill individuals with 'exorcisms'. Staewen though did not suggest that any beatings occurred during therapeutic ceremonies, but still described the practices as being conducted with considerable force.

> They get drugs that whip up all their senses. By forcing the sick to dance for days or weeks, one tries to drive out the 'evil spirits'. Or they are tied up in a pit so that they can only see a piece of heaven and their food is thrown down. And often it is only then, when the local medicine man has to acknowledge that he is powerless, that the patient is taken to hospital. Maybe the 'docteur' will help him...[94]

For Staewen, the inevitable culmination of the local quest for therapy was treatment at the Albert Schweitzer Hospital. He did not provide any details on where he had obtained his information, but mentioned having exchanged with Ruth Breitenstein, who served at the hospital on seven occasions from 1957 to 1966 and was responsible for caring for the psychiatric patients during her later stays. In her memoir, Breitenstein would use almost identical words when describing how the mentally ill were treated in their villages, also without disclosing her sources.[95]

A number of female staff members from the hospital who secretly attended dance events in the 1960s recalled them in a similar manner and were fascinated by their 'aggressive' side. Some perceived them as healing rituals,[96] while others did not.[97] Louise Jilek-Aall provides an especially detailed account of such an event. One day, she observed 'noticeable excitement among the Africans at the hospital'. In response to her persistent requests for information, they told her of 'a big feast at a village' and a 'famous medicine man who was expected to come'. The auxiliary Gustave Manyihou invited her to 'come and

---

93 Staewen, *Kulturelle und psychologische Bedingungen der Zusammenarbeit mit Afrikanern*.

94 Staewen, 'Die geistes- und gemütskranken Patienten des Spitals Lambarene 1964', AMS. A translated and abridged version of this text was subsequently published as: Staewen, 'Les malades mentaux de l'hôpital de Lambaréné'.

95 Breitenstein, 'Meine Arbeit mit den geistes- und gemütskranken Menschen in Lambarene', 71. Breitenstein had not undergone formal nursing training, but had worked with mentally ill patients in Switzerland.

96 Group Interview Speicherschwendi. The nurse Anderegg referred to the ceremony as a 'death dance'. She found it 'frightening', because all the participants were drunk and aggressive. Interview Elisabeth Anderegg.

97 Stocker, 'Diary 1961–63', 18.

see for yourself [...] you could observe a medicine man at work'.[98] Together
with Eric, the hospital's carpenter, Jilek-Aall stole away on the night of the
event and canoed to the village. Believing that she had spotted Manyihou,
'oblivious' to their presence, among the dancers, Jilek-Aall described a transformation: he was no longer the 'submissive orderly', but now a 'wild man, un-
restrained and disinhibited in his emotional expressions; strangely fearsome'.[99]
The 'medicine man' appeared in a mask and approached the visitors, clearly
making a point of indicating their presence. When the dancing and singing
intensified, Jilek-Aall became 'really scared'. A young man, 'obviously seriously
ill', appeared in the middle of the circle of dancers that had formed.[100] The
man in the mask proceeded to touch the sick man, after which the latter
seemed to fall into a state of unconsciousness. He was then taken into a 'compound' out of Jilek-Aall's sight, after which she and Eric were asked to leave.[101]
Manyihou came to work at the hospital the following day, but made no mention of the previous night's events.

For Jilek-Aall, the episode betrayed 'how little did we actually know'; she saw
a 'different world [...] of which I could never be a part'.[102] However, her description reveals her fascination with the strangeness of the event. Moreover, violence pervades her narrative to a much lesser extent than in other accounts;
instead, she draws attention to the communitarian aspects of local therapeutic
practices. For a more detailed interpretation of such practices, we can turn to
a text by Dr. Munz in which he describes another local treatment method.

Munz was in regular contact with Marcelline Nyndounge, a Fang woman
who ran a 'traditional hospital village' some two hours by rowing boat from the
Albert Schweitzer Hospital. This 'hospital village' was called 'Meteghe', which
Munz translates as 'earth' or 'soft'. Contrary to this name, he observed 'extremely hard phases of treatment' there.[103] A patient's stay, which typically lasted for
several weeks, culminated in him or her being laid into a ritual grave that the
patient then destroyed. All the other patients participated in this ceremony,
singing and dancing throughout. Thereafter, Nyndounge talked to the patient
for several hours. The goal of this consultation, 'during which (the patient) is
soon beaten by Marcelline in the face, soon quietly and motherly cheered up
and comforted', was to find the cause of the illness. Munz did not list what
causes were considered, but he suspected that, unlike for other healers he had

---

98   Jilek-Aall, *Working with Dr. Schweitzer*, 117. No information could be obtained on Eric.
99   Ibid., 120.
100   Ibid., 123.
101   Ibid., 124.
102   Ibid., 127.
103   Munz, *Albert Schweitzer im Gedächtnis der Afrikaner und in meiner Erinnerung*, 127.

heard of, blaming someone else was not Nyndounge's central concern; hence her ways were 'soft'.[104] When the cause was eventually discovered, the other patients resumed their singing and dancing.[105] The fundamental importance attached to finding the cause of a disorder was also emphasized by anthropologists studying the Mitsogho people of southern Gabon, who insisted that most local therapies were to bring about an 'individual and social re-equilibrium'.[106] Nyndounge, in contrast, was primarily concerned with ensuring that her patients returned home in a cured state.

These more detailed accounts of Jilek-Aall and Munz, as well as the following one by the anthropologist Fernandez, suggest a different interpretation of beatings during treatment than the one put forward by European visitors such as Staewen. African healers, family members, and patients shared another conception of such therapeutic violence. They regarded beatings administered in the context of treatment as fundamentally distinct from those committed as acts of wanton violence. They were aware that 'the struggle against evil and the combating of misfortune is nowhere a child's play', to use Munz' words.[107]

Many of the motifs identified in the above accounts – chains and ropes, beatings, spirits, but not dancing – also make an appearance in Fernandez's detailed description of Antoine, a Fang man who would have been considered a psychiatric case by Europeans. Antoine's example, which reveals much about Fang conceptions of (mental) health, provides a basis of comparison for the patients whom we will encounter later in this chapter. A key difference between Antoine's story and comparable accounts in sources relating to the Albert Schweitzer Hospital is that he was never admitted to a hospital. In his case, this option appears to have not even been considered, suggesting that it was reserved for specific afflictions.

Antoine started to jump on rooftops and to babble incomprehensibly. He expected mail arriving from France, wanted to build a European-style house, and predicted that he would become 'as rich as a white man'. He annoyed and ridiculed almost everyone in his village, but his fellow villagers remained curious about his repeated prophecies. When he started to swing a long stick at people in the village, his brother tied him up and confined him to bed for a day.[108] Villagers agreed that Antoine was '"heartsick" [...] the concept of general application to those disturbed in their thinking about themselves, about

---

104   Ibid., 140.
105   Ibid., 131.
106   Otto Gollnhofer and Roger Sillans, 'Phénoménologie de la possession chez les Mitsogho (Gabon). Rites et techniques', 742.
107   Munz, *Albert Schweitzer im Gedächtnis der Afrikaner und in meiner Erinnerung*, 128.
108   Fernandez, *Bwiti*, 188. Fernandez also provides valuable information in his footnotes.

others, and about the visible world in which men lived'.[109] According to Fernandez, this was a state that manifested itself in either an 'excess of activity' or
an 'excess of tranquility',[110] either way representing a malfunction of the heart,
'the Fang organ of perception, intellection, and balanced judgment'.[111] Proper
functioning of the heart was considered crucial, Fernandez argues, because
Fang individual and societal well-being derived from the state of 'oneheartedness', namely 'an orderly preparation in the discharge of all things' that manifested itself in 'general integrity of feeling and thought in human affairs'.[112] The
categorization of Antoine's illness, as well as its cause, was disputed among
villagers. As often occurred in relation to other illnesses, some believed that
Antoine may have been the target of somebody else's spiritual aggression. Alternatively, other villagers suspected that the disorder might have been caused
by Antoine's own aggression, such as his breaking of a taboo, or him challenging his own *Evu*.[113]

As long as Antoine did not disturb the sense of peace and order in the village, he enjoyed considerable freedom to indulge in his extraordinary behavior. As soon as he threatened the village's calm though, he was forced to undergo treatment. This was, according to Fernandez aimed at 'reunification,
knitting together, the making as one', which was achieved by 'returning men,
and the village affected by their actions, to appropriate activity or tranquility
by calming or animating demons or ancestral spirits, whichever be involved'.[114]
Antoine's brother enlisted the help of a 'woman herbalist from a nearby village'. She 'determined that his witchcraft spirit was twisting his heart, and she
treated him with a concoction to calm it. She beat him with leaf branches
dipped in hot herbal infusions'.[115] Antoine's therapy did not have immediate
effect. He did, however, manage to go to Oyem, where he resumed his former
job as a tailor. He would return to his village one year later in an 'apparently
normal' state.[116]

Woodbury and his colleagues likewise noted that the impact of a person's
mental state on social life was decisive in local diagnoses. 'As in most primitive
cultures, a person is considered mentally ill only when his defense mechanisms

---

109   'Nkukwan nlem' (N) and 'Nkôkôm nlem' (F) were the Fang concepts that Fernandez rendered as 'heartsick', 190.
110   Ibid., 194.
111   Ibid., 190.
112   Ibid., 192.
113   Ibid., 190.
114   Ibid., 195.
115   Ibid., 189.
116   Ibid.

are threatening or burdensome to the community', they wrote, further specifying that 'insanity is classified by the Gabonese into two broad categories: fou furieux and fou doux'.[117] This classification recalls Fernandez's dichotomy between 'excess of activity' and 'excess of tranquility'.[118] These categories found their equivalent at the Albert Schweitzer Hospital in the form of the 'loud' and 'quiet' wards in which psychiatric patients were segregated. As discussed in Chapter 1 and suggested by Munz, the idea of balance, so persistent in these psychiatric cases of the early 1960s, might misrepresent local conceptions of disease. Psychiatric cases at the hospital prove that mechanisms of attack and defence were also at play.

3   Treating the Mentally Ill at the Albert Schweitzer Hospital: Drugs and Community

The 1961 case of Leo, a kitchen servant at the Albert Schweitzer Hospital, illustrates many facets of psychiatric care at the institution. His story, as narrated by Dr. Jilek-Aall, started when his wife suffered a miscarriage after he had beaten her.[119] Her brother then demanded money from Leo to compensate for the death of his unborn nephew. After Leo refused to pay, his brother-in-law placed a curse upon him. Seeking protection, Leo relocated to the hospital grounds, but soon started to behave strangely. After claiming that he was being attacked by the Devil, Leo was moved to one of the bare cells for 'loud' patients in the psychiatric compound. By this stage, his state was such that 'no amount of medicine could pacify him and it was such a battle to subdue him for an injection that we gave it up, since it did not seem to help'.[120] When Leo eventually calmed down, the doctors were compelled to force-feed him because he refused to eat for fear of being poisoned. Jilek-Aall was curious about the cause of Leo's condition and sought the opinions of African personnel. She did not specify with whom she spoke, but the answers that she received varied. Some people believed that the Devil was responsible; others thought that

> Leo might have been poisoned and worried that in-laws might try to sneak in harmful substances; others assumed ancestral spirits were taking revenge for the unborn child whose death he had caused; some

---

117   Woodbury et al., 'Psychiatric Care at the Albert Schweitzer Hospital', 148.
118   Fernandez, *Bwiti*, 194.
119   Jilek-Aall, *Working with Dr. Schweitzer*, 154–62.
120   Ibid., 164.

believed that Leo was bewitched and that an evil spirit possessed him.
They told me that such a spirit had the shape of a bird and would
lodge in a person's chest.[121]

Fearing that Leo would die, his relatives, including his brother-in-law, appeared
to encourage and forgive him, but to no avail.[122] Ultimately, however, a cure did
arrive in the form of what Jilek-Aall described as a sort of miracle healing.
Schweitzer, reminding the reader of Jesus, simply talked to Leo, after which the
latter recovered and soon returned to work. 'When later asked about his illness,
he would give us an embarrassed smile and answer that he could not remem-
ber anything of it at all', Jilek-Aall concluded the story.[123]

The treatment for psychiatric patients at the Albert Schweitzer Hospital
consisted of three key pillars. Patients were individually confined in small and
solid single cells, particularly when they were severely agitated; they received
drugs to reduce the number of such episodes; and, unlike Leo, they took part in
what can be considered to have been a form of occupational therapy. The latter
aimed to recreate a sense of community and belonging, the loss of which was
assumed to be an essential cause of their mental illness.

In Gabon, some missionaries had used drugs to calm down mentally ill patients before Schweitzer's arrival in Lambaréné.[124] During his first stay,
Schweitzer administered tranquilizers to keep psychiatric patients quiet at
night; it had annoyed him that they had disturbed the other patients and that
he had had to get up at night to administer these injections.[125] The first mentally ill person he treated features prominently in Schweitzer's writings. Three
months after his arrival, he had been called to a village, where he found the
woman tied to a tree:

> I gave the order to untie her; people obeyed only reluctantly and with
> fear. As soon as the woman felt free, she threw herself on me to tear off
> my lantern and break it. The people around us ran away screaming. I took
> the woman by the wrists and succeeded in having her sit and calm her

---

121   Ibid., 165. The bird-shaped spirit is possibly a reference to the *Evu*. See also Chapter 2.

122   Ibid., 167.

123   Ibid., 170.

124   Morel, 'Au Gabon avant l'arrivée du Docteur Schweitzer', 187. Morel was a missionary with
       the PEMS. He arrived in Lambaréné in 1908 and reported administering 'a potion of bro-
       mide and chloral'.

125   Schweitzer, 'Notes et Nouvelles de la part du prof. Albert Schweitzer. Deuxième rapport', 18.

down. She lent her arm to a shot of scopolamine and morphine and soon fell asleep.[126]

She was subsequently taken to the hospital, where she received further doses of scopolamine and morphine. Schweitzer diagnosed her with a 'manic excitation, which came back periodically', treating her with bromide and fortifiers, in response to which the woman 'calmed down very quickly and was cured – for a time at least – after a few days'.[127] Schweitzer thus acknowledged that this method might not deliver long-term results and admitted the probability of relapses. Moreover, he learned shortly thereafter that it did not always work. Having declared the woman cured, he attempted to treat a man exhibiting similar symptoms by employing the same methods. But Schweitzer's first auxiliary, Joseph Azoawanié, suspected poisoning, predicting that the patient would die, as indeed he did after fifteen days.[128] Scopolamine and morphine were still used at the hospital in the late 1940s to treat mental illness, at least in cases of 'extreme necessity',[129] but no further details on their application are provided in the sources.

Drugs remained an important instrument in the treatment of mentally ill patients at the hospital. In 1955, Schweitzer placed high hopes in Plexonal Forte, a barbiturate manufactured by the Swiss pharmaceutical company Sandoz. In words that recalled his enthusiasm for drugs used to treat infectious diseases, he wrote to Sandoz that 'it will be a redemption for them (*the mentally ill*) as it will be for us if we can calm them down with these new medicines. In the heat that reigns here, one cannot keep the mentally ill trapped, as in Europe'.[130] When Francis Catchpool, an English doctor who served two terms in the late 1950s, ordered a supply of medications two years later, he requested paraldehyde for psychiatric patients, a standard sedative.[131] Neither Schweitzer nor Catchpool listed among their orders any of the new antipsychotics, which had become the preferred treatment across the world for a wide range of psychiatric illnesses by the mid-1950s.[132]

---

126 Ibid., 19.
127 Ibid.
128 Ibid., 20.
129 Schweitzer to Alliez, 27 November 1948, AMS.
130 Schweitzer to Sandoz, 17 January 1955, AMS. Italics mine.
131 Catchpool to Schweitzer, undated, probably 1957, AMS.
132 The first antipsychotics, chlorpromazine, was officially released onto the French market at the end of 1952. See: Ban, 'Fifty Years Chlorpromazine'; López-Muñoz et al., 'History of the Discovery and Clinical Introduction of Chlorpromazine'.

Schweitzer first mentioned these in March 1960, when he thanked Sandoz for having delivered a supply of Melleril. The company had sent this anti-psychotic two years after its launch as a 'test preparation' to Lambaréné, with Schweitzer replying that it 'has proven to be excellent'.[133] When Andrews visited in June of the following year, he noted that the hospital had several antipsychotics in stock, but that the staff had never been sufficiently confident to administer them without the advice of a specialist. Now, under Andrews' expert supervision, they were willing to test these drugs. On the trials, Andrews wrote:

> It was conceived essentially as an experiment to see how the native patients would react to the medication and whether it would be possible to quiet the agitated enough to permit some or all of them to join the others outside during the day for the purpose of returning them sooner to the community.[134]

When Woodbury and his colleagues visited the hospital in December 1964, they claimed that Melleril was the only antipsychotic in use.[135]

This short overview of the drugs used to treat mentally ill patients at the hospital suggests that the doctors adopted a trial-and-error approach in line with those described in the previous chapter in relation to leprosy and dysentery. This approach also corresponds to the history of antipsychotics in Europe.[136] Medical personnel at the Albert Schweitzer hospital administered these drugs in order to tranquilize patients and ensure their own safety as well as that of other patients. Pharmaceutical treatment, it was argued, would enable psychiatric patients to leave their cells occasionally. It was also hoped that it would facilitate the introduction of forms of occupational therapy based on community-building. The sedative effects of the drugs were appreciated by staff and patients' relatives alike, but patients frequently resisted their application, as we have seen in the case of Leo. In the 1960s, African auxiliaries

---

133   Schweitzer did not specify when the hospital had received the drug, nor did he provide any details on subsequent trials. Schweitzer to Sandoz, 20 March 1961, AMS. The letter might be archived among the correspondence of Fritz Dinner. On Melleril, see:; Zeller, *Globalisierungsstrategien – Der Weg von Novartis*, 314.

134   Andrews, 'Psychiatric Facilities at the Albert Schweitzer Hospital', 525. Marplan, an antidepressant, was given to five patients who 'appeared depressed', Trilafon to five supposedly 'disturbed patients'. After four days, Andrews was cautiously optimistic about the results, but did acknowledge that the trials were of little wider value given their limited extend.

135   Woodbury et al., 'Psychiatric Care at the Albert Schweitzer Hospital', 146.

136   Meier et al., *Testfall Münsterlingen*.

employed the following 'trick' whenever psychiatric patients attempted to evade an injection:

> They would arm themselves with patience and chat with the patient to calm him down. Then they would ask him to put his hand through a hole to grab an object that interested him. One of them took the opportunity to hold this arm and the other to do the injection.[137]

African auxiliaries had a crucial role to play in the care of psychiatric patients. This was because the doctor responsible for psychiatric cases was required to spend a large amount of time in other wards, and it was not until the early 1960s that a European nurse was assigned the dedicated role of caring for the mentally ill.[138] Most frequently discussed in the sources is Jean Mendoume, who began working at the hospital in 1924 (see Illustration 39).[139] European nurses who worked with Mendoume praised him on several occasions. Jeanette Siefert, for example, claimed that he noticed 'earlier than anyone else when a seizure of raving madness was coming; he managed that the already somewhat rebellious man handed him the knife and let himself be locked up in his chamber'.[140] Besides illustrating that safety measures were not always strictly enforced at the hospital, this statement demonstrates the critical function fulfilled by African auxiliaries as middle figures in this transcultural setting. Ironically, Mendoume himself would be confined in one of the hospital's cells for psychiatric patients after an episode of 'senseless drunkenness', as Schweitzer explained to his secretary.[141] The way in which Schweitzer narrated this story suggests that this was not the first time that Mendoume had committed such misdemeanor; nevertheless, he played too crucial a role in the psychiatric unit for Schweitzer and his team to consider dismissing him from his job.

Staff's main responsibility in the psychiatric unit was, after administering drugs and keeping them calm, to ensure that their patients had enough work

---

137 Nyama, 'La dame tout de blanc vêtue et son trousseau de clés', 48.
138 Woodbury et al., 'Psychiatric Care at the Albert Schweitzer Hospital', 146. In the 1930s, the one nurse responsible for caring for the mentally ill was also required to dress ulcers, monitor the women who manufactured palm oil, buy and distribute food, and oversee the maintenance of general hygiene at the hospital. See: Schweitzer, 'Briefe aus dem Lambarene Spital November 1935', 5–6.
139 See the 1962 'liste des employés les plus anciens, proposés pour une décoration', which is kept in a folder entitled 'affaires concernant le personnel indigene' in a box labeled 'divers' in the cellar of the AMS.
140 Siefert, *Meine Arbeitsjahre in Lambarene 1933–1935*, 57.
141 Schweitzer to Martin, 27 June 1937, AMS.

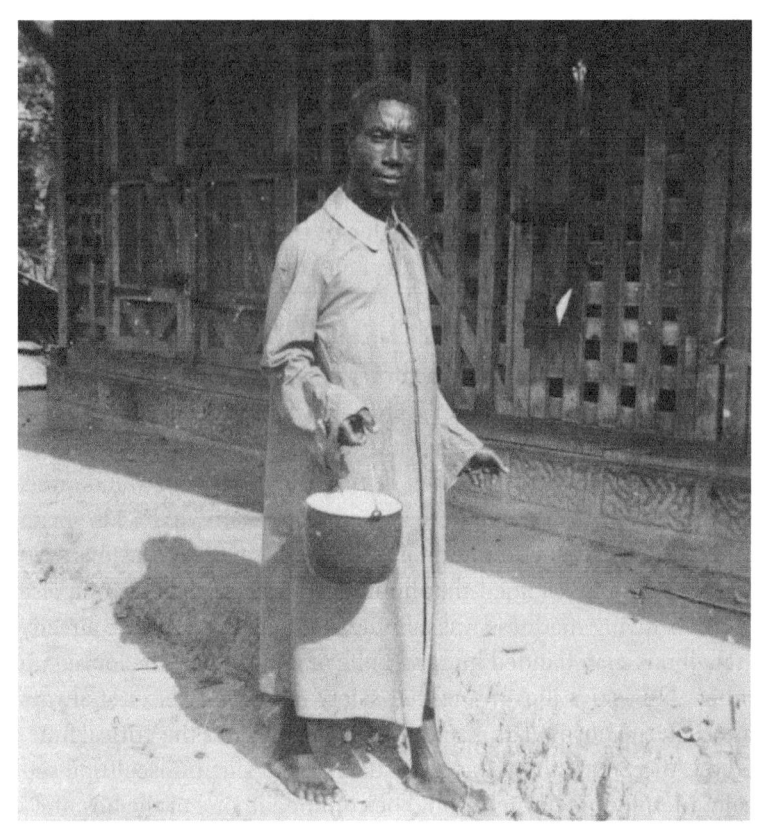

ILLUSTRATION 39   Jean Mendoume in front of the psychiatric ward, ca. 1934
© ARCHIVES CENTRALES ALBERT SCHWEITZER GUNSBACH

to keep them occupied. This form of occupational therapy, which represented a key pillar of what Schweitzer perceived as his 'civilizing mission', was consistent with the hospital-wide practice of engaging everyone in labor, patients and their relatives or visitors alike. For Schweitzer, work ethic and an ethics-based sense of community – the latter, however, under threat from the spread of individualistic materialism – were standout features of 'Western civilization'.

Fostering a communal work ethic, he believed, was thus the logical remedy for those who had been negatively affected by other aspects of this very 'civilization'. In 1927, Mombo, 'an epileptic who also often has seizures of mental disorder', worked as one of Emma Haussknecht's assistants. She was unimpressed by the efforts of the two psychiatric patients who were her assistants, bemoaning that 'I can hardly count on them when it comes to work, especially not on Mombo'.[142] Five years later, the nurse Emilie Spoerri was more satisfied with the work performed by Antoine, a psychiatric patient who assisted her

---

142   Albert Schweitzer, 'Neues von Albert Schweitzer Juli 1927', 2.

with the distribution of food and other unspecified tasks.[143] In the 1930s, mentally ill patients who were categorized as 'quiet' produced wood carvings on a regular basis.[144] None of these activities was sufficiently productive to play an important role in the hospital economy; psychiatric patients were put to work to keep them occupied.

By the 1960s, occupational therapy formed a more integral part of the hospital's psychiatric treatment regime, now also incorporating more productive tasks such as the manufacturing of rope from pineapple fiber or the making of fishing nets.[145] The main activity for psychiatric patients, however, had become working in the hospital's vegetable garden, which provided food for European staff and patients (see Illustrations 40, 41, and 42).[146] In this way, mentally ill patients acquired some economic importance and partly replaced the wage laborers whom Schweitzer had employed during World War Two.[147]

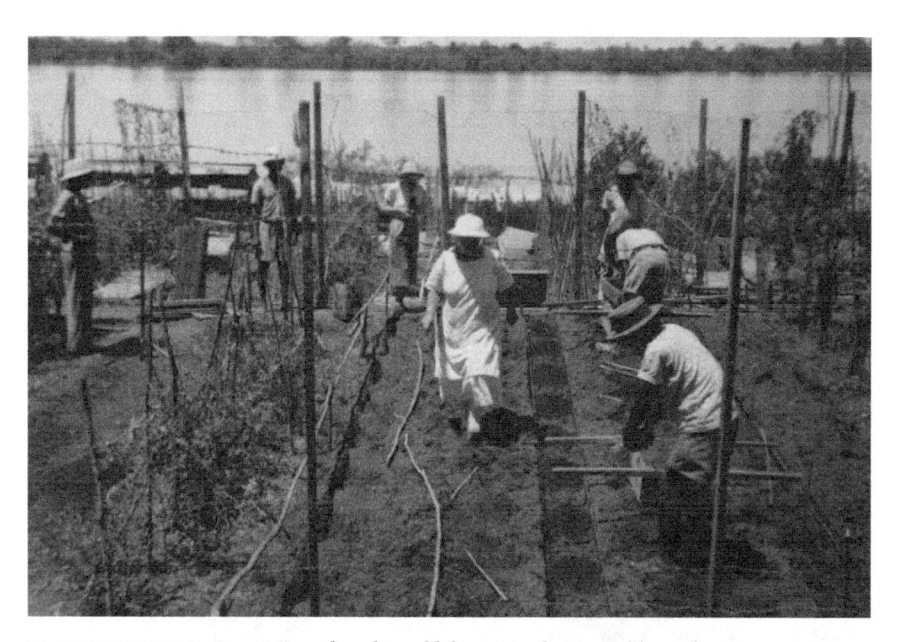

ILLUSTRATION 40   Emma Haussknecht and laborers in the vegetable garden, ca. 1950
© ARCHIVES CENTRALES ALBERT SCHWEITZER GUNSBACH

143   Spoerri to Schweitzer, 6 June 1932, AMS.
144   Siefert, *Meine Arbeitsjahre in Lambarene 1933–1935*, 57.
145   Andrews, 'Psychiatric Facilities at the Albert Schweitzer Hospital', 525; Group Interview Speicherschwendi. It is unclear what happened to these objects.
146   Breitenstein, 'Meine Arbeit mit den geistes- und gemütskranken Menschen in Lambarene', 72; Interview Marianne Stocker.
147   Schweitzer to Seaver, 'Notes Sur l'Hôpital 1939–1945', AMS. In this letter, Schweitzer provides a detailed overview of the hospital at the time of World War Two. Verena Schmid,

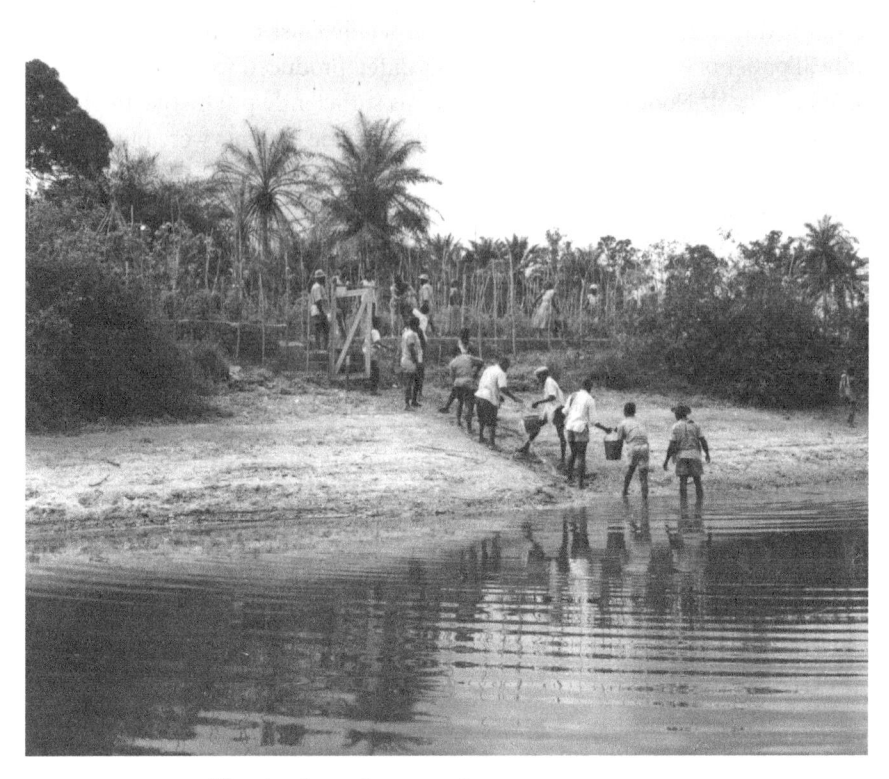

ILLUSTRATION 41   Watering the garden, ca. 1958
                   © ARCHIVES CENTRALES ALBERT SCHWEITZER GUNSBACH

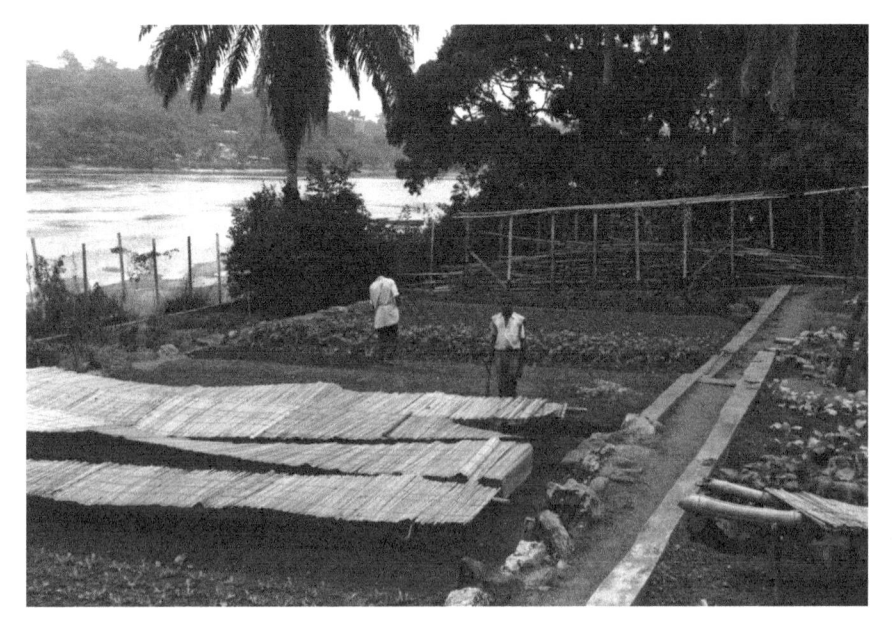

ILLUSTRATION 42   The vegetable garden and two workers, undated
                   © ARCHIVES CENTRALES ALBERT SCHWEITZER GUNSBACH

In accordance with the theory that the trend towards individualization imposed by 'Western civilization' made Africans mentally ill, treatment of psychiatric patients at the hospital aimed to restore their sense of belonging by recreating a new community for them. Many patients who came to the hospital
with a mental disorder lived in the somewhat urbanized area of Lambaréné,
where they worked for the colonial administration or in the capitalist economy, for example as traders or wage laborers. Psychiatrists posited that these
patients had lost the connections to their communities in this rapidly changing environment, which disturbed their personal identity and inner peace.

The one case study provided by Woodbury and his colleagues demonstrates
this argument. A successful businessman from Cameroon whom the authors
called J.D. was treated at the hospital for malaria, intestinal worms, amoebic
dysentery, and for gonorrhea, the disease that had led his wife to leave him. J.D.
continued to complain of 'aches all over'. He also had dreams of having sexual
intercourse with European women or being chased by a man with a gun. He
was eventually diagnosed with a 'psychoneurotic depressive reaction', which
Woodbury and his co-authors attributed to 'a longing for the tribal clan and
family ties', a state that he apparently rediscovered at the hospital. They argued
that he 'was loath to give up the physical symptoms that were his admission
ticket, so to speak, to the hospital community'.[148] J.D. exemplifies many of the
issues discussed in the historiography of mental illness in colonial Africa. He
'surfaced up' as a result of living near Europeans; he was also 'insufficiently
other' due to his participation in the capitalist economy as a businessman and
his desires for European women. At the Albert Schweitzer Hospital, he was
thus to be reintegrated into a community of Africans incorporating mentally ill
patients from all local ethnic groups. Unlike the relatives of other patients, psychiatric patients' family members were not welcome to stay at the hospital and
form part of treatment.[149]

J.D. was not the only patient undergoing treatment for a mental disorder
who reportedly expressed a wish to remain at the hospital. In his 1964 text,
Staewen discussed a number of patients, one of whom was Mongale, a former
'medicine man'.[150] The 'initial drug- and age-related state of confusion' for
which he was originally treated soon diminished, in Staewen's view chiefly as a

---

who was responsible for the vegetable garden in the early 1950s, wrote extensively about
her successful harvests, but never mentioned having any assistants.

148   Woodbury et al., 'Psychiatric Care at the Albert Schweitzer Hospital', 150.

149   Ibid., 146–47. The visiting psychiatrists received the following explanation for this: 'relatives were suspected of giving the patients 'bitter root', a potion containing an alkaloid
with effects similar to LSD-25, as the patients frequently became psychotic again after a
visit'.

150   Staewen, 'Die geistes- und gemütskranken Patienten des Spitals Lambarene', AMS, 3.

result of occupational therapy.[151] Mongale soon felt at ease at the hospital. 'I am at home here', he said according to Staewen, 'where should I go? My brothers and sisters are no longer alive and my children hardly know me anymore. I want to stay here and work'.[152] Following Staewen's narrative, the hospital provided mentally ill Africans with a second family that stood in for the village communities whose absence from their lives had made many of them sick in the first place. In this analogy, the European nurse in the psychiatric ward, a role fulfilled by Ruth Breitenstein at the time of Staewen's visit, acted as a substitute mother:

> Under her empathetic guidance, which can and must sometimes be quite firm, the patients form a real group. They become a family with their 'mother', although they are thrown together from very different races, tribes and ways of life. Despite being deeply affected by their own illness, the sick develop a very simple but very effective sense of togetherness which cannot be observed in Europe among comparable patients.[153]

Staewen expanded on these claims by recounting the story of another agitated patient, a woman who had been brought to the hospital tied up in ropes. The patient had been immediately confined in a cell – 'so she can't damage herself or escape into the nearby jungle' – where she received an unspecified first dose of drugs. After two days, she was allowed to leave her cell to join her fellow psychiatric patients for a meal. They welcomed her warmly and offered her food, which she accepted despite her fear of being poisoned.[154] According to Woodbury, the 'cooperative preparation of breakfast and lunch' was the 'main activity' that fostered this familial community spirit.[155] When Staewen's patient got upset again, refused her medication, and stripped naked, her peers were more successful in calming her down than Breitenstein.[156]

These Western observers imagined the existence of a community within the hospital, especially among African psychiatric patients and their European staff. As a key component of the hospital's psychiatric treatment regime, community-building was an adaptation of the colonial 'civilizing mission' to the circumstances and requirements of psychiatric care. It was aimed at spreading specific aspects of European 'civilization', such as an appreciation

---

151   Ibid., 2.
152   Ibid.
153   Ibid., 2–3.
154   Ibid., 3.
155   Woodbury et al., 'Psychiatric Care at the Albert Schweitzer Hospital', 146.
156   Staewen, 'Die geistes- und gemütskranken Patienten des Spitals Lambarene', AMS, 3.

for the virtues of manual labor, but at the same time it also sought to prevent the individualization that was thought to accompany the imposition of European values and which was believed to be harmful to Africans' mental health.

The 'psychiatric family' at the Albert Schweitzer Hospital was not thought suitable for Europeans. They would disturb the dynamics and would not bear it. Schweitzer explained to his friend Arthur Stoll that European psychiatric patients were not to be attended to by Africans, 'because it would depress and agitate them'.[157] In 1925, a French war veteran with 'nervous disorders' was brought to the hospital from a nearby lumber camp. Schweitzer believed that his condition was due to an old war wound that had been aggravated once again by sun stroke. Schweitzer demanded that the local colonial administrator pay for the patient's journey home to France, back to his own family so to speak, because 'he complicates my service a lot'.[158] This repatriation did not occur, and the patient passed away shortly after Schweitzer had sent this request. Schweitzer's fixation with the dangers of sunlight is frequently referred to by visitors and staff.[159] According to one anecdote, when Schweitzer did not feel well for a number of weeks in 1924, he explained his own condition with reference to holes in the ceiling through which the sun could penetrate.[160]

Another European psychiatric case that is described in detail in the sources is that of Roger Ghigo. After Ghigo was repatriated to France in 1948, Schweitzer related the patient's case history to his doctor in Marseille. Ghigo had come to the hospital with a 'strong mania', which included hallucinations as well as episodes of great agitation and sadness. Schweitzer ordered to keep him away from African staff and patients at the hospital, and to treat him with morphine and scopolamine. When his condition improved, Ghigo ate at the table for European staff in an attempt to provide him with a feeling of community. Once again, Schweitzer suspected that the sun might have had an influence in causing Ghigo's illness, since it shone directly onto the desk where he usually worked. In addition, as in a number of similar cases that he had experienced, Schweitzer believed that the malaria drug Atebrine might also have been to blame for Ghigo's condition. Schweitzer hoped that in Europe Ghigo's 'electroshock treatment will have good effects'.[161]

---

157   Schweitzer to Stoll, 29 June 1948, AMS.

158   Schweitzer to Garnier, 9 March 1925, AMS.

159   Siefert, *Meine Arbeitsjahre in Lambarene 1933–1935*, 138; Mai, *Albert Schweitzer und seine Kranken*, 10; Munz-Boddingius, 'Meine Chance und Freude, Hebamme in Lambarene gewesen zu sein'.

160   Schweitzer, 'Mitteilungen aus Lambarene. Erstes Heft, 1924', 61–62.

161   Schweitzer to Alliez, 27 November 1948, AMS.

Schweitzer's belief in the superiority of European 'civilization' – or, at the very least, its uniqueness – is rendered obvious in these examples. However, in contrast to the diagnoses of doctors in other colonies when Europeans fell mentally ill, Schweitzer did not directly link mental disorders among Europeans to a longing for their own 'civilization'. Nevertheless therapy for European psychiatric patients was, as for Africans, partly intended to restore their sense of belonging. This objective was to be achieved by ultimately sending mentally ill Europeans back home, where they could also be treated with electroconvulsive therapy, a technology that had never been considered worthy of acquiring in Lambaréné.

4   Accommodating the Mentally Ill at the Hospital: Perspectives on Safety

During his first stay in Lambaréné, Schweitzer wrote of agitated psychiatric patients and that 'if I keep them at the station, they fill it with their screams'.[162] When one such individual was brought to the hospital for treatment, Schweitzer resolved this issue by ordering the patient and his family to camp on a sandbank some distance away, where he paid them several visits per day.[163] In 1924, when the hospital's buildings were still made out of bamboo and brickwork from leaves, a sleeping sickness patient suddenly developed 'states of excitement' and became 'dangerous'. A more solid wooden cell was subsequently built to accommodate cases like him.[164] It was still not possible, however, to house 'loud insane persons' for an extended period of time, even in this new cell, 'because the other patients can't bear it next to them'.[165] Furthermore, the new structure had not been sufficiently secured. In March 1926, 'a madman [...] tears down the cell for the mentally ill and breaks out, spreading terror everywhere in the hospital'.[166] In the following months, Schweitzer rejected a number of 'dangerous' mentally ill people.[167] As he explained to Maud Royden, his contact person at the Guildhouse congregation, 'I don't have the desired number of solid wooden huts to lock them up safely'.[168]

---

162   Schweitzer, 'Notes et Nouvelles de la part du prof. Albert Schweitzer. Deuxième rapport', 18.
163   Ibid., 18–19.
164   Schweitzer, 'Mitteilungen aus Lambarene. Erstes Heft, 1924', 56.
165   Schweitzer, 'Mitteilungen aus Lambarene. Zweites Heft, 1924–1925', 157.
166   Schweitzer, *Mitteilungen aus Lambarene. Drittes Heft, 1925–1927*, 24.
167   Ibid., 24–25.
168   Schweitzer to Royden, Juillet 1926, AMS.

At the hospital's new site, which opened in early 1927, psychiatric patients were housed in cells with wooden floors rather than the 'moist soil' used in its previous accommodation for the mentally ill.[169] This unit, financed by donations from the Guildhouse, had to be vacated in January 1930 to make space for dysentery patients to be quarantined,[170] but a fund from a deceased member of the Guildhouse congregation provided further money to construct a new building for psychiatric patients (see Illustration 43). It contained seven cells, which had all been constructed so as to ensure that the patients would be 'locked up, but it has air and light, like it's outside'. When this unit was opened in September 1930, representatives from the both missions and from neighboring villages attended the ceremony, suggesting that psychiatric care was regarded as an important issue by a wide range of actors in the area.[171]

Psychiatric patients, however, continued to present problems for the hospital personnel. The nurse Elsa Lauterburg-Bonjour voiced staff members' concerns about the security risks that they posed:

> Since we do not have the necessary security measures, it is not uncommon for a lunatic to break out. Although they are imprisoned in thick-walled single cells during episodes of raving madness, if the seizure outbreaks unexpectedly, scary scenes can occur.[172]

A main challenge for the staff was to ensure peace and quiet for other patients. In late 1933, an additional building for mentally ill patients was constructed. Schweitzer justified this expense with reference not only to the need for more space to accommodate psychiatric patients, but also to the fact that 'we have so many noisy insane people, who cause sleepless days and nights to the others and upset them'. According to Schweitzer's proud report, the six new cells were 'even bigger and airier' than the ones in the building from 1930.[173]

In August 1934, the French doctor Roger le Forestier painted a radically different picture of the living conditions experienced by psychiatric patients at the hospital:

> The nurses' good hearts are saddened when they look at our fools behind the wooden bars of the designated huts. They wonder if it is more

---

169 Schweitzer, *Mitteilungen aus Lambarene. Drittes Heft, 1925–1927*, 49.
170 Schweitzer to Rieder, 19 January 1930, AWHS. Emily Rieder, Noel Gillespie's mother, was also linked to the Guildhouse congregation.
171 Schweitzer to Royden, 30 September 1930, AMS.
172 Lauterburg-Bonjour, *Lambarene: Erlebnisse einer Bernerin im afrikanischen Urwald*, 16.
173 Schweitzer to Royden, 27 January 1933, AMS.

humane to treat fools by caging them like wild animals, or to let them live and die freely in the forest? Perhaps we could find a way, for example by building an isolated acclimatization area like the hut of the dysenterics.[174]

To improve their situation, Le Forestier further proposed measures to occupy psychiatric patients in the wider hospital. These were, however, already partly in effect, as revealed in the examples of Mombo and others, and would be intensified over the course of the following three decades. Le Forestier had arrived in Lambaréné to serve at the hospital for the usual two-and-a-half-year term approximately six weeks before writing this letter, which was already the second that he had composed to Schweitzer with suggestions on what could be improved at the institution.[175] This 'urge to continuous reforms and changes',[176] a characteristic to which Schweitzer and the personnel who were loyal to him did not take kindly, led to Le Forestier's departure only three months after his arrival.

Le Forestier believed, unlike Schweitzer, that 'our indigenous fools are very different from the European fools'.[177] Le Forestier's rather progressive argument for the time that psychiatric patients in Lambaréné required more space did follow a racial logic. 'Keeping the natives, born for the wide open spaces, in a wooden cage, seems to me to be a psychological fault', he wrote. As proof of the ineffective or even harmful nature of the treatment for psychiatric patients at the hospital, Le Forestier added that 'by the way, one of them killed himself in his cage'.[178] This incident was also described by his colleague Dr. Goldschmid:

> One of our insane men (you didn't know him anymore, he was here since January 1934) hung himself in his cell a few days ago. He made a strong noose out of his loincloth and strangled himself in an almost kneeling position. Jean Mendoume and Miss Alice saw him at 10 o'clock in the morning and wanted to bathe him at 11 o'clock. In the meantime the thing happened.[179]

---

174   Le Forestier to Schweitzer, 23 August 1934, AMS.
175   The first letter consisted of eighteen pages. See: Le Forestier to Schweitzer, 5 August 1934, AMS.
176   These are the words of Dr. Goldschmid, who was very loyal towards Schweitzer. See: Goldschmid to Schweitzer, 22 August 1934, AMS. See also Schweitzer's letters to his secretary, Emmy Martin, from the same period.
177   Le Forestier to Schweitzer, 23 August 1934, AMS.
178   Ibid.
179   Goldschmid to Schweitzer, 31 July 1934, AMS.

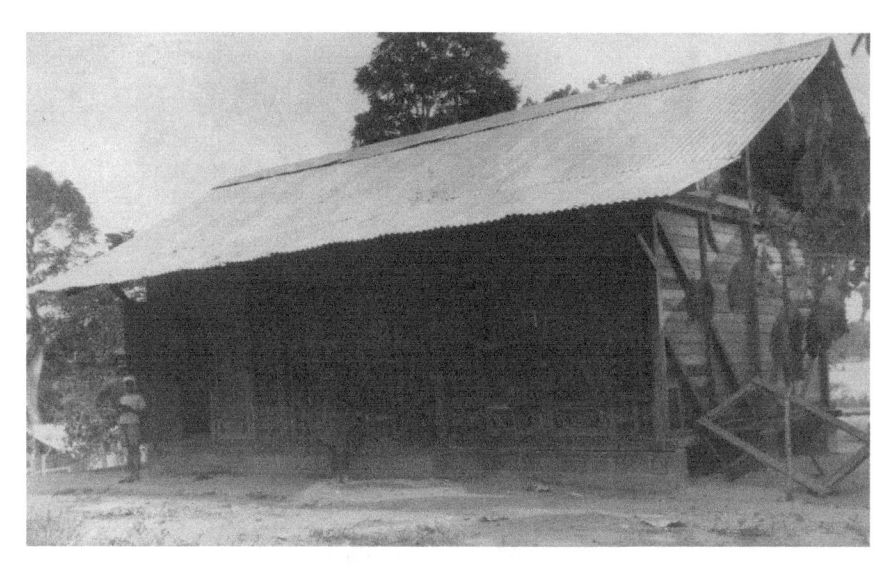

ILLUSTRATION 43 The psychiatric ward, 1931
© ARCHIVES CENTRALES ALBERT SCHWEITZER GUNSBACH

Goldschmid did not comment further on this episode, which represented the most dramatic dent to the harmonious image normally invoked by the hospital staff to characterize the treatment of psychiatric patients. Not only did this suicide clearly demonstrate the limits of psychiatric therapy, it also showed that not even patient safety could be guaranteed at the hospital.

By the 1960s, the psychiatric cells stood completely empty without even a bed, but were still arranged according to the mental state of their occupants, specifically their degree of agitation (see illustration 44). One building consisting of six rooms was reserved for the 'least disturbed individuals', while two other buildings, also with six cells each, were designed to ensure 'maximum security'.[180]

Both the accommodation and the treatment of psychiatric patients were not devised primarily according to their needs, but with those of the hospital staff and other patients in mind. Breitenstein recalled that her twenty patients lived as an isolated group on the margins of the hospital grounds, where they 'disturbed the others as little as possible'.[181] Dr. Friedman, who supervised Breitenstein, admitted that often the only option open to him and his fellow doctors when treating psychiatric patients was to administer 'tranquilizers so

---

180   Andrews, 'Psychiatric Facilities at the Albert Schweitzer Hospital', 524.
181   Breitenstein, 'Meine Arbeit mit den geistes- und gemütskranken Menschen in Lambarene', 71.

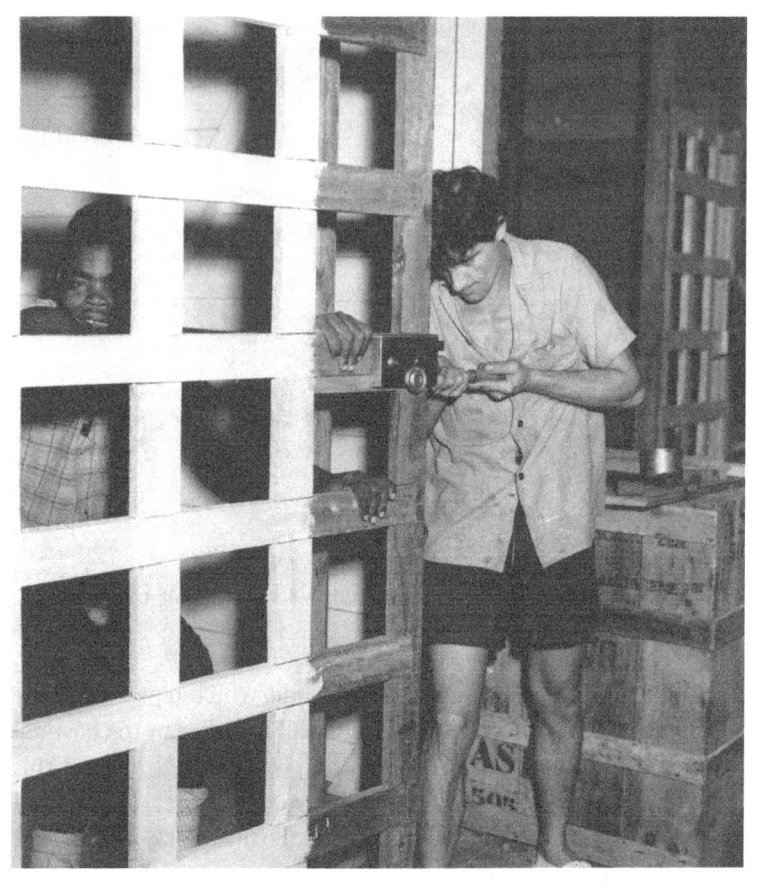

ILLUSTRATION 44   The carpenter Erwin Mathis renovating what might be a psychiatric cell,
early 1950s
© ARCHIVES CENTRALES ALBERT SCHWEITZER GUNSBACH

that they would not become too dangerous'.[182] Once again, Friedman displayed his therapeutic pessimism here, while also revealing staff members' anxieties about the potential for psychiatric patients to become violent.

A different set of safety concerns worried patients and their families, as three examples demonstrate. In 1961, Dr. Friedman informed visitor Götting about a man who felt haunted by spirits. As the Christian son of a catechist, the victim formed part of the modernized Gabonese middle class. When his father died, he was convinced that the protection that he believed his father had provided had vanished. Maintaining that spirits were now instructing him to unbury his family's 'fetish', he followed their orders, but 'he neglected [...] to

182   Günther and Götting, *Was heisst Ehrfurcht vor dem Leben?*, 169.

worship' it. Subsequently, his business worsened. At the spirits' command, he then broke into his neighbor's house, where he destroyed the porcelain. This, he claimed, awoke his neighbor's spirits, which started to fight against his own. Finally, the neighbor woke up, subdued him and brought him to the hospital in ropes. 'Now he is here, and ponders how he could possibly win the terrible fight eventually', Götting concluded the story.[183] For his part, Friedman again believed that this patient was beyond his medical competencies. This case suggests that Gabonese regarded spiritual and physical safety as interconnected and multidimensional concepts. While hospital staff organized psychiatric care and accommodation in a way that would protect themselves and other patients from the aggressions of the mentally ill, psychiatric patients felt that the hospital provided them with safety from the aggressions of malicious forces.

The second example on local safety concerns is the story of Eugène, a businessman who lived in Lambaréné, which was recounted by Staewen in 1964. Eugène and his wife had been unable to have children together. He had thus resolved to take another wife, a decision that so infuriated his first wife that she had threatened to poison him if he married a second time. Ignoring her warning, Eugène married a second wife, in response to which his first wife left him. Two years later, he began to believe that his family was plotting to kill him. His 'persecution mania' and 'agitation' subsequently intensified to such an extent that, after several months, he was brought to the hospital by these very relatives. There, according to Stawaen, Eugène was not cured – '(this persecutional disease is unfortunately often incurable)', the author explained – but he felt safe: "'Nothing can happen to me here", he says, "I can feel safe in Doctor Schweitzer's hospital. Evil people can't achieve anything here"'.[184] Eugène's story contains a number of familiar elements: the partly Europeanized protagonist, the involvement of his family, the fear of being poisoned. Eugène was in a state of constant fear, presumably of his family to poison him, which was why Staewen considered him sick. Significantly, this case provides us with a glimpse into patients' imaginations and motivations: from Eugène's perspective, he was not the cause of danger, but the one in danger.

It was not only patients with acute symptoms who appreciated the sense of safety that the hospital provided. Staewen cited the example of a recovering psychiatric patient whose father requested that she stay on at the hospital as an aide. He had brought her there after a 'wild bout of ravaging madness', which she had experienced a few months after getting married in Libreville.

---

183   Ibid., 172–73.
184   Staewen, 'Die geistes- und gemütskranken Patienten des Spitals Lambarene', AMS, 1.

Her father feared that she would experience a relapse if she returned there, a view with which she agreed. As she reportedly emphasized, 'I'd like to stay here very much. Here everyone is friendly to me, and they have said that I work well',[185] thereby subscribing to Schweitzer's rhetoric of work as salvation. Moreover, she and her father both hoped that she would find a sufficient degree of shelter from the intimidations of modernity in Libreville, as well as protection from an intimidating individual, her husband. Still fearing herself to be in danger and her mental health under threat, she sought the continued protection of the Albert Schweitzer Hospital.

Schweitzer showed some awareness of psychiatric patients' conceptions of the hospital as a place of safety. He wrote that most patients considered the hospital, just like mission stations, as a place where 'taboos, curses, and magic were powerless'; they came not so much to benefit from medical care, but to be somewhere where 'the sinister powers, to which they feel exposed to, have no reach'.[186] Augustin Emane's interviewees confirmed this interpretation. They regarded the Albert Schweitzer Hospital as a place of safety from 'all the schemings that are part of the world and cosmogony' and a site that was marked by the absence of any sort of conflict.[187] Many Gabonese considered the area to be a zone of powerful spirits. The fact that Schweitzer maintained his hospital on these specific grounds, where the Galoa king Nkombe had resided, contributed to this perception and to the sense of permanence attributed to the work of both men. According to Emane, the hospital thus became a place where 'the encounter between the world of whites and that of the blacks' occurred 'without the usual conflicts'.[188]

Njambi, our introductory case, stayed at the hospital some three decades before most of the other patients referred to in this chapter (see Illustration 45). Concluding his story allows us to recap many of the chapter's key tropes. Njambi became a familiar member of the hospital community; indeed, he may well be the most talked about patient in the hospital's history. As the story goes, however, he was constantly afraid of being sent away.[189] Although he was usually considered a 'quiet' patient who needed to be protected from his 'loud' counterparts,[190] he was known to display (self-) destructive tendencies and to

---

185   Ibid., 2.

186   Schweitzer, *Afrikanische Geschichten*, 61.

187   Emane, *Docteur Schweitzer: une icône africaine*, 105–6.

188   Ibid., 109–12.

189   Schweitzer, *Mitteilungen aus Lambarene. Drittes Heft, 1925–1927*, 53; Lauterburg-Bonjour, *Lambarene: Erlebnisse einer Bernerin im afrikanischen Urwald*, 16.

190   Schweitzer, 'Briefe aus dem Lambarene Spital Pfingsten 1931', 8; Bähr, *Albert Schweitzer: Leben, Werk und Denken*, 129.

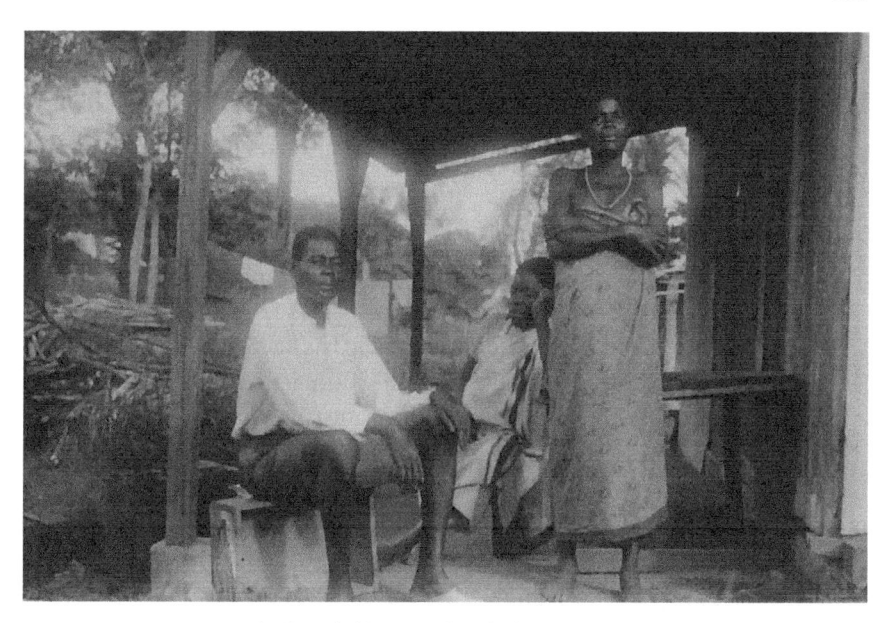

ILLUSTRATION 45   Njambi (front left), an unidentified nurse, and a sleeping sickness patient, early 1930s
© ARCHIVES CENTRALES ALBERT SCHWEITZER GUNSBACH

experience 'loud' emotional outbursts. Elsa Lauterburg-Bonjour described one of those, which occurred in early 1931:

> Last Sunday, while my husband was performing an emergency operation and the doctor was on a mission station, N'Jambi, a tall, strong lad who has been doing light work in the hospital for three years, suddenly suffered an outburst of rage. He had locked himself in his cell with petrol and matches and uttered loud threats. In order to prevent a hospital fire, my husband, who had been called here, tore open the locked door by force. At that moment bottles and open knives rushed towards him, but they missed their target.[191]

This account illustrates why hospital staff were so concerned about safety. Given all the dangerous objects that Njambi wielded in this anecdote, staff members appear to have exhibited an almost naïve trust in a man who had killed his wife, 'in the delirium' as Schweitzer, who had known him since 1913, insisted towards the Guildhouse congregation who symbolically adopted him

---

191   Lauterburg-Bonjour, *Lambarene: Erlebnisse einer Bernerin im afrikanischen Urwald*, 16.

in 1930.[192] Medical personnel were repeatedly required to subdue Njambi; in Lauterburg-Bonjour's account, for example, an unnamed auxiliary, probably Jean Mendoume, played a decisive role in restraining him. Drugs would then be used to calm him down further:

> A brave helper courageously threw himself at the possessed man and after a hot struggle could take another knife from him, but carried a bad blow. Calmed by morphine, the lunatic soon sat in his cell, praised France and Napoleon and begged for chocolate. The next day he whimpered ashamed and contrite through the small air hole: 'Moi honte, moi beaucoup honte', and begged for the mercy of the Christian god.[193]

Following this episode, Njambi remained incarcerated in his cell for four months, after which he was allowed to go for short walks under the escort of two auxiliaries.[194] Apart from Mendoume, drugs, and confinement, Schweitzer himself was key to pacifying Njambi. Indeed, Siefert identified Njambi as proof of Schweitzer's special knack with psychiatric patients. 'Dr Schweitzer often went to the insane, and you could observe how soothing he was to them, for example when he stood with the raving mad Tschambi and chatted with him', she wrote:[195]

Njambi illustrates how much attention and value were given to the care of mentally ill people at the Albert Schweitzer Hospital. He was provided with escorts to enable him to leave his cell, even though this in turn allowed him to continue to threaten staff and patients and left them feeling unsafe. He shows how staff aimed to regulate the movements of their psychiatric patients, but was not able to fully control their moods. Schweitzer reported in 1933 how the personnel had learned to deal with Njambi's outbursts, a strategy in which Mendoume played an important role:

> Yesterday evening, Tschambi [...], after having been well enough to move around in freedom for months, suddenly began to make confused and dangerous speeches again. Fortunately, his guard Mendume heard it and had the presence of mind to immediately clear his cell (in which he had piled up dangerous tools and empty bottles to be used as projectiles). So we could lock him up there without him being able to resist when he,

---

192   Schweitzer to Rieder, 5 April 1930, AWHS.
193   Lauterburg-Bonjour, *Lambarene: Erlebnisse einer Bernerin im afrikanischen Urwald*, 16.
194   Schweitzer to Schweitzer Comittee, 2 July 1931, AWHS.
195   Siefert, *Meine Arbeitsjahre in Lambarene 1933–1935*, 57.

after his habit, entered it as soon as the evening bell rang. For this presence of mind Mendume received a fine gift.[196]

Given the menacing acts that Njambi committed, it is notable that Schweitzer chose to emphasize his supposedly dangerous monologues. Despite the threat that he posed, Njambi's freedom appears to have remained considerable; however, his outbursts did no longer come completely unexpectedly, with staff members, especially Mendoume, learning to anticipate their arrival.

On 24 September 1936, Dr. Goldschmid predicted that Njambi would die the following night of the 'galloping consumption' that he had acquired. 'The poor man was completely lucid in the last few days and not confused at all', Goldschmid explained.[197] In the letter in which the doctor confirmed Njambi's passing, he remarked that 'for him it was a relief, we no longer have the heavy sorrow with him, yet we felt sorry for him'.[198]

5   Conclusion

Colonial doctors in general and psychiatrists who visited the Albert Schweitzer Hospital posited that the stresses of modernity triggered mental illness among Africans. The case histories that they presented in their texts, such as those of the businessmen Eugène and J.D., support this interpretation. Part of the reason why such patients were considered mentally ill was that they were judged to be 'insufficiently other'.[199] This dimension is emphasized less in sources written by hospital insiders. In these documents, which discuss patients like Leo and Njambi, the authors focus on more universal human character flaws, such as a violent temperament or an extreme feeling of guilt. Patients displaying such traits 'surfaced up'[200] after committing a serious crime or when working for Europeans. In many of the cases described from the hospital, it were relationship problems that triggered psychiatric symptoms. In these instances, however, it was usually husbands who were treated at the hospital, while wives remained 'hidden patients'.[201]

---

196   Schweitzer, 'Briefe aus dem Lambarene Spital Juli 1933', 8.
197   Goldschmid to Schweitzer, 24 September 1936, AMS.
198   Goldschmid to Schweitzer, 10 October 1936, AMS. In this letter, Goldschmid confirmed that Njambi had died on 26 September 1936.
199   Vaughan, *Curing Their Ills*, 101.
200   Jackson, *Surfacing Up*.
201   Studer, *The Hidden Patients*.

The frequent reports of mentally ill individuals who were brought to the hospital in chains or ropes, as well as the relatively low number of psychiatric cases who were treated there, suggest that only mentally ill persons who exhibited certain symptoms ended up at the hospital. The numerous accounts of local healing methods not only indicate how these fascinated European observers, but also suggest that the number of mentally ill Gabonese must have been substantially larger than the total of patients who underwent hospital treatment. European observers, including staff from the hospital, perceived local treatment methods as violent, ostensibly so in order to overcome the malicious powers that were often considered by Gabonese to be the cause of mental illness. It was from such forces that patients, usually supported by their relatives, sought protection at the Albert Schweitzer Hospital. The institution thus acted as a relief station for communities unable to cope with particular manifestations of mental illness.

Visiting doctors offered a positive assessment of the hospital's combined treatment regime of drugs and occupational therapy, a strategy that aimed to cure psychiatric patients rather than simply confine them. While the hospital's approach to pharmaceutical treatment was consistent with that which it applied in relation to other diseases, its focus on putting patients to work conformed to Schweitzer's conception of the 'civilizing mission'. Labor was the feature of Western 'civilization' that Schweitzer believed was most worthy of being spread, a conviction by which he justified his interference in the everyday lives and values of his patients. In psychiatric care, this practice took on a therapeutic dimension as staff sought to recreate the sense of community that they believed the mentally ill had lost. In many ways, psychiatric care encapsulated the morals and practices championed at the Albert Schweitzer Hospital: treatment was improvised, but the days of patients, *gardiens*, staff, and visitors were highly structured, with labor their central feature.

CHAPTER 6

Conclusions

How can we make sense of medical practices that aim to comprehend patients' psyches while ignoring their obstetric practices? How are we to understand a medicine that strives for control in surgery, but performs trial-and-error tests when it comes to pharmaceuticals? Analyzing the daily routines and practices of biomedicine exposes these inconsistencies, which run the risk of remaining concealed when one focuses either on biomedicine's spectacular and domineering elements or on its interactive and hybrid aspects. Such incoherences defy a simple story and reveal the inherently improvised quality of biomedicine.

Improvised practices illustrate how biomedicine adapts to and is adapted by unexpected circumstances and local challenges. Practitioners are confronted daily not only with challenges to biomedical ideals and norms, but also with contradictions to their personal ideas and preconceptions. Improvisations are the result of the complexity of everyday medical practice, a theme that is not sufficiently captured in medical theory. At the Albert Schweitzer Hospital, one result of such improvisations was that therapy and care were rather individualized, which comes as a surprise when compared to the population medicine of colonial governments. Given the institution's curative focus, however, an individualized approach is less surprising. While the concept of improvisation might be romanticized, it enables us to analytically join the domineering and the interactive sides of biomedicine.

To further evaluate how these two aspects are (dis)connected, it is illuminating to analyze how the different notions and themes evoked in each chapter of this book relate to other wards. After this, the question remains of how a specific historical case study can be situated within biomedicine in general and within colonial medicine and its successor, global health, in particular.

1 Connecting Concepts: the Incoherence of Biomedical Practices

Chapter 1 illustrated that the tension between the rules in place at the Albert Schweitzer Hospital and their lax or inconsistent implementation was characteristic of most aspects of hospital life, including those beyond the strictly medical. The following chapters then examined ideas and improvisations of the biomedicine practiced at the institution; my focus on practices revealed a number of contradictions between ideas and actions, as well as between different practices. Two of these contradictions are worth highlighting now in order to illustrate the standing of the hospital in Gabon and to illuminate its main practices and ideologies.

The sterility and strict organization of the operating theater contrasts clearly with the unsanitary conditions, disorder and ad hoc solutions that often prevailed elsewhere in the hospital. The operating theater was a retreat where staff could feel comfortable executing their medical duties and in which Schweitzer could enforce his version of control. Patients' living quarters, meanwhile, represented a space in which patients could feel at ease, at least according to Schweitzer's somewhat paternalistic conception. In this sense, surgery's standing at the hospital mirrors Schweitzer's place within Gabon, where the institution appeared conspicuously detached from its surrounding environment. This detachment, and its underlying policy of noninterference, is connected to Schweitzer's ethical reasoning, to his version of the 'civilizing mission'.

Highlighting contradictions in the care of mentally ill patients is instructive because these illustrate the connections between medical practices, conceptions of health, the idea of a 'civilizing mission', and improvisations. In relation to diagnostics, doctors labeled patients' fear of being poisoned delusional even as they attributed to poison symptoms or deaths that seemed inexplicable from their biomedical perspective. Identifying the causes of mental illnesses, doctors assumed that the pressures of modernity imposed by colonization and capitalism left Africans mentally ill, as did their 'backward' beliefs in spirits that threatened to attack them. When it came to therapy, the focus on manual labor corresponded to Schweitzer's conception of the 'civilizing mission' and to the manner in which he thought it worth spreading. In this sense, psychiatric care best illustrates that labor was the field in which Schweitzer most deeply interfered in the everyday lives and values of his patients, not only psychiatric ones. In another sense, the psychiatric unit with its numerous and detailed stories of individual patients and their incongruous treatment exemplifies the improvised side of the biomedicine practiced at the hospital.

In order to further reveal the degree of improvisation at the hospital, and what I mean by this term, I will now provide thoughts on how practices at different wards related to one other. Procedural control, as defined in Chapter 2, can be traced in varying degrees to all units of the hospital, but it was most pronounced in the operating theater. In order to achieve their aim of healing patients, surgeons were required to maintain a high degree of control, not only in Western hospitals, but also in colonial facilities, such as the Albert Schweitzer Hospital. Many Gabonese men, and some women, were prepared to subject themselves to this medical practice and its correspondingly strict measures of control.

Most Gabonese women remained reluctant to deliver their babies at hospitals until the late 1950s. This was despite the fact that childbirth practices, at least at Schweitzer's facility, did not allow for the same levels of procedural control as surgical interventions, as the numerous complicated births and deliveries outside of the labor room illustrated. Pregnant women and their unborn babies had many more opportunities to exert their agency than surgical patients under anesthesia. The fact that people frequently sought surgical treatment but that mothers rarely chose to deliver their babies at hospitals suggests that patients and doctors equally valued biomedical practices that promised controlled treatments, procedures, and results.

Doctors at the Albert Schweitzer Hospital meticulously recorded the treatment of infectious diseases with pharmaceuticals, illustrating their desire to maintain procedural control. The practice of forcibly isolating patients, not only in order to hinder the spread of infections throughout the hospital, but also to monitor what they ate and therewith minimize side effects, is the most extreme illustration of this determination to ensure control. However, the practice of trial-and-error testing of new drugs demonstrates that doctors could not constantly uphold control; drugs and patients did not necessarily interact as they expected. The increase in leprosy sufferers who sought treatment at the hospital after sulfones became available demonstrates that patients weighed the potential efficacy of a treatment before subjecting themselves to its methods. If their health promised to improve, they were willing to accept adverse side effects and yield some control over their bodies.

The treatment of mentally ill persons demanded similar levels of procedural control, which was achieved by confining them in cells or by tranquilizing them with drugs. However, regular violent or loud episodes reveal that complete control was impossible to maintain in the psychiatric unit, although there are no reports of psychiatric patients who escaped. Indeed, some even expressed a desire to remain at the hospital indefinitely, despite the fact that many had been brought there initially against their will.

Ignorance, as defined in Chapter 3, can be observed in three dimensions at the Albert Schweitzer Hospital. First, European medical personnel shared the colonial habit of blaming Africans for being ignorant of proper biomedical practices. It should be noted here that doctors across the world regularly bemoaned patient ignorance. In Lambaréné, these accusations of ignorance were especially persistent in urgent obstetric cases. Doctors and nurses at the hospital also complained of surgical patients seeking treatment when it was already too late for them to undergo an operation or, more rarely, that they had undergone non-biomedical interventions. Medical personnel blamed dysentery patients, European and African alike, for underestimating the possibility of contracting the disease and the probability of infecting others. Gabonese communities were accused of treating their mentally ill members with particularly unsuitable methods, including being placed in chains or fed stimulating substances. This was despite the fact that forced isolation and drugs were key elements of psychiatric treatment at the hospital. Allegations of ignorance were also directed against African auxiliaries, who were entrusted with only minor organizational responsibilities and were prevented from freely accessing certain rooms and supplies by locked doors and cupboards.

On the other two levels, ignorance operated as a strategy at the hospital. For one, Schweitzer and his personnel intentionally ignored colonial discourses and practices. Through careful selection, Schweitzer recruited only personnel who were capable of practicing such 'unknowing'. Instead of framing maternity care around common colonial and missionary discourses of depopulation or domesticity, it was presented purely as a medical service. Hospital staff did not indoctrinate local women who came to the hospital to give birth in the prevailing ideas on reproduction or the mother's role in the family. Pregnant women seemed indifferent as to whether hospitals followed a colonial ideology or not; the government hospital in Lambaréné hosted approximately the same number of deliveries as the Albert Schweitzer Hospital. To make more informed claims in this regard, however, would require a closer analysis of the obstetric ward at the former. In contrast, Gabonese came in greater numbers to Schweitzer's hospital, as compared to the government facility, for surgery and the treatment of infectious diseases. In these areas its medical personnel did not ignore relevant colonial discussions and did adhere to contemporary global biomedical trends. In psychiatry, Schweitzer and his staff subscribed to a certain degree to the discourse that assumed that 'modernity' had rendered the 'pre-modern' colonial subject mentally ill. A more persistent idea among doctors and nurses who cared for psychiatric patients at the hospital, however, was that the latter's 'superstitions', such as their belief in spirits or fears of being poisoned, were to blame for their condition. The psychiatric unit was relatively progressive in its focus on therapy, rather than confinement, as its preferred means of treatment, a strategy that also incorporated manual labor as a form of occupational therapy. Moreover, some especially invasive contemporary therapeutic techniques that were widespread in other colonies, such as electric convulsive therapy or lobotomies, were never applied.

'Unknowing' local practices was a second strategy of ignorance consciously applied at the Albert Schweitzer Hospital. For example, doctors argued that surgery was the only suitable approach to repairing large hernias or injuries suffered in animal attacks; they did not consider alternative therapies. Schweitzer and his staff worked to ignore local delivery practices and implied that local methods would be of no help in potentially difficult deliveries. In general, medical personnel at the hospital largely ignored local methods of treatment, especially when only ineffective biomedical therapies were available. When, for instance, new drugs became available, staff started to become interested in local medical treatments. The fate of leprosy sufferers in their communities caught the attention of biomedical personnel precisely at the time when leprosy patients were flocking to the hospital in significantly greater numbers due to the availability of sulfones. Correspondingly, the hospital staff's interest in the nature and local treatment of mental illness grew when new biomedical drugs in the form of antipsychotics promised more efficacious therapies. The production of ignorance is thus most obvious in domains in which biomedical therapies appeared to be less effective than local forms of treatment.

Doctors did not only apply the trial-and-error approach to testing drugs for leprosy and dysentery, as described in Chapter 4. The contrast between the fixed regulations that doctors aimed to establish for administering drugs and the rapidity with which these were reconfigured also arose when attempting to find the most useful antipsychotics, for example. Moreover, the treatment regimes that doctors adopted for psychiatric patients like Njambi can also be characterized as fundamentally trial-and-error in nature. While doctors repeatedly granted him some freedoms in the hope that this would improve his condition, they had to be prepared to respond quickly to his unpredictable behavior.

Surgical patients benefited from similar laissez-faire rules, which left doctors and nurses hoping that their patients would not be exposed to any infections during the recovery process. It was perhaps these freedoms in particular that attracted patients to the hospital. Indeed, patients did tend to prefer Schweitzer's institution for longer stays, while choosing the government clinic across the Ogooué for ambulant treatment. Fittingly, it can thus be said that patients, as a social group, reached this conclusion by 'trialing' each institution and learning from each other's 'errors'.

In obstetrics, trial-and-error methods took a different form than in the treatment of infectious diseases, as each delivery posed its own challenges and required a somewhat unique approach. Furthermore, unlike a patient suffering from leprosy or dysentery, a woman in childbirth could not undergo more than one trial. Staff errors could be fatal, but medical personnel would typically blame patients and their relatives for any complications. While conducting experiments during a delivery was difficult, doctors tested various emergency methods such as craniotomies or cesareans, albeit on a very limited scale.

Useful technological artifacts, such as forceps or vacuum extractors, were introduced after some testing to facilitate regular but difficult births.

Trial-and-error methods, which are closely linked to the idea of improvisation in medicine, also had their limits at the hospital. Some administrative matters, such as organizing the mail, were carefully planned and executed. In the medical field, the approach in the surgical ward was diametrically opposed to a trial-and-error method, as procedures were carefully planned and innovations remained minimal. The two most important units at the Albert Schweitzer Hospital corresponded to the most prestigious domains of biomedicine, surgery and the treatment of infectious diseases. In light of my argument about the improvised nature of biomedicine, it is illuminating that they were based on contrasting clinical principles.

A central concern of Chapter 5 was to illuminate the ways in which Schweitzer and his staff attempted to 'civilize' or 'educate' patients at the hospital. These efforts stand in contrast to the social freedoms that patients enjoyed at the institution. Generally, patients' movements were not controlled, except when they were inside the Grande Pharmacie. They were free to visit friends and indulge in personal habits, such as bathing in the river or going fishing, even when sick. This applied to most patients; exceptions were the mentally ill or those on drugs whose diet was strictly monitored. Schweitzer and his personnel also largely refrained from enforcing typical colonial measures that imposed domesticity upon women.

The 'civilizing mission' at the hospital had a strong focus on manual labor. Schweitzer attached great importance to this aspect of colonial social control, which becomes apparent when examining the way in which the institution was organized and its daily routines. People staying at the hospital – including *gardiens,* recovering and mildly ill patients, and visitors from all over the world – were controlled in the sense that they were supposed to provide labor during much of their stay. This practice reflects Schweitzer's belief that manual labor represented the foundation of 'cultural advancement'. However, numerous patients and *gardiens* did resist this command, as the regular complaints by staff members who acted as their supervisors demonstrate.

Labor was usually not envisaged as a form of therapy. While work was a central feature of the newly established leprosy village, doctors did not attach any medical benefits to patients' labor. Instead, work represented a means to keep them busy and introduce them to what staff believed to be one of the central tenets of Western 'civilization'. Only in psychiatric care was work in the form of occupational therapy considered an essential feature of patients' path to recovery.

Schweitzer's 'civilizing mission' had another dimension. Hospital residents were expected to behave in a manner reflecting Schweitzer's 'Reverence for Life'; in contrast to colonial governments or missions, though, Schweitzer had no wider public health agenda and did not aim to convert hospital residents to Christianity. In order to elucidate the complex relationship between social control and procedural control and between biomedical practice and the 'civilizing mission', a deeper analysis of the ways in which biopolitical ideas diffuse through societies, and of the role that procedural control in biomedicine plays in this process, offers a fruitful avenue for future research.

At various points in this book, I have emphasized that all staff members at the Albert Schweitzer Hospital – doctors, nurses, and auxiliaries alike – had to be able and willing to carry out a wide variety of tasks. Alongside their medical duties, doctors had to repair lamps and engines. They had to remove animals from operation sites or ignore their presence in the consultation rooms. Surgeons had to attend difficult deliveries, as well as conduct trials with leprosy drugs. Nurses had to acquire materials for their wards, plastics for the delivery table, or rust-free instruments for the operating theater, while they were also expected to work in the kitchens, in the laundry, in the gardens, and on the plantations. Indeed, even while enjoying a 'carte blanche' in terms of medical care,[1] nurses still had to supervise African laborers and look after birds or apes as pets. Despite these diverse responsibilities, a strict routine was demanded of staff in many areas of hospital life, an expectation that was especially pronounced for African auxiliaries. Like nurses, auxiliaries were also expected to perform a variety of tasks that required a wide range of skills, but given their relatively lowly position in the hospital hierarchy, historians face greater difficulty in identifying the improvisations that they employed in the process. Their key role as intermediaries, however, was by its very nature improvised, as exhibited most obviously in the act of translating, for which auxiliaries constantly switched not only between languages, but also between medical systems.

Schweitzer believed that Lambaréné needed a specific sort of biomedicine and a specific sort of biomedical practitioner. The former had to be adapted to local circumstances and to his specific demands. The latter had to deal with contradictory practices by, among other things, maintaining great flexibility. This was pivotal because, even as physicians had to perform controlled surgeries in a universal and uniform manner, they also had to try out different treatments for different individuals affected by infectious diseases. Similarly, practitioners at

---

1   Sixt, 'Krankenschwester bei Albert Schweitzer', 64. Sixt's German original term is 'Narrenfreiheit'.

the hospital had to adhere to a defined 'civilizing mission', which was not limited to mentally ill patients, and simultaneously refuse to interfere in local social arrangements and practices, not limited to those of mothers.

Patients also had to improvise during their stays at the hospital, which usually represented exceptional experiences in their biographies. They were expected to find ways to occupy and entertain themselves, an issue that merits further historical attention. They had to adapt to the food that was provided by the hospital, which was not necessarily what they ate at home. They also had to accustom themselves to not using toilets. Nevertheless, some patients seem to have grown so used to life at the Albert Schweitzer Hospital that, once healed, they chose to remain there to serve as auxiliaries.

2   The Practice of Global Biomedicine: Schweitzer and the Value of the Local

The fact that patients came to the hospital only for certain diseases reminds us that Africans improvised on a regular basis by selecting treatments from a range of possibilities. While the vast majority of mentally ill Gabonese people were never taken to a hospital, afflictions that necessitated surgery, such as hernias, were regularly treated in biomedical institutions. By the early 1960s, doctors acknowledged the existence of medical pluralism among Gabonese. Dr. Walter Munz actively sought to cooperate with a local healer who ran her own 'little forest hospital', as he called it, in order to identify cases that he thought could be cured at the Albert Schweitzer Hospital.[2] For his part, Schweitzer believed that he had to accept that medical pluralism could not be eradicated in Gabon. 'The blacks now select beforehand: "that's something for the doctor, and that's something for the fetish man"', he told a visitor in 1961, continuing that 'there's nothing I can do about it. I have to take what remains. We have become colleagues again, the fetish man and I'.[3]

Schweitzer and Munz, like most Western doctors, failed to realize that African pluralism might have equivalents in Europe. In this manner, they created a somewhat problematic African exceptionalism, just as research on the matter later risked doing. At the same time, historians of medicine in the West have largely ignored findings by Africanists, even though both groups were interested

---

2   Munz, *Albert Schweitzer im Gedächtnis der Afrikaner und in meiner Erinnerung*, 139. This local healer was not Marcelline Nyndounge, who was mentioned in Chapter 5, but Cathérine Andone, who practiced near Lac Zilé.

3   Günther and Götting, *Was heisst Ehrfurcht vor dem Leben?*, 160–61.

in questions of power, choice, and affect. Closer attention to issues of pluralism, for example by interrogating the role of the 'therapy management group' or similar questions and concepts from African contexts,[4] would certainly enrich our understanding of medicine in the West from the patient's perspective, as researchers frequently demand. Thus, instead of calling for more interdisciplinary exchanges, I would suggest looking more seriously at the geographical and institutional margins of one's own discipline.

Another matter that Africanists increasingly examine in connection with medicine is its interconnectedness to other domains of power, areas that Western scholars would distinguish as religion, politics, or economics. The role of biomedicine specifically and of its practitioners in this interconnection remains obscure. Augustin Emane has explained the ever-increasing number of patients seeking care at Schweitzer's hospital and the high esteem he enjoyed in local communities as the result of a series of 'productive misunderstandings', to borrow Julie Livingston's useful term.[5] According to Emane, these misunderstandings went far beyond the hospital's self-conception as a space for strictly medical encounters.[6] As my evidence also underscores, Emane agrees with findings from ongoing research on figures similar to Schweitzer, such as Eugène Jamot in Cameroon or Albert Ruskin Cook in Uganda. Their local influence, authority, and reputation exceeded their roles as medical researchers or practitioners.[7] Like research on medical pluralism, the study of such figures can readily partake in the construction of African exceptionalism, which recent research cautions us against doing. In Gabon, Florence Bernault has identified 'a colonial encounter in which each side mixed notions of human and superhuman power'.[8] How and to what extent medicine, religion, economics, and politics are entangled merits further attention in the West as well. An examination of healing and harming in Western medical practice is one possibility to do so, as Claire Wendland has suggested.[9] Our understanding of the issue would also profit from further analyses of the roles of the pharmaceutical

---

4   Janzen, *The Quest for Therapy*, 150.

5   Livingston, 'Productive Misunderstandings'.

6   Emane, *Docteur Schweitzer: une icône africaine*, 44–5, 65–69.

7   I am grateful to Neil Kodesh and Guillaume Lachenal for pointing this out and for sharing this information about their respective ongoing research projects. Conversation in Madison, March 2017. See also: Geissler et al., *Traces of the Future*, especially 62–105 on Ayos, where Jamot is still present in many ways.

8   Frederick Cooper's words about Bernault, *Colonial Transactions*. https://www.dukeupress. edu/colonial-transactions (2 June 2020).

9   Wendland, *A Heart for the Work*, 211–12.

industry, of Christian beliefs, and of insurance imperatives in medical practice and treatment choice.

Schweitzer and his hospital in Gabon are oddly placed in this aggregate of power and ideas. He regularly referred to God, but not as a form of superhuman power, and certainly not one with healing powers. For Schweitzer, God was an ethical principle, with Jesus as a model and guide. In line with his Christian convictions, Schweitzer aimed to keep out what he labeled 'superstitious' medical practices. While it is illusory to believe that he completely managed to do so, the lack of information about such matters tells us something about the degree of his efforts and the secrecy of these practices. It may also suggest that he was relatively successful. At the same time, Schweitzer and many of his personnel acknowledged the existence of practices and beliefs in the region that they considered fundamentally different from their own and did not attempt to eradicate them.

Within these dynamics of medical pluralism and colonial entanglements, which have been studied all over the globe, missions and governments were the two main providers of biomedicine. Medical interventions by colonial governments, especially during the interwar period, often focused on specific diseases within a broad region. In this sense, these operations were transnational; they crossed territorial boundaries and were sometimes trans-colonial endeavors. In any case, they were organized on a top-down basis; knowledge from local experts was usually dismissed. This dismissal of vernacular knowledge comes as no surprise. Yet many government officials stationed in the colonies also suspected that health had a significant social and economic dimension.[10] It was less expensive and less complex, however, to orchestrate campaigns that targeted only a particular affliction. In some ways, these campaigns were preventive; they certainly had a very technical and universal approach to medicine and its practice. They conceived of disease among the colonized as something collective; whole populations were regarded as unhealthy and targeted with biomedical interventionist practices. The health campaigns of colonial governments thus often exemplified the domineering side of biomedicine.

Missionary medicine, by comparison, was curative and local.[11] While missions' staff might have been transnational, their idea and practice of biomedicine often significantly differed from those of government personnel.

---

10   This is a central point of many of the contributions in Widmer and Lipphardt, *Health and Difference*. For the Gabonese context, see: Headrick, *Colonialism, Health and Illness in French Equatorial Africa*, 187–88.

11   Jennings, 'Healing of Bodies, Salvation of Souls'; Prince, 'Situating Health and the Public in Africa', 16–18.

Missionaries and medical practitioners at their stations had a broader notion of health, one that was not exclusively based on biologically traceable processes, even though these were important aspects for them too. Often, but by no means always, their notion of health included a spiritual or religious dimension. More basically and practically, medical missionaries contrasted with their government counterparts in that the former placed a stronger emphasis on well-being, rather than disease. They connected ideas about health with ideas about how to lead a proper social life within a community. The responsibilities and possibilities of the individual were central to the missionary conception of health and disease and to their practices of medicine. Thus, these practices often exemplified the interactive side of biomedicine.

With regard to its practice of biomedicine, the Albert Schweitzer Hospital leaned toward the latter of these ideal types. In comparison to government practitioners, Schweitzer's colonial network was minimal. He did not seek transnational cooperation; in fact, he preferred to recruit doctors with no work experience in the colonies. For Schweitzer and his personnel, the individual and his or her acute afflictions were at the center of their daily medical practice. Like the medical specialists of colonial governments, they placed greater emphasis on disease than on health, but the hospital did not target whole populations in a preventive manner. For Schweitzer, like for many missionary doctors, being healthy included a specific way of living.

3   Taxonomies of Global Health and the Albert Schweitzer Hospital

After Albert Schweitzer's death in 1965, his daughter Rhena and Dr. Walter Munz took over the direction of the hospital. They soon started planning to remodel its facilities and buildings, which were not considered modern enough.[12] In 1974, after a series of difficulties and with closure looming, the 'Fondation Internationale de l'Hôpital du Docteur Albert Schweitzer à Lambaréné' was founded. With the financial help of the Gabonese state, the new amenities were opened for patients in 1981, located a short walk uphill from where Schweitzer had erected his second hospital. The national government gained influence with regard to the hospital's structure and strategy, as exemplified by the research station and laboratory that were attached to the hospital at the state's request.[13] The system of cooperation between the state and the

---

12   Interview Munz and Munz.
13   Mabika, 'L'hôpital Albert Schweitzer de Lambaréné', 211–14. See also: https://www.cermel. org/history.php (2 June 2020).

Fondation still takes place and requires repeated negotiations of interest and power to secure the hospital's offers. During my six years of working on this project, rumors about the institution closing down made their way to my office on three different occasions. Donations and doctors from abroad remain central pillars to ensure that biomedicine continues to be practiced at the Albert Schweitzer Hospital. The history of the hospital hence illustrates numerous developments of biomedicine in the global context.

In discussions on global health, practitioners and theoreticians with some historical awareness often draw a line from colonial medicine to tropical medicine to international health to present-day global health.[14] They stress continuities in power structures inherent in many historical and current health programs and also identify continuities in practices, such as transnational cooperation or the disregard of local realities. Scholars of global health typically identify two distinct approaches, which can be traced throughout the twentieth century and which echo my own characterization of biomedicine's domineering and interactive sides.[15]

The dominant approach to global health remains a vertical one. Proponents consider disease as something mainly biological and thus universal. Hence, they believe in technical solutions. This approach is exemplified by organizations such as Médecins sans Frontières or the Rockefeller Foundation and lies behind many programs of the World Health Organization. Earlier in the century, the medical interventions of colonial governments shared many of these characteristics. Today's non-governmental organizations, like colonial administrations before them, normally are aware of the social and economic roots of many health problems. Nevertheless, their focus was and is on programs that target specific diseases, which has the advantages of producing somewhat measurable outcomes and of being politically acceptable. In theory, such an approach does not require advanced knowledge of the societies for which interventions are planned. Local realities and practices gain importance only when they threaten the success of the program.

At the other pole of the global health spectrum, a holistic approach has always placed greater emphasis on general well-being and primary healthcare. It conceives of health within the context of global challenges, such as migration

---

14   Anderson, 'Making Global Health History'; Geissler, 'Introduction: A Life Science in Its African Para-State'; Greene et al., 'Colonial Medicine and Its Legacies'; Webb, Jr and Giles-Vernick, 'Global Health in Africa, Introduction'.

15   Packard, *A History of Global Health*, 337–39; Prince, 'Situating Health and the Public in Africa'. See also: Bruchhausen, 'Reviews of V. Adams, "Metrics. What Counts in Global Health" and R. Packard, "A History of Global Health. Interventions into the Lives of Other Peoples"'.

or climate change. It aims to address the social and economic roots of disease and thus calls for taking into account historical and anthropological knowledge. In some ways, this type of practice is an heir of missionary medicine, which is today exemplified by Partners in Health. In general, this approach was and is considered too costly, too difficult to measure, and politically suspect.

In this taxonomy of global health ideal types, it is less obvious that the Albert Schweitzer Hospital leaned towards the more holistic vision, as it incorporated elements from both approaches. The practice of medicine there can be characterized as top-down, for Schweitzer established clear rules and determined limits with regard to innovations. However, his approach was not strictly vertical, as he placed greater emphasis, if only implicitly, on sustainability. A more obvious difference from the vertical approach is that the hospital did not only address single diseases. Personnel treated whatever illness patients came to the institution for. In this sense, they delivered primary healthcare, as demanded by a holistic approach to global health.

Schweitzer and his personnel sometimes adopted a technical attitude toward medicine and disease. The procedural control enacted in surgery is a prime example thereof. The individual care provided for mentally ill persons, on the other hand, illustrates a practice that puts humans at the center. The warm reception of patients more clearly suggests that, by certain measures, staff had a non-technical approach to medicine, in accordance with Schweitzer's 'Reverence for Life'. This ethical principle and the laissez-faire policy connected to it directed personnel to accept medical pluralism in the region and hence acknowledge the limits not only of their techniques, but also of their responsibilities. Trial-and-error methods, for example, depended by definition on the situation, the locale, and the individual, but only as long as the patient was on the hospital grounds. In this sense, medical practitioners at the Albert Schweitzer Hospital did not consider biomedicine something neutral and universally applicable.

Like the more holistic approach to global health, Schweitzer and his personnel took into account local realities and demands. The hospital's main medical offers, surgery and the treatment of infectious diseases, were responses to the most salient local health problems that biomedicine was able to cure. This does not mean that external factors had no influence on what the hospital offered or what Gabonese demanded. The example of leprosy illustrates that the development of more efficacious drugs could lead to an influx of patients. The quickly growing number of mothers choosing to give birth at the hospital in the late 1950s similarly suggests an external reason for an increase in demand and service. In this way, Schweitzer and his personnel were interested in satisfying people's basic health needs; they treated patients for what they wanted treated.

However, as with today's vertical approach to global health, neither Schweitzer nor any of his staff showed an interest in solving African health problems on a social or economic level. Their actions were largely confined to the hospital grounds and thus remained vastly curative and apolitical. The few times when doctors or nurses left the institution, they often did so to treat people in lumber camps. They thus supported the existing economic system that exploited people and their environment. This system accelerated the spread of a variety of diseases that were treated at the hospital, such as hernias or dysentery, and its existence certainly did not contribute to the general well-being of individuals or populations. And whenever Schweitzer voiced political opinions on local issues, which he rarely did in written form, he usually defended the colonial status quo.

I argue not only that the Albert Schweitzer Hospital was peculiarly placed within these taxonomies of global health, but also that any medical institution is bound to be. This peculiarity is a central aspect of biomedicine, in Africa and beyond; it is at once domineering and interactive. The improvised and incoherent nature of biomedicine becomes plainly visible through an analytical focus on medical practices and attention to how these were executed on a daily basis. One precondition for studying medical practices historically, as opposed to via anthropological or sociological participative research, is the availability of detailed narrative sources. Analyzing official colonial government and mission documents such as annual reports or dispatches from surveys conveys the impression that medical campaigns and treatments were well planned and seamlessly conducted. The findings of my study thus contribute to a growing scholarship that places the rationality of the colonial project at large in doubt; while biomedical endeavors and European ventures in the colonies may have been driven by a grand plan, their underlying ideas were rarely fully applicable in practice.

In order to reach an understanding of biomedicine that is both broad and deep, it is essential to take into account more than one domain of biomedicine, to conduct research on different aspects of medical care and its relationship to society, and to study the same setting from more than one point of view and with more than one analytical lens. If I had examined only surgery at the Albert Schweitzer Hospital, I might have concluded that the hospital was a highly structured and rational place with a relatively neutral mission; I might also have concluded that patients came mainly from lumber camps, to which they would return after being rather informally accommodated. If I had examined solely the treatment of leprosy, I might have concluded that the hospital was a therapeutically random institution that focused on a relatively insignificant disease and on providing accommodation to patients; I might have seen its main mission as spreading the art of manual labor among Gabonese patients, who would rarely return to their communities. The Albert Schweitzer Hospital was none of these things and all of these things; it was the microhistorical 'normal exception'. It was, like any medical place, a place full of ideas, but also full of incoherence and improvisations.

Bibliography

Archival Sources

Archives of the Maison Albert Schweitzer, Gunsbach (AMS)

– Letters from the correspondence between Albert Schweitzer and the following individuals or organizations (as listed in the catalogue):

Abelmann, Arthur.
Alliez, Joseph.
Barasch, Heinz.
Bayer, Aktiengesellschaft.
Bernoulli, Eugen.
Bonnema, Barend.
Bonnema, Lies.
Boyard, James.
Catchpool, Francis.
Chesterman, Clement.
De Pulligny, Jean.
Degen & Kuhn, Drs.
Dubourg, Docteur.
Elise, Stalder.
Elise, Vogel.
Friedmann, Richard.
Garnier, Administrateur.
Gauss, Werner.
Giemsa, Gustav.
Goldschmid, Ladislav.
Hediger, Karl.
Houget, Docteur.
Hume, Edward.
Irrmann, Docteur.
Israël, Paul.
Juillard, Edouard.
Kik, Richard.
Kopp, René.

Lagendijk, Maria.
Lambaréné, Administrateur.
Langhorn, Docteur.
Le Forestier, Roger.
Mandel, Georges.
Martin, Emmy (*transcribed by Walter Schriber*).
Naegele, Jean-Pierre.
Percy, Emeric.
Rieder, Emily.
Röthlisberger, Emmy.
Royden, Maud.
Russell, Lilian.
Sandoz, AG.
Seaver, George.
Spiro, Karl.
Spoerri, Emilie.
Stalder, Elise.
Stoll, Arthur.
Stolz, Pierre.
Strassburger Comitee.
Szabo, André.
Thiébaud, Marcel.
Van der Kreek, Greet
Weber, Alice.
Weiss, Robert.
Wildikann, Anna.

Note: Sometimes Schweitzer's secretaries, Mathilde Kottmann or Emma Haussknecht, actually wrote his letters, which he always signed.

– Notebooks of Albert Schweitzer are kept at Syracuse University. The AMS holds copies, which were also digitized. I have quoted from the following two:
'Medizinische Notizen, Albert Schweitzer Lambarene 1953'.
'1930 Therapeutische Notizen'.

– Hospital records were digitized and codified for this project. I have quoted from the following:
Appels mensuels; 1932–1976, L – P – AM1–13.
Cahiers des patients (also include appels mensuels); 1913–1917 & 1925–1929/31, L – P – C1–16.
Cahiers des patients (Européens); 1928–1931, L – P – E1.
Protocols des accouchements; 1937–1941 & 1958–1965, L – P – A1–8.
Protocols des opérations; 1925–1977, L – P – O1–23.
Statistiques de l'Hôpital: 1926–1931 (L – A – S1); 1932–1936 (L – A – S 2); 1937–1943, 1946, 1950, 1966 (L – A – S3).

– Medical manuscripts from personnel and visitors are uncatalogued. The following were brought to my attention by the archivist:
Anonymous, 'Leprosan Patienten', dated 14 February 1958.
Anonymous, 'Lepra Medikamente', undated (possibly 1958).
Goldwyn, Robert M. 'Diary of November and December 1960, at the Albert Schweitzer Hospital, Lambaréné, Gabon'.
Naegele, Jean-Pierre. 'Traitement des malades lépreux à l'Hôpital du Docteur Albert Schweitzer, à Lambaréné au cours de l'année 1950'.
Naegele, Jean-Pierre 'Rapport Medical sur l'HAS 1951'.
Naegele, Jean-Pierre 'Streiflichter aus Lambarene. 1951 III Um die Lepra', 1951.
Schoenfeld, Eugen. Draft of 'A Summer at Dr. Schweitzer's Hospital: Smith, Kline, and French Foreign Fellowship Report', 1961.
Staewen, Christoph. 'Die geistes- und gemütskranken Patienten des Spitals Lambarene', 1964.

Archives of the Wisconsin Historical Society, Madison (AWHS)
Noel A. Gillespie Papers.
  Call Number: Wis Mss UR; Micro 447;
    Box 2 (1922–1926),
    Box 7 ('Albert Schweitzer').

Archives Nationales du Gabon, Libreville (ANG)
Archives Coloniales: Santé et Assistance PR(H), 'Services Sanitaires'.
  1 H 226.1: Région Sanitaire du Moyen Ogooué. Centre Médical de Lambaréné 1961;

1 H 235.3: Région sanitaire du Moyen-Ogooué. Hôpital Schweitzer – Lépreux re-
    cencés depuis 1947;

1 H 235.4: Région sanitaire du Moyen-Ogooué. Hôpital Schweitzer. Rapport annuel
    1955;

1 H 254.1: Lèpre. – Organisation de la lutte contre la lèpre en A.E.F. et au Gabon
    1951–55;

1 H 254.4: Lèpre. – Instructions, dépistages, traitements, pensions, statistiques 1953.
Rubriques des Archives de Lambarene 2 DC(1), 'Services Sanitaries'.

   44.11: Rapports Annuels (1953, 1954).

Archives Nationales d'Outre-Mer, Aix-en-Provence (ANOM)

Fonds Territoriaux, Afrique Équatoriale Française, Gouvernement Général de l'Afrique
    Équatorial Française, Série D – Politique et administration générale 1883/1959,
    4 D Rapports politiques et administratifs 1889/1959,
        4(1)D – Gabon 1894/1953,
            4(1)D 36–38 (1930–32);
            4(1)D 44 (1936).

Archives du Service Historique de la Défense, Toulon (SHD)

Série F 'Service de santé', (sous série 2F4);
    Missions Gabon, 2013 ZK,
        005–174 (1939, 1948, 1953);
    Rapports annuels Gabon, 2013 ZK,
        005–127 (1931–34), 005–005 (1945, 1952–57), 005–128 (1946–51);
    Rapports annuels AEF, 2013 ZK,
        005–121 (1933–36), 005–160 (1939–44), 005–89 (1945–47), 005–91 (1949–50),
        005–92 (1951), 005–97 (1952), 005–93 (1952–53), 005–94 (1952), 005–16 (1954–55),
        005–95 (1955–56).

Interviews

I have conducted semi-structured interviews in either French or Swiss German. They
were digitally recorded with the agreement of the interviewee. The following persons
were so kind to speak to me:

Anderegg, Elisabeth, Waldstatt, 16 October 2014.

Azizet-Mburu, Daudette, Libreville, 14 September 2015.

Bouassa, Albert, Lambaréné, 18 September 2015.

Boucah, Jacques, Libreville, 15 September 2015.

Bunch, Ursula, Brittnau, 29 October 2014.

Munz, Walter and Jo, St. Gallen, 3 December 2014; interview conducted together with Hines Mabika and Hubert Steinke.

Ndiaye-Boucah, Marie-Joséphine, Libreville, 14 September 2015.

Nsowe, Léontine, Lambaréné, 18 September 2015; Nsowe did not want to be recorded.

Padje-Poabalou, Anne-Marie, Lambaréné, 18 September 2015.

Rolagho, Jacques-Adrien, Libreville 12 September 2015.

Stocker, Marianne, Richterswil, 21 January 2015.

In addition, I have conducted the following two group interviews, which were recorded with the agreement of the interviewees:

Group Interview Speicherschwendi, 3 November 2014. Interview partners: Hedwig Schnee, Marianne Stocker, Myrtha Suhner, Anna-Maria Heer; interview conducted together with Hines Mabika.

Group Interview Port-Gentil, 17 September 2015. Interview partners: Benoit Moussavou-Wora, Yanja Marthe Rembendambja, Ngouawiri Suzanne Rembendambja, Didier Faustin.

Published References

Achebe, Chinua. *The Education of a British-Protected Child: Essays*. New York: Alfred A. Knopf, 2009.

Addae, Stephen. *The Evolution of Modern Medicine in a Developing Country: Ghana 1880–1960*. Edinburgh: Durham Academic Press, 1997.

Akyeampong, Emmanuel, Allan Hill, and Arthur Kleinman. 'Introduction: Culture, Mental Illness, and Psychiatric Practice in Africa'. In *Culture of Mental Illness and Psychiatric Practice in Africa*, edited by Emmanuel Akyeampong, Allan Hill, and Arthur Kleinman, 24–49. Bloomington: Indiana University Press, 2015.

Alexandre, Pierre, and Jacques Binet. *Le groupe dit Pahouin* (*Fang, Boulou, Beti*). Paris: Presses Universitaires de France, 1958.

Allman, Jean. 'Making Mothers: Missionaries, Medical Officers and Women's Work in Colonial Asante, 1924–1945'. In *History Workshop Journal*, 38:23–47. Oxford University Press, 1994.

Ambouroue-Avaro, Joseph. *Un peuple gabonais à l'aube de la colonisation : le Bas-Ogowe au 19e siècle*. Paris: Karthala, 1981.

Anderegg, Elisabeth. 'Operationssaal und Sterilisation'. In *Mit dem Herzen einer Gazelle und der Haut eines Nilpferds: Albert Schweitzer in seinen letzten Lebensjahren und die Entwicklung seines Spitals bis zur Gegenwart*, edited by Jo Munz and Walter Munz, 55–57. Frauenfeld: Huber, 2005.

Anderson, Warwick. 'Making Global Health History: The Postcolonial Worldliness of Biomedicine'. *Social History of Medicine* 27, no. 2 (2014): 372–84.

Andrews, George R. 'Psychiatric Facilities at the Albert Schweitzer Hospital'. *American Journal of Psychiatry* 118, no. 6 (1961): 524–28.

Arnold, Matthieu. '"Vous les noirs, nous les blancs…" L'opposition entre Européens et Africains dans les sermons de Schweitzer à Lambaréné (1913–1931)'. *Revue d'histoire et de philosophie religieuses* 83, no. 4 (2003): 421–441.

Au, Sokhieng. 'Cutting the Flesh: Surgery, Autopsy and Cannibalism in the Belgian Congo'. *Medical History* 61, no. 2 (2017): 295–312.

Audoynaud, André. *Le docteur Schweitzer et son hôpital à Lambaréné: l'envers d'un mythe*. Paris: L'Harmattan, 2005.

Aujoulat, Pierre. 'Albert Schweitzer, médecin de brousse 1935 et 1965'. In *Rayonnement d'Albert Schweitzer: 34 études et 100 témoignage*, edited by Robert Minder, 220–24. Colmar: Ed. Alsatia, 1975.

Bado, Jean-Paul. *Médecine coloniale et grandes endémies en Afrique 1900–1960 : lèpre, trypanosomiase humaine et onchocercose*. Paris: Ed. Karthala, 1996.

Bado, Jean-Paul. 'Histoire, maladies et médecines en Afrique Occidentale XIXe-XXe siècles'. *Revue française d'histoire d'outre-mer* 86, no. 322–323 (1999): 237–268.

Bähr, Hans Walter, ed. *Albert Schweitzer: Leben, Werk und Denken 1905–1965: Mitgeteilt in seinen Briefen*. Heidelberg: Lambert Schneider, 1987.

Balandier, Georges. *Sociologie actuelle de l'Afrique Noire: changements sociaux au Gabon et au Congo*. Paris: Presses Universitaires de France, 1955.

Balandier, Georges. *Afrique ambiguë*. Paris: Plon, 1957.

Balandier, Georges, and Jean-Claude Pauvert. *Les villages gabonais: aspects démographiques, économiques, sociologiques, projets de modernisation*. Montpellier: Imprimerie Charité, 1952.

Balsiger, Greti. 'Ein helles Band und ein Sonntag'. In *Wir halfen dem Doktor in Lambarene: Festgabe zum 85. Geburtstag von Albert Schweitzer*, edited by Olga Fausel-Wieber, Ilse Schnabel, and Gertrud Koch, 139–50. Zürich: Schweizer Druck- und Verlagshaus, 1960.

Ban, Thomas A. 'Fifty Years Chlorpromazine: A Historical Perspective'. *Neuropsychiatric Disease and Treatment* 3, no. 4 (August 2007): 495–500.

Barthélemy, Guy. *Wie ich Lambarene erlebte: Ein junger Mensch besucht Albert Schweitzer*. München: C.H. Beck, 1953.

Barthélemy, Guy. *Lettre à Albert Schweitzer*, 1966.

Barthélemy, Pascale. 'Sages-femmes africaines diplômées en AOF des années 1920 aux années 1960. Une redéfinition des rapports sociaux de sexe en contexte colonial'. In *Histoire des femmes en situation coloniale: Afrique et Asie, XXe siècle*, edited by Anne Hugon, 119–44. Paris: Karthala, 2004.

Baudoux, Raymond. *La situation psychiatrique au Congo et au Ruanda-Urundi en 1950–1951*. Institut royal colonial belge, 1952.

Becht, Jean-Claude. 'Témoignage d'une chirurgien, Mme Le Docteur Greet Barthélémy'. In *Schweitzer, le médecin*, edited by Jean-Paul Sorg, 170–75. Strasbourg: Editions Oberlin, 1995.

Bell, Heather. *Frontiers of Medicine in the Anglo-Egyptian Sudan, 1899–1940*. Oxford: Clarendon Press, 2004.

Berman, Edgar. *In Africa with Schweitzer: A Remarkable Memoir by the U.S. Surgeon Who Worked with Schweitzer*. New York: Harper & Row, 1986.

Bernault, Florence. 'Dévoreurs de la nation: Les migrations fang au Gabon'. *Être étranger et migrant en Afrique au XX e siècle*, edited by Catherine Coquery-Vidrovitch and Issiaka Mandé 169–187, Paris: L'Harmattan, 2003.

Bernault, Florence. 'Body, Power and Sacrifice in Equatorial Africa'. *The Journal of African History* 47, no. 02 (2006): 207–239.

Bernault, Florence. 'De la modernité comme impuissance. Fétichisme et crise du politique en Afrique équatoriale et ailleurs'. *Cahiers d'études africaines*, no. 3 (2009): 747–774.

Bernault, Florence. 'Carnal Technologies and the Double Life of the Body in Gabon'. *Critical African Studies* 5, no. 3 (2013): 175–194.

Bernault, Florence. 'Witchcraft and the Colonial Life of the Fetish'. In *Spirits in Politics: Uncertainties of Power and Healing in African Societies*, edited by Barbara Meier and Arne S. Steinforth, 49–70. Frankfurt: Campus Verlag, 2013.

Bernault, Florence. *Colonial Transactions: Imaginaries, Bodies, and Histories in Gabon*. Durham: Duke University Press, 2019.

Bernault, Florence, and Joseph Tonda. 'Dynamiques de l'invisible en Afrique'. *Politique Africaine*, no. 3 (2000): 5–16.

Bessuges, Jacques. *Lambaréné à l'ombre de Schweitzer*. Limoges: Dessagne, 1968.

Bhabha, Homi K. 'Signs Taken for Wonders: Questions of Ambivalence and Authority under a Tree Outside Delhi, May 1817'. *Critical Inquiry* 12, no. 1 (1985): 144–165.

Bijker, Wiebe E., Thomas Peter Hughes, and Trevor J. Pinch, eds. 'General Introduction'. In *The Social Construction of Technological Systems: New Directions in the Sociology and History of Technology*, 1–6. Cambridge (Mass.): MIT Press, 1987.

Bonneuil, Christophe. 'Development as Experiment: Science and State Building in Late Colonial and Postcolonial Africa, 1930–1970'. *Osiris*, 2000, 258–281.

Borck, Cornelius. 'Quo vadis, Krankenhausgeschichte? Plädoyer für ihre Fortführung als Umbaugeschichte'. In *Krankenhausgeschichte heute: was heißt und zu welchem Ende studiert man Hospital- und Krankenhausgeschichte?*, edited by Gunnar Stollberg, Christina Vanja, and Ernst Kraas, 17–22. Berlin: Lit-Verlag, 2011.

Boundzanga, Noël Bertrand, and Wilson-André Ndombet, eds. *Le Malentendu Schweitzer*. Paris: L'Harmattan, 2014.

Breitenstein, Ruth. 'Meine Arbeit mit den geistes- und gemütskranken Menschen in Lambarene'. In *Mit dem Herzen einer Gazelle und der Haut eines Nilpferds: Albert Schweitzer in seinen letzten Lebensjahren und die Entwicklung seines Spitals bis zur Gegenwart*, edited by Jo Munz and Walter Munz, 71–74. Frauenfeld: Huber, 2005.

Bruchhausen, Walter. '"Practising Hygiene and Fighting the Natives' Diseases". Public and Child Health in German East Africa and Tanganyika Territory, 1900–1960'. *Dynamis: Acta Hispanica Ad Medicinae Scientiarumque. Historiam Illustrandam* 23 (2003): 085–113.

Bruchhausen, Walter. 'Heil und Unheil aus dem Leib. Körpereingriffe in der ostafrikanischen Medizin.' *Würzburger medizinhistorische Mitteilungen* 24 (2005): 82–98.

Bruchhausen, Walter. *Medizin zwischen den Welten: Geschichte und Gegenwart des medizinischen Pluralismus im südöstlichen Tansania.* Göttingen: V&R unipress, 2006.

Bruchhausen, Walter. 'Medicine between Religious Worlds: The Mission Hospitals of South-East Tanzania during the Twentieth Century'. In *From Western Medicine to Global Medicine. The Hospital beyond the West*, edited by Mark Harrison, Margaret Jones, and Helen Sweet. Hyderabad: Orient BlackSwan, 2009.

Bruchhausen, Walter. '"Biomedizin" in sozial-und kulturwissenschaftlichen Beiträgen'. *NTM Zeitschrift für Geschichte der Wissenschaften, Technik und Medizin* 18, no. 4 (2010): 497–522.

Bruchhausen, Walter. 'Medical Pluralism as a Historical Phenomenon: A Regional and Multi-Level Approach to Health Care in German, British and Independent East Africa'. In *Crossing Colonial Historiographies: Histories of Colonial and Indigenous Medicines in Transnational Perspective*, edited by Anne Digby, Waltraud Ernst, and Projit B. Mukharji, 99–110. Newcastle upon Tyne: Cambridge Scholars Publishing, 2010.

Bruchhausen, Walter. 'Reviews of V. Adams, 'Metrics. What Counts in Global Health' (2016) and R. Packard, 'A History of Global Health. Interventions into the Lives of Other Peoples' (2016)'. *NTM. Zeitschrift für Geschichte der Wissenschaften, Technik und Medizin* 25, no. 2 (2017): 257–63.

Brydan, David. 'Mikomeseng: Leprosy, Legitimacy and Francoist Repression in Spanish Guinea'. *Social History of Medicine* 31, no. 3 (2017): 627–647.

Carleton Paget, James. 'Albert Schweitzer and Africa'. *Journal of Religion in Africa* 42, no. 3 (2012): 277–316.

Carleton Paget, James, and Michael J. Thate. 'Introduction: Questioning the Relevance of Albert Schweitzer'. In *Albert Schweitzer in Thought and Action: A Life in Parts*, edited by James Carleton Paget and Michael J. Thate, 1–23. New York: Syracuse University Press, 2016.

Chakrabarti, Pratik. *Medicine and Empire, 1600–1960.* Basingstoke: Palgrave Macmillan, 2014.

Cinnamon, John M. 'Missionary Expertise, Social Science, and the Uses of Ethnographic Knowledge in Colonial Gabon'. *History in Africa* 33, no. 1 (2006): 413–32.

Cinnamon, John M. 'Colonial Anthropologies and the Primordial Imagination in Equatorial Africa'. In *Ordering Africa: Anthropology, European Imperialism and the Politics of Knowledge*, edited by Helen Tilley, 225–51. Manchester: Manchester University Press, 2010.

Cinnamon, John M. 'Counting and Recounting: Dislocation, Colonial Demography, and Historical Memory in Northern Gabon'. In *The Demographics of Empire: The Colonial Order and the Creation of Knowledge*, edited by Karl Ittmann, 130–56. Athens: Ohio University Press, 2010.

Cinnamon, John M. 'Of Fetishism and Totemism: Missionary Ethnology and Academic Social Science in Early-Twentieth-Century Gabon'. In *The Spiritual in the Secular: Missionaries and Knowledge about Africa*, edited by David Maxwell and Patrick Harries, 100–134. Grand Rapids: William B. Eerdmans, 2012.

Cinnamon, John M. 'Spirits, Power and the Political Imagination in Late-Colonial Gabon'. *Africa* 82, no. 02 (2012): 187–211.

Coghe, Samuël. 'Inter-Imperial Learning and African Health Care in Portuguese Angola in the Interwar Period'. *Social History of Medicine* 28, no. 1 (2015): 134–154.

Coghe, Samuël, and Alexandra Widmer. 'Colonial Demography. Discourses, Rationalities, Methods'. In *Twentieth Century Population Thinking: A Critical Reader in Primary Sources*, edited by Heinrich Hartmann, 37–64. London: Routledge, 2016.

Cole, Jonathan. 'Engendering Health: Pronatalist Politics and the History of Nursing and Midwifery in Colonial Senegal, 1914–1967'. In *Routledge Handbook of the History of Nursing*, edited by Patricia D'Antonio, Julie A. Fairman, and Jean C. Whelan, 114–30. London: Routledge Taylor & Francis Group, 2013.

Collignon, René. 'Some Aspects of Mental Illness in French-Speaking West Africa'. In *Culture of Mental Illness and Psychiatric Practice in Africa*, edited by Emmanuel Akyeampong, Allan Hill, and Arthur Kleinman, 163–85. Bloomington: Indiana University Press, 2015.

Comaroff, John L., and Jean Comaroff. *Christianity, Colonialism and Consciousness in South Africa*. Chicago: The University of Chicago Press, 1997.

Condrau, Flurin. 'The Patient's View Meets the Clinical Gaze'. *Social History of Medicine* 20, no. 3 (2007): 525–540.

Conklin, Alice L. *A Mission to Civilize: The Republican Idea of Empire in France and West Africa, 1895–1930*. Stanford: Stanford University Press, 2003.

Cooper, Frederick. 'Conflict and Connection: Rethinking Colonial African History'. *The American Historical Review* 99, no. 5 (1994): 1516–45.

Cooper, Frederick, and Ann Laura Stoler. 'Introduction Tensions of Empire: Colonial Control and Visions of Rule'. *American Ethnologist* 16, no. 4 (1989): 609–621.

Cordell, Dennis D., Karl Ittman, and Gregory H. Maddox. 'Counting Subjects: Demography and Empire'. In *The Demographics of Empire: The Colonial Order and the Creation of Knowledge*, edited by Karl Ittmann, 1–21. Athens: Ohio University Press, 2010.

Cousins, Norman. *Dr. Schweitzer of Lambaréné*. New York: Harper, 1960.

Craig, Charles Franklin. *The Etiology, Diagnosis, and Treatment of Amebiasis*. Williams & Wilkins, 1944.

Crozier, Anna. *Practising Colonial Medicine: The Colonial Medical Service in British East Africa*. London: I.B. Tauris, 2007.

Crozier, Anna. 'What Was Tropical about Tropical Neurasthenia? The Utility of the Diagnosis in the Management of British East Africa'. *Journal of the History of Medicine and Allied Sciences* 64, no. 4 (2009): 518–548.

Cunningham, Andrew, and Bridie Andrews, eds. *Western Medicine as Contested Knowledge*. Manchester: Manchester University Press, 1997.

Davin, Anna. 'Imperialism and Motherhood'. In *History Workshop* (1978), 9–65.

Debusmann, Robert. 'Médicalisation et pluralisme au Cameroun allemand: autorité médicale et stratégies profanes'. *Outre-mers* 90, no. 338–339 (2003): 225–246.

Deschamps, Hubert. *Traditions orales et archives au Gabon : contribution à l'ethno-histoire*. Paris: Berger-Levrault, 1962.

Digby, Anne. *Diversity and Division in Medicine: Health Care in South Africa from the 1800s*. Oxford: Peter Lang, 2006.

Digby, Anne, and Howard Phillips. *At the Heart of Healing: Groote Schuur Hospital, 1938–2008*. Auckland Park: Jacana, 2008.

Dilley, Roy, and Thomas G. Kirsch, eds. 'Regimes of Ignorance: An Introduction'. In *Regimes of Ignorance: Anthropological Perspectives on the Production and Reproduction of Non-Knowledge*. New York: Berghahn Books, 2015.

Dinges, Martin. 'Arztpraxen 1500–1900. Zum Stand der Forschung'. In *Arztpraxen im Vergleich: 18.–20. Jahrhundert*, edited by Elisabeth Dietrich-Daum, Martin Dinges, Robert Jütte, and Christine Roilo, 23–61. Innsbruck: StudienVerlag, 2008.

Dinges, Martin, Kay Peter Jankrift, Sabine Schlegelmilch, and Michael Stolberg, eds. *Medical Practice, 1600–1900: Physicians and Their Patients*. Leiden: Brill, 2015.

Dinges, Martin, and Michael Stolberg. 'Introduction'. In *Medical Practice, 1600–1900: Physicians and Their Patients*, edited by Martin Dinges, Kay Peter Jankrift, Sabine Schlegelmilch, and Michael Stolberg, 1–7. Leiden: Brill, 2015.

Dirar, Uoldelul Chelati. 'Curing Bodies to Rescue Souls: Health in Capuchin's Missionary Strategy in Eritrea, 1894–1935'. In *Healing Bodies, Saving Souls: Medical Missions in Asia and Africa*, edited by David Hardiman, 251–80. Amsterdam: Rodopi, 2006.

Donzé, Pierre-Yves. *L'ombre de César: les chirurgiens et la construction du système hospitalier vaudois 1840–1960*. Lausanne: Bibliothèque d'Histoire de la médecine et de la Santé, 2007.

Doyle, Shane. *Before HIV: Sexuality, Fertility and Mortality in East Africa 1900–1980*. Oxford: Oxford University Press, 2013.

Dreier, Marcel. '"Europäisch gebären". Katholische Mission, Mutterschaft und Moderne im ländlichen Tansania 1930–1960'. In *Der schwarze Körper als Missionsgebiet:*

Medizin, Ethnologie und Theologie in Afrika und Europa 1880–1960, edited by Siegfried Weichlein and Linda Ratschiller, 153–74. Köln: Böhlau Verlag, 2016.

Duffin, Jacalyn. *Langstaff: A Nineteenth-Century Medical Life*. Toronto: University of Toronto Press, 1993.

Ebang, Emmanuel. 'De la diversité des itinéraires thérapeutiques au Gabon : essai d'analyse des logiques de la quête de guérison en milieu urbain africain'. In *Le Gabon: approche pluridisciplinaire*, edited by Gilchrist Anicet Nzenguet Iguemba, 22–35. Paris: L'Harmattan, 2006.

Eckart, Wolfgang U. *Medizin und Kolonialimperialismus: Deutschland 1884 – 1945*. Paderborn, Zürich: Ferdinand Schöningh, 1997.

Eckart, Wolfgang U. 'The Colony as Laboratory: German Sleeping Sickness Campaigns in German East Africa and in Togo, 1900–1914'. *History and Philosophy of the Life Sciences*, 2002, 69–89.

Edington, Claire. *Beyond the Asylum: Colonies Agricoles and the History of Psychiatry in French Indochina, 1918–1945*. Ann Arbor: Michigan Publishing, University of Michigan Library, 2011.

Emane, Augustin. *Docteur Schweitzer: une icône africaine*. Paris: Fayard, 2013.

Ernst, Waltraud, ed. *Plural Medicine, Tradition and Modernity, 1800–2000*. London: Routledge, 2002.

Fabian, Johannes. *Out of Our Minds: Reason and Madness in the Exploration of Central Africa*. Berkeley: University of California Press, 2000.

Faget, G.H., R.C. Pogge, and F.A. Johansen. 'Present Status of Diasone in the Treatment of Leprosy: Brief Clinical Note'. *Public Health Reports (1896–1970)*, 1946, 960–963.

Feierman, Steven. 'Struggles for Control: The Social Roots of Health and Healing in Modern Africa'. *African Studies Review* 28, no. 2–3 (1985): 73–147.

Feierman, Steven, and John M. Janzen. 'Introduction'. In *The Social Basis of Health and Healing in Africa*. Berkeley: University of California Press, 1992.

Fernandez, James W. 'Christian Acculturation and Fang Witchcraft'. *Cahiers d'études Africaines* 2, no. 6 (1961): 244–270.

Fernandez, James W. 'The Sound of Bells in a Christian Country: In Quest of the Historical Schweitzer'. *The Massachusetts Review* 5, no. 3 (1964): 537–562.

Fernandez, James W. 'Symbolic Consensus in a Fang Reformative Cult'. *American Anthropologist* 67, no. 4 (1965): 902–929.

Fernandez, James W. *Bwiti: An Ethnography of the Religious Imagination in Africa*. Princeton: Princeton University Press, 1982.

Franck, Frederick. *Days with Albert Schweitzer: A Lambaréné Landscape*. London: Peter Davies, 1959.

Franck, Frederick. *My Friend in Africa*. London: Peter Davies, 1961.

Friedl-Meyer, Martha. *Lehrbuch der Chirurgie für das Pflegepersonal*. Zürich: Schulthess, 1943.

Füllemann, Emmy. 'Aus jüngster Zeit'. In *Wir halfen dem Doktor in Lambarene: Festgabe zum 85. Geburtstag von Albert Schweitzer*, edited by Olga Fausel-Wieber, Ilse Schnabel, and Gertrud Koch, 160–64. Zürich: Schweizer Druck- und Verlagshaus, 1960.

Gardinier, David E. *Historical Dictionary of Gabon*. 2nd ed. African Historical Dictionaries, No. 58. Metuchen: Scarecrow Press, 1994.

Gaulme, François. *Le pays de Cama : un ancien état côtier du Gabon et ses origines*. Paris: Karthala, 1981.

Geissler, Paul W., Guillaume Lachenal, John Manton, and Noémi Tousignant, eds. *Traces of the Future: An Archaeology of Medical Science in Africa*. Bristol: Intellect, 2016.

Geissler, Paul Wenzel. 'Public Secrets in Public Health: Knowing Not to Know While Making Scientific Knowledge'. *American Ethnologist* 40, no. 1 (2013): 13–34.

Geissler, Wenzel, ed. 'Introduction: A Life Science in Its African Para-State'. In *Para-States and Medical Science: Making African Global Health*. Critical Global Health. Durham: Duke University Press, 2015.

Giles-Vernick, Tamara. *Cutting the Vines of the Past: Environmental Histories of the Central African Rain Forest*. Charlottesville: University Press of Virginia, 2002.

Giles-Vernick, Tamara, and James L.A. Webb Jr, eds. *Global Health in Africa: Historical Perspectives on Disease Control*. Athens: Ohio University Press, 2013.

Gillespie, Noel. 'With Schweitzer in Lambarene: Noel Gillespie's Letters from Africa'. Edited by W.C. Haygood. *Wisconsin Magazine of History* 54 (1971): 166–203.

Ginzburg, Carlo. *The Cheese and the Worms: The Cosmos of a Sixteenth-Century Miller*. Baltimore: Johns Hopkins University Press, 1980.

Gollnhofer, Otto, and Roger Sillans. 'Phénoménologie de la possession chez les Mitsogho (Gabon). Rites et techniques'. *Anthropos*, 1979, 737–752.

Good, Charles M. *The Steamer Parish: The Rise and Fall of Missionary Medicine on an African Frontier*. Chicago: The University of Chicago Press, 2004.

Gouda, Frances. 'Mimicry and Projection in the Colonial Encounter: The Dutch East Indies/Indonesia as Experimental Laboratory, 1900–1942'. *Journal of Colonialism and Colonial History* 1, no. 2 (2000).

Gould, Tony. *A Disease Apart : Leprosy in the Modern World*. New York: St. Martin's Press, 2005.

Graboyes, Melissa. *The Experiment Must Continue: Medical Research and Ethics in East Africa, 1940–2014*. Athens: Ohio University Press, 2015.

Granshaw, Lindsay. 'The Rise of the Modern Hospital in Britain'. In *Medicine in Society: Historical Essays*, edited by Andrew Wear, 197–218. Cambridge: Cambridge University Press, 1998.

Gray, Christopher J. *Colonial Rule and Crisis in Equatorial Africa: Southern Gabon, ca. 1850–1940*. Rochester: University of Rochester Press, 2002.

Gray, Christopher, and François Ngolet. 'Lambaréné, Okoume and the Transformation of Labor along the Middle Ogooue (Gabon), 1870–1945'. *The Journal of African History* 40, no. 01 (1999): 87–107.

Grébert, Fernand. *Au Gabon (Afrique équatoriale française)*. Paris: Société des Missions évangéliques, 1922.

Greene, Jeremy, Marguerite Thorp Basilico, Heidi Kim, and Paul Farmer. 'Colonial Medicine and Its Legacies. J. Greene. M. Thorp Basilico, H. Kim, P. Farmer'. In *Reimagining Global Health: An Introduction*, edited by Paul Farmer, Jim Yong Kim, Arthur Kleinman, and Matthew Basilico. Berkeley: University of California Press, 2013.

Greenwood, Anna, ed. *Beyond the State: The Colonial Medical Service in British Africa*. Manchester: Manchester University Press, 2016.

Greenwood, Anna, ed. 'The Colonial Medical Service and the Struggle for Control of the Zanzibar Maternity Association, 1918–47'. In *Beyond the State: The Colonial Medical Service in British Africa*, edited by Anna Greenwood, 85–104. Manchester: Manchester University Press, 2016.

Groß, Matthias, and Linsey McGoey, eds. 'Introduction'. In *Routledge International Handbook of Ignorance Studies*. London New York: Routledge,Taylor and Francis Group, 2015.

Günther, Siegwart-Horst, and Gerald Götting. *Was heisst Ehrfurcht vor dem Leben? Begegnung mit Albert Schweitzer*. Berlin: Neues Leben, 2005.

Hardiman, David, ed. *Healing Bodies, Saving Souls: Medical Missions in Asia and Africa*. Amsterdam: Rodopi, 2006.

Hardiman, David, ed. *Missionaries and Their Medicine: A Christian Modernity for Tribal India*. Manchester: Manchester University Press, 2014.

Hardimann, David. 'The Mission Hospital, 1880–1960'. In *From Western Medicine to Global Medicine. The Hospital beyond the West*, edited by Mark Harrison, Margaret Jones, and Helen Sweet, 198–220. Hyderabad: Orient BlackSwan, 2009.

Harries, Patrick. 'From the Alps to Africa: Swiss Missionaries and Anthropology'. In *Ordering Africa: Anthropology, European Imperialism and the Politics of Knowledge*, edited by Helen Tilley, 201–24. Manchester: Manchester University Press, 2010.

Harris, Ruth. 'The Allure of Albert Schweitzer'. *History of European Ideas* 40, no. 6 (2014): 804–825.

Harris, Ruth. 'Schweitzer and Africa'. *The Historical Journal* 59, no. 4 (2016): 1107–1132.

Harrison, Mark, Margaret Jones, and Helen Sweet, eds. *From Western Medicine to Global Medicine: The Hospital beyond the West*. Hyderabad: Orient BlackSwan, 2009.

Haussknecht, Emma *Emma Haussknecht, 1895–1956: 30 Jahre mit Albert Schweitzer in Lambaréné. Eine Biographie zusammengetragen von Almut und Hermann Reichenbecher*. Edited by Almut Reichenbecher and Herman Reichenbecher. 2nd edition. Berlin: Pro Business, 2007.

Havik, Philip J. 'Reconsidering Indigenous Health, Medical Services and Colonial Rule in Portuguese West Africa'. *O Colonialismo Português: Novos Rumos Para a Historiografia Dos PALOP*, 2013, 233–66.

Havik, Philip J. 'Public Health, Social Medicine and Disease Control: Medical Services, Maternal Care and Sexually Transmitted Diseases in Former Portuguese West Africa (1920–63)'. *Medical History* 62, no. 4 (2018): 485–506.

Headrick, Rita. *Colonialism, Health and Illness in French Equatorial Africa, 1885–1935*. Atlanta: African Studies Association Press, 1994.

Heaton, Matthew M. *Black Skin, White Coats: Nigerian Psychiatrists, Decolonization, and the Globalization of Psychiatry*. Athens: Ohio University Press, 2013.

Hess, Volker. 'Krankenakten als Gegenstand der Krankenhausgeschichtsschreibung'. In *Krankenhausgeschichte heute: was heißt und zu welchem Ende studiert man Hospital- und Krankenhausgeschichte?*, edited by Gunnar Stollberg, Christina Vanja, and Ernst Kraas, 43–52. Berlin: Lit-Verlag, 2011.

Hess, Volker, Laura Hottenrott, and Peter Steinkamp. *Testen im Osten: DDR-Arzneimitelstudien Im Auftrag Westlicher Pharmaindustrie, 1964–1990*. Berlin: be.bra wissenschaft verlag, 2016.

Hess, Volker, and Sabine Schlegelmilch. 'Cornucopia Officinae Medicae: Medical Practice Records and Their Origin'. In *Medical Practice, 1600–1900: Physicians and Their Patients*, edited by Martin Dinges, Kay Peter Jankrift, Sabine Schlegelmilch, and Michael Stolberg, 1–7. Leiden: Brill, 2015.

Hirschauer, Stefan. 'The Manufacture of Bodies in Surgery'. *Social Studies of Science* 21, no. 2 (1991): 279–319.

Hokkanen, Markku. 'Quests for Health and Contests for Meaning: African Church Leaders and Scottish Missionaries in the Early Twentieth Century Presbyterian Church in Northern Malawi'. *Journal of Southern African Studies* 33, no. 4 (2007): 733–750.

Hokkanen, Markku. *Medicine, Mobility, and the Empire: Nyasaland Networks, 1859–1960*. Manchester: Manchester University Press, 2017.

Hölzl, Richard. 'Lepra als entangled disease. Leidende afrikanische Körper in Medien und Praxis der katholischen Mission in Ostafrika 1911–1945'. In *Der schwarze Körper als Missionsgebiet: Medizin, Ethnologie und Theologie in Afrika und Europa 1880–1960*, edited by Siegfried Weichlein and Linda Ratschiller, 95–122. Köln: Böhlau Verlag, 2016.

Horwitz, Simonne. *Baragwanath Hospital, Soweto: A History of Medical Care, 1941–1990*. Johannesburg: Wits University Press, 2013.

Howell, Joel D. *Technology in the Hospital: Transforming Patient Care in the Early Twentieth Century*. Baltimore: Johns Hopkins University Press, 1995.

Howell, Joel D. 'Hospitals'. In *Medicine in the Twentieth Century*, edited by Roger Cooter and John Pickstone, 503–18. Amsterdam: Harwood Academic Publishers, 2000.

Hugon, Anne. 'La redéfinition de la maternité en Gold Coast, des années 1920 aux années 1950 : projet colonial et réalités locales'. In *Histoire des femmes en situation coloniale: Afrique et Asie, xxe siècle*, edited by Anne Hugon, 145–71. Paris: Karthala, 2004.

Hugon, Anne. 'Les sages-femmes africaines en contexte colonial. Auxiliaires de l'accouchement ou agent de la médicalisation? Le cas du Ghana des années 1930 aux années 1950'. In *Les nouvelles pratiques de santé: acteurs, objets, logiques sociales (XVIIIe–XXesiècles)*, edited by Patrice Bourdelais and Olivier Faure. Belin. Paris: Belin, 2005.

Hugon, Anne. 'L'historiographie de la maternité en Afrique subsaharienne'. *Clio. Femmes, Genre, Histoire*, no. 21 (2005): 212–229.

Hunt, Nancy Rose. '"Le Bebe en Brousse": European Women, African Birth Spacing and Colonial Intervention in Breast Feeding in the Belgian Congo'. *The International Journal of African Historical Studies* 21, no. 3 (1988): 401–432.

Hunt, Nancy Rose. *A Colonial Lexicon of Birth Ritual, Medicalization, and Mobility in the Congo*. Durham: Duke University Press, 1999.

Hunt, Nancy Rose. 'Health and Healing'. In *The Oxford Handbook of Modern African History*, edited by John Parker and Richard Reid, 378–95. Oxford: Oxford University Press, 2013.

Hunt, Nancy Rose. *A Nervous State: Violence, Remedies, and Reverie in Colonial Congo*. Durham: Duke University Press, 2016.

Iliffe, John. *East African Doctors: A History of the Modern Profession*. Kampala: Fountain Publishers, 2002.

Israël, Jeanette. 'Schweitzer, le médecin que nous avons connu'. In *Schweitzer, le médecin*, edited by Jean-Paul Sorg, 176–79. Strasbourg: Editions Oberlin, 1995.

Jackson, Lynette A. *Surfacing up : Psychiatry and Social Order in Colonial Zimbabwe, 1908–1968*. Ithaca: Cornell University Press, 2005.

Janzen, John M. *The Quest for Therapy in Lower Zaire*. Berkeley: University of California Press, 1978.

Jean-Baptiste, Rachel. '"A Black Girl Should Not Be With a White Man": Sex, Race, and African Women's Social and Legal Status in Colonial Gabon, c. 1900–1946'. *Journal of Women's History* 22, no. 2 (2010): 56–82.

Jennings, Michael. '"A Matter of Vital Importance"; the Place of the Medical Mission in Maternal and Child Healthcare in Tanganyika, 1919–39'. In *Healing Bodies, Saving Souls: Medical Missions in Asia and Africa*, edited by David Hardiman, 227–50. Amsterdam: Rodopi, 2006.

Jennings, Michael. '"Healing of Bodies, Salvation of Souls": Missionary Medicine in Colonial Tanganyika, 1870s–1939'. *Journal of Religion in Africa* 38, no. 1 (2008): 27–56.

Jilek-Aall, Louise. *Working with Dr. Schweitzer : Sharing His Reverence for Life*. Blaine: Hancock House, 1990.

Jolly, Margaret. 'Introduction'. In *Maternities and Modernities: Colonial and Postcolonial Experiences in Asia and the Pacific*, edited by Margaret Jolly and Kalpana Ram. Cambridge, New York: Cambridge University Press, 1998.

Joy, Charles Rhind, Melvin Arnold, and Albert Schweitzer. *The Africa of Albert Schweitzer*. London: Black, 1949.

Kalusa, Walima T. 'Christian Medical Discourse and Praxis on the Imperial Frontier: Explaining the Popularity of Missionary Medicine in Mwinilunga District, Zambia, 1906–1935'. In *The Spiritual in the Secular: Missionaries and Knowledge about Africa*, edited by David Maxwell and Patrick Harries, 245–66. Grand Rapids: William B. Eerdmans, 2012.

Kalusa, Walima T. 'Medical Training, African Auxiliaries, and Social Healing in Colonial Mwinilunga, Northern Rhodesia (Zambia), 1945–1964'. In *Public Health in the British Empire: Intermediaries, Subordinates, and the Practice of Public Health, 1850–1960*, edited by Ryan Johnson and Amna Khalid. New York: Routledge, 2012.

Kalusa, Walima T. 'Missionaries, African Patients, and Negotiating Missionary Medicine at Kalene Hospital, Zambia, 1906–1935'. *Journal of Southern African Studies* 40, no. 2 (2014): 283–294.

Kalusa, Walima Tuesday, and Megan Vaughan. *Death, Belief and Politics in Central African History*. Lusaka: Lembani Trust, 2013.

Kanogo, Tabitha. 'The Medicalization of Maternity in Colonial Kenya'. In *African Historians and African Voices: Essays Presented to Bethwell Allan Ogot on His Seventieth Birthday*, edited by Bethwell A. Ogot and E.S. Atieno Odhiambo. Basel: P. Schlettwein Publishing, 2001.

Keller, Richard. 'Madness and Colonization: Psychiatry in the British and French Empires, 1800–1962'. *Journal of Social History* 35, no. 2 (2001): 295–326.

Keller, Richard. 'Taking Science to the Colonies: Psychiatric Innovation in France and North Africa'. In *Psychiatry and Empire*, edited by Sloan Mahone and Megan Vaughan, 17–40. London: Palgrave Macmillan, 2007.

Kik, Richard. *Beim Oganga von Lambarene: Geschichten aus dem Leben Albert Schweitzers*. Reutlingen: Ensslin & Laiblin Verlag, 1954.

Kinzelbach, Annemarie, Stephanie Neuner, and Karen Nolte. 'Medicine in Practice: Knowledge, Diagnosis and Therapy'. In *Medical Practice, 1600–1900: Physicians and Their Patients*, edited by Martin Dinges, Kay Peter Jankrift, Sabine Schlegelmilch, and Michael Stolberg, 1–7. Leiden: Brill, 2015.

Klausen, Susanne Maria. *Race, Maternity, and the Politics of Birth Control in South Africa, 1910–39*. Basingstoke: Palgrave Macmillan, 2004.

Klee, Ernst. *Das Personenlexikon Zum Dritten Reich: Wer War Was Vor Und Nach 1945?* Frankfurt am Main: S. Fischer, 2003.

Kleinman, Arthur. 'What Is Specific to Western Medicine'. In *Companion Encyclopedia of the History of Medicine*, edited by William F. Bynum and Roy Porter, 15–23. London: Routledge, 1994.

Klingmüller, Victor, and Kristian Grön. *Die Lepra: Handbuch der Haut- und Geschlechtskrankheiten, Bd. 10*. Berlin: Verlag von Julius Springer, 1930.

Knorr-Cetina, Karin. *Wissenskulturen: ein Vergleich naturwissenschaftlicher Wissensformen*. Frankfurt: Suhrkamp, 2002.

Koch, Gertrud. 'Lieber grand Docteur!' In *Wir halfen dem Doktor in Lambarene: Festgabe zum 85. Geburtstag von Albert Schweitzer*, edited by Olga Fausel-Wieber, Ilse Schnabel, and Gertrud Koch, 164–68. Zürich: Schweizer Druck- und Verlagshaus, 1960.

Körtner, Ulrich H.J. '"Ehrfurcht vor dem Leben" – Zur Stellung der Ethik Albert Schweitzer in der ethischen Diskussion der Gegenwart'. In *Albert Schweitzer. Facetten einer Jahrhundertgestalt Referate einer Vorlesungsreihe des Collegium generale der Universität Bern im Frühjahrssemester 2013*, edited by Angela Berlis, Hubert Steinke, Fritz von Gunten, and Andreas Wagner, 99–136. Bern: Haupt Verlag, 2013.

Kumwenda, Linda B. *The Development of UMCA Medical Work in Northern Rhodesia, 1910–1950, with Special Reference to the African Medical Personnel*. Basel: Basler Afrika Bibliographien, 2000.

Kumwenda, Linda B. 'African Medical Personnel of the Universities' Mission to Central Africa in Northern Rhodesia'. In *Healing Bodies, Saving Souls: Medical Missions in Asia and Africa*, edited by David Hardiman, 193–226. Amsterdam: Rodopi, 2006.

Lachenal, Guillaume. 'Franco-African Familiarities: A History of the Pasteur Institute of Cameroon, 1945–2000'. In *From Western Medicine to Global Medicine. The Hospital beyond the West*, edited by Mark Harrison, Margaret Jones, and Helen Sweet, 411–44. Hyderabad: Orient BlackSwan, 2009.

Lachenal, Guillaume. 'Le médecin qui voulut être roi. Médecine coloniale et utopie au Cameroun'. *Annales. Histoire, sciences sociale*. 65, no. 1 (2010): 121–56.

Lachenal, Guillaume. *Le médicament qui devait sauver l'Afrique: Un scandale pharmaceutique aux colonies*. Paris: La Découverte, 2014.

Lachenal, Guillaume, Joseph Owona Ntsama, Daniel Ze Bekolo, Thomas Kombang Ekodogo, and John Manton. 'Neglected Actors in Neglected Tropical Diseases Research: Historical Perspectives on Health Workers and Contemporary Buruli Ulcer Research in Ayos, Cameroon'. *PLoS Neglected Tropical Diseases* 10, no. 4 (2016): e0004488.

Lachenal, Guillaume, and Bertrand Taithe. 'Une généalogie missionnaire et coloniale de l'humanitaire : le cas Aujoulat au Cameroun, 1935–1973'. *Le Mouvement Social* n° 227, no. 2 (2009): 45–63.

Lammel, Hans-Uwe. 'Das Hospital als Raum dazwischen – Fragen einer postkolonialen Krankenhausgeschichte'. In *Krankenhausgeschichte heute: was heißt und zu welchem Ende studiert man Hospital- und Krankenhausgeschichte?*, edited by Gunnar Stollberg, Christina Vanja, and Ernst Kraas, 125–30. Berlin: Lit-Verlag, 2011.

Landau, Paul S. 'Explaining Surgical Evangelism in Colonial Southern Africa: Teeth, Pain and Faith'. *The Journal of African History* 37, no. 02 (1996): 261–281.

Landau, Paul Stuart. *The Realm of the Word: Language, Gender, and Christianity in a Southern African Kingdom*. Portsmouth, London, Cape Town: Heinemann James Currey David Philip, 1995.

Langwick, Stacey A. *Bodies, Politics, and African Healing: The Matter of Maladies in Tanzania*. Bloomington: Indiana University Press, 2011.

Last, Murray. 'The Importance of Knowing about Not Knowing: Observations from Hausaland'. In *The Social Basis of Health and Healing in Africa*, edited by Steven Feierman and John M. Janzen, 393–406, 1992.

Last, Murray. 'Non-Western Concepts of Disease'. In *Companion Encyclopedia of the History of Medicine*, edited by William F. Bynum and Roy Porter, Reprinted ed., 634–60. London: Routledge, 1994.

Latour, Bruno. *Reassembling the Social: An Introduction to Actor-Network-Theory*. Oxford: Oxford University Press, 2007.

Lauterburg-Bonjour, Elsa. *Lambarene: Erlebnisse einer Bernerin im afrikanischen Urwald*. Bern: Haupt, 1931.

Lauterburg-Bonjour, Markus. 'Man stellt sich um'. In *Wir halfen dem Doktor in Lambarene: Festgabe zum 85. Geburtstag von Albert Schweitzer*, edited by Olga Fausel-Wieber, Ilse Schnabel, and Gertrud Koch, 18–44. Zürich: Schweizer Druck- und Verlagshaus, 1960.

Lavignotte, Henri. *L'évur: croyance des Fañ du Gabon*. Paris: Société des Missions évangéliques, 1952.

Lehmann, Bethli. 'Meine Erinnerung an das Frischoperiertenhaus, die Case Bouka'. In *Mit dem Herzen einer Gazelle und der Haut eines Nilpferds: Albert Schweitzer in seinen letzten Lebensjahren und die Entwicklung seines Spitals bis zur Gegenwart*, edited by Jo Munz and Walter Munz, 59–60. Frauenfeld: Huber, 2005.

Lehmann, Heinrich, and Eugen Bernoulli, eds. *Übersicht der gebräuchlichen und neueren Arzneimittel für Ärzte, Apotheker und Zahnärzte*. 8th edition. Basel: Schwabe, 1955.

Lehmann, Heinrich, and Eugen Bernoulli, eds. *Übersicht der gebräuchlichen und neueren Arzneimittel für Ärzte, Apotheker und Zahnärzte*. 9th edition. Basel: Schwabe, 1959.

Levin, Miriam R. 'Contexts of Control'. In *Cultures of Control*, edited by Miriam R. Levin, 13–39. Studies in the History of Science, Technology, and Medicine, v. 9. Amsterdam: Harwood Academic Publishers, 2000.

Livingston, Julie. 'Productive Misunderstandings and the Dynamism of Plural Medicine in Mid-Century Bechuanaland'. *Journal of Southern African Studies* 33, no. 4 (2007): 801–810.

Livingston, Julie. *Improvising Medicine: An African Oncology Ward in an Emerging Cancer Epidemic*. Durham: Duke University Press, 2012.

López-Muñoz, Francisco, Cecilio Alamo, Eduardo Cuenca, Winston Shen, Patrick Clervoy, and Gabriel Rubio. 'History of the Discovery and Clinical Introduction of Chlorpromazine'. *Annals of Clinical Psychiatry* 17, no. 3 (1 July 2005): 113–35.

Löwy, Ilana. 'Historiography of Biomedicine: 'Bio', 'Medicine', and in Between'. *Isis* 102, no. 1 (2011): 116–122.

Lyons, Maryinez. 'The Power to Heal: African Auxiliaries in Colonial Belgian Congo and Uganda'. In *Contesting Colonial Hegemony: State and Society in Africa and India*, edited by Dagmar Engels and Shula Marks, 202–23. London: British Academic Press, 1994.

Lyons, Maryinez. *The Colonial Disease: A Social History of Sleeping Sickness in Northern Zaire, 1900–1940*. Cambridge: Cambridge University Press, 2002.

Mabika, Hines. 'Médicalisation de l'Afrique centrale. Le Cas du Gabon, 1890–1970: diagnostic, stratégies et résultats'. Aix-En-Provence, 2008.

Mabika, Hines. 'L'hôpital Albert Schweitzer de Lambaréné, 1913–2013'. In *Albert Schweitzer. Facetten einer Jahrhundertgestalt Referate einer Vorlesungsreihe des Collegium generale der Universität Bern im Frühjahrssemester 2013*, edited by Angela Berlis, Hubert Steinke, Fritz von Gunten, and Andreas Wagner. Bern: Haupt Verlag, 2013.

Mabika, Hines. 'La famine dans les Nouvelles de l'hôpital Albert Schweitzer de Lambaréné: archéologie de la médiatisation des crises alimentaires africaines au 20e siècle?' *Itinera* 37, no. 37 (2014): 75–94.

Mabika Ognandzi, Hines. *Médicaliser l'Afrique: Enjeux, Processus et Stratégies d'introduction de La Médecine Occidentale Au Gabon (XIXe–XXe Siècle)*. Paris: L'Harmattan, 2017.

Mabika Ognandzi, Hines, Hubert Steinke, and Tizian Zumthurm. *Schweitzer's Lambaréné: A Hospital in Colonial Africa (Working Title)*, in preparation.

MacGaffey, Wyatt. 'Changing Representations in Central African History'. *The Journal of African History* 46, no. 02 (2005): 189–207.

Mahone, Sloan. 'East African Psychiatry and the Practical Problems of Empire'. In *Psychiatry and Empire*, edited by Sloan Mahone and Megan Vaughan, 41–66. Cambridge Imperial and Post-Colonial Studies Series. London: Palgrave Macmillan, 2007.

Mai, Hermann. *Albert Schweitzer und seine Kranken: ein Beitrag zur Geschichte der Tropenmedizin*. Tübingen: Verlag Tübinger Chronik, 1992.

Malloy, Patrick. 'Research Material and Necromancy: Imagining the Political-Economy of Biomedicine in Colonial Tanganyika'. *The International Journal of African Historical Studies* 47, no. 3 (2014): 425.

Malowany, Maureen. 'Unfinished Agendas: Writing the History of Medicine of Sub-Saharan Africa'. *African Affairs* 99, no. 395 (2000): 325–349.

Manderson, Lenore. 'Women and the State: Maternal and Child Welfare in Colonial Malaya, 1900–1940'. In *Women and Children First: International Maternal and Infant*

Welfare 1870–1945, edited by Valerie A. Fildes, Lara Marks, and Hilary Marland, 154–77. London: Routledge, 1992.

Manning, Patrick. 'African Population: Projections, 1850–1960'. In *The Demographics of Empire: The Colonial Order and the Creation of Knowledge*, edited by Karl Ittmann, 245–76. Athens: Ohio University Press, 2010.

Manson-Bahr, Philip. 'Amoebic Dysentery and Its Effective Treatment'. *British Medical Journal* 2, no. 4207 (1941): 255.

Manton, John. 'Mission, Clinic, and Laboratory: Curing Leprosy in Nigeria, 1945–67'. In *The Spiritual in the Secular: Missionaries and Knowledge about Africa*, edited by David Maxwell and Patrick Harries, 313–34. Grand Rapids: William B. Eerdmans, 2012.

Manton, John. 'Trialing Drugs, Creating Publics: Medical Research, Leprosy Control, and the Construction of a Public Health Sphere in Post-1945 Nigeria'. In *Para-States and Medical Science: Making African Global Health*, edited by Wenzel Geissler, 78–99. Durham, N.C: Duke University Press, 2015.

Marie, Chelsea, and William Arthur Petri Jr. 'Amoebic Dysentery'. *BMJ Clinical Evidence* 2013 (30 August 2013).

Marks, Harry M. *The Progress of Experiment: Science and Therapeutic Reform in the United States, 1900–1990*. Cambridge: Cambridge University Press, 1997.

Marland, Hilary. 'Childbirth and Maternity'. In *Medicine in the Twentieth Century*, edited by Roger Cooter and John Pickstone, 559–74. Amsterdam: Harwood Academic Publishers, 2000.

Martinelli-Stettler, Ida. 'Colmar weckte Erinnerungen'. In *Wir halfen dem Doktor in Lambarene: Festgabe zum 85. Geburtstag von Albert Schweitzer*, edited by Olga Fausel-Wieber, Ilse Schnabel, and Gertrud Koch, 120–22. Zürich: Schweizer Druck- und Verlagshaus, 1960.

Mary, André. 'L'alternative de la vision et de la possession dans les sociétés religieuses et thérapeutiques du Gabon'. *Cahiers d'Études africaines*, 1983, 281–310.

Mbondobari, Sylvère. *Archäologie eines modernen Mythos: Albert Schweitzers Nachruhm in europäischen und afrikanischen Text- und Bildmedien*. Frankfurt am Main: Lang, 2003.

McCulloch, Jock. *Colonial Psychiatry and the African Mind*. Cambridge: Cambridge University Press, 1995.

McKnight, Gerald. *Verdict on Schweitzer: The Man behind the Legend of Lambaréné*. London: Muller, 1964.

Mebiame Zomo, Maixant. 'Le travail des missions chrétiennes au Gabon pendant la colonisation'. In *Colonisation et colonisés au Gabon*, edited by Fabrice Nguiabama-Makaya, 49–76. Paris: L'Harmattan, 2007.

Meier, Marietta, Mario König, Magaly Tornay, and Ursina Klauser. *Testfall Münsterlingen: klinische Versuche in der Psychiatrie, 1940–1980*. Zürich: Chronos, 2019.

Mekodiomba, Romain. 'Rôle et influence des églises missionnaires dans la mission civilisatrice au Gabon'. In *Colonisation et colonisés au Gabon*, edited by Fabrice Nguiabama-Makaya, 77–108. Paris: L'Harmattan, 2007.

Melamed, Steven E.G., and Antonia Melamed. 'Albert Schweitzer in Gabon'. In *Culture, Ecology, and Politics in Gabon's Rainforest*, edited by Michael Charles Reed and James F. James, 165–92. Lewiston: Edwin Mellen Press, 2003.

Merlet, Annie. *Légendes et histoire des Myéné de l'Ogooué*. Libreville: Centre Culturel Français St-Exupéry, 1990.

Metegue N'Nah, Nicolas. *Histoire du Gabon: des origines à l'aube du XXIe siècle*. Paris: L'Harmattan, 2006.

Minko Mve, Bernardin. *Gabon entre tradition et post-modernité: dynamique des structures d'accueil Fang*. Paris: L'Harmattan, 2003.

Moll, Sebastian. *Albert Schweitzer: Meister der Selbstinszenierung*. Berlin: Berlin University Press, 2014.

Monnais, Laurence. *Médicaments coloniaux: l'expérience vietnamienne, 1905–1940*. Paris: Les Indes Savantes, 2014.

Moore-Sheeley, Kirsten. 'The Products of Experiment: Changing Conceptions of Difference in the History of Tuberculosis in East Africa, 1920s–1970s'. *Social History of Medicine* 31, no. 3 (2017): 533–554.

Morel, Léon. 'Au Gabon avant l'arrivée du Docteur Schweitzer'. In *Rayonnement d'Albert Schweitzer: 34 études et 100 témoignage*, edited by Robert Minder, 185–88. Colmar: Ed. Alsatia, 1975.

Moscucci, Ornella. *The Science of Woman: Gynaecology and Gender in England, 1800–1929*. Cambridge: Cambridge University Press, 1990.

Mudimbe, Valentin Y. *The Invention of Africa: Gnosis, Philosophy, and the Order of Knowledge*. Bloomington: Indiana University Press, 1988.

Müller, Rolf. '50 Jahre Albert-Schweitzer-Spital in Lambarene'. *Münchner Medizinische Wochenschrift* 105, no. 51 (1963): 2–29.

Munz, Jo, and Walter Munz. *Mit dem Herzen einer Gazelle und der Haut eines Nilpferds: Albert Schweitzer in seinen letzten Lebensjahren und die Entwicklung seines Spitals bis zur Gegenwart*. Frauenfeld: Huber, 2005.

Munz, Jo, and Walter Munz. *Albert Schweitzers Lambarene: Zeitzeugen berichten zum 100 Jährigen Jubiläum des Urwaldspitals 1913–2013*. Eglisau: elfundzehn Verlag, 2013.

Munz, Walter. *Albert Schweitzer im Gedächtnis der Afrikaner und in meiner Erinnerung*. Bern: Paul Haupt, 1991.

Munz-Boddingius, Jo. 'Meine Chance und Freude, Hebamme in Lambarene gewesen zu sein'. In *Mit dem Herzen einer Gazelle und der Haut eines Nilpferds: Albert Schweitzer in seinen letzten Lebensjahren und die Entwicklung seines Spitals bis zur Gegenwart*, edited by Jo Munz and Walter Munz, 65–70. Frauenfeld: Huber, 2005.

Myscofski, Carole A. 'Against the Grain: Learning and Teaching', 2001. http://digitalc ommons.iwu.edu/cgi/viewcontent.cgi?article=1003&context=teaching_excellence.

Naipaul, V.S. *The Masque of Africa : Glimpses of African Belief.* London: Picador, 2010.

Ndao, Mor. 'Colonisation et politique de santé maternelle et infantile au Sénégal (1905–1960)'. *French Colonial History* 9, no. 1 (2008): 191–211.

Nessmann, Victor. *Avec Albert Schweitzer de 1924 à 1926. Lettres de Lambaréné.* Strasbourg: Editions Oberlin, 1994.

Nestel, Sheryl. '(Ad) Ministering Angels: Colonial Nursing and the Extension of Empire in Africa'. *Journal of Medical Humanities* 19, no. 4 (1998): 257–277.

Neukirch, Siegfried. 'Bananeneinkauf und Transporte'. In *Mit dem Herzen einer Gazelle und der Haut eines Nilpferds: Albert Schweitzer in seinen letzten Lebensjahren und die Entwicklung seines Spitals bis zur Gegenwart*, edited by Jo Munz and Walter Munz, 41–44. Frauenfeld: Huber, 2005.

Ngalamulume, Kalala. 'The Regulation of Madness in Sénégal, 1890–1914'. In *Medicine and Health in Africa: Multidisciplinary Perspectives*, edited by Paula Viterbo and Kalala Ngalamulume. Münster: Lit, 2010.

Ngalamulume, Kalala. *Colonial Pathologies, Environment, and Western Medicine in Saint-Louis-Du-Senegal, 1867–1920.* New York: Peter Lang, 2012.

Nguema Minko, Emanuelle. 'L'évangélisation comme forme religieuse de la conquête politique du Gabon'. In *Colonisation et colonisés au Gabon*, edited by Fabrice Nguia-bama-Makaya, 25–48. Paris: L'Harmattan, 2007.

Nies-Berger, Edouard. *Albert Schweitzer as I Knew Him.* Hillsdale: Pendragon Press, 2003.

Nüesch-Wohlfender, Elisabeth. 'Hausfrauliches'. In *Wir halfen dem Doktor in Lambarene: Festgabe zum 85. Geburtstag von Albert Schweitzer*, edited by Olga Fausel-Wieber, Ilse Schnabel, and Gertrud Koch, 150–60. Zürich: Schweizer Druck- und Verlagshaus, 1960.

Nyama, Albert. 'La dame tout de blanc vêtue et son trousseau de clés'. In *Akewa: Ali Silvers Weg für Albert Schweitzers Werk veröffentlicht zum 70. Geburtstag Ali Silvers*, edited by Makoto Abé and Ali Silver, 45–50. Tübingen: Friedrich C. Braun Verlag, 1984.

Nzenguet Iguemba, Gilchrist Anicet. *Colonisation, fiscalité et mutations au Gabon, 1910–1947.* Paris: L'Harmattan, 2005.

Oermann, Nils Ole. *Albert Schweitzer 1875–1965: Eine Biographie.* München: C.H. Beck, 2010.

Ohls, Isgard. *Improvisationen der Ehrfurcht vor allem Lebendigen – Albert Schweitzers Ästhetik der Mission: mit zeitgeschichtlichem Dokumentenanhang.* Göttingen: V&R unipress, 2008.

Ohls, Isgard. *Der Arzt Albert Schweitzer: weltweit vernetzte Tropenmedizin zwischen Forschen, Heilen und Ethik.* Göttingen: V&R unipress, 2015.

Olumwullah, Osaak A. *Dis-Ease in the Colonial State: Medicine, Society, and Social Change among the AbaNyole of Western Kenya*. Westport: Greenwood Press, 2002.

Ombigath, Pierre Romuald. 'La Crise économique de 1930 et ses répercussions sur l'industrie forestière du Gabon, 1930–1939'. In *Le Gabon: approche pluridisciplinaire*, edited by Gilchrist Anicet Nzenguet Iguemba, 143–71. Paris: L'Harmattan, 2006.

Ombongi, Kenneth S. 'The Historical Interface between the State and Medical Science in Africa: Kenya's Case'. In *Evidence, Ethos and Experiment: The Anthropology and History of Medical Research in Africa*, edited by Wenzel Geissler and Catherine Molyneux, 353–71. New York: Berghahn Books, 2011.

Østergaard Christensen, Lavrids. *At Work with Albert Schweitzer*. London: George Allen & Unwin, 1962.

Oswald, Suzanne. *Mein Onkel Bery: Erinnerungen an Albert Schweitzer*. Zürich: Rotapfel-Verlag, 1972.

Ott, Emma. 'Kleine Steine im grossen Mosaik'. In *Wir halfen dem Doktor in Lambarene: Festgabe zum 85. Geburtstag von Albert Schweitzer*, edited by Olga Fausel-Wieber, Ilse Schnabel, and Gertrud Koch, 105–13. Zürich: Schweizer Druck- und Verlagshaus, 1960.

Ott, Emma. 'Natur, Mensch und Tier'. In *Wir halfen dem Doktor in Lambarene: Festgabe zum 85. Geburtstag von Albert Schweitzer*, edited by Olga Fausel-Wieber, Ilse Schnabel, and Gertrud Koch, 133–39. Zürich: Schweizer Druck- und Verlagshaus, 1960.

Packard, Randall M. *A History of Global Health: Interventions into the Lives of Other Peoples*. Baltimore: Johns Hopkins University Press, 2016.

Parle, Julie, and Vanessa Noble. '"The Hospital Was Just Like a Home": Self, Service and the "McCord Hospital Family"'. *Medical History* 58, no. 2 (2014): 188–209.

Parle, Julie, and Vanessa Noble. *The People's Hospital: A History of McCords, Durban 1890s–1970s*. Pietermaritzburg: Occasional Publications of the Natal Society Foundation, 2017.

Patterson, K. David. *Health in Colonial Ghana: Disease, Medicine, and Socio-Economic Change, 1900–1955*. Waltham: Crossroad Press, 1981.

Pearson, Jessica Lynne. *The Colonial Politics of Global Health: France and the United Nations in Postwar Africa*. Cambridge: Harvard University Press, 2018.

Pedersen, Jean Elisabeth. '"Special Customs": Paternity Suits and Citizenship in France and the Colonies, 1870–1912'. In *Domesticating the Empire: Race, Gender, and Family Life in French and Dutch Colonialism*, edited by Julia A. Clancy-Smith and Frances Gouda, 43–64. Charlottesville: University Press of Virginia, 1998.

Peltonen, Matti. 'Clues, Margins, and Monads: The Micro–Macro Link in Historical Research'. *History and Theory* 40, no. 3 (2001): 347–359.

Penn, Jack. 'A Visit to Albert Schweitzer'. *Plastic and Reconstructive Surgery* 18, no. 3 (1956): 161–168.

Pernick, Martin S. *A Calculus of Suffering: Pain, Professionalism, and Anesthesia in Nineteenth-Century America.* New York: Columbia University Press, 1985.

Pickering, Andrew. *The Mangle of Practice: Time, Agency, and Science.* Chicago: University of Chicago Press, 1995.

Pickstone, John V. *Ways of Knowing: A New History of Science, Technology and Medicine.* Chicago: University of Chicago Press, 2001.

Porter, Roy. 'Madness and Its Institutions'. In *Medicine in Society: Historical Essays*, edited by Andrew Wear, 277–301. Cambridge, 1992.

Pounah, Paul-Vincent. *Notre passé : étude historique.* Paris: Société d'Impressions Techniques, 1970.

Pourtier, Roland. *Le Gabon: espace, histoire, société.* Vol. 1. Paris: Ed. l'Harmattan, 1989.

Pourtier, Roland. *Le Gabon: état et developpement.* Vol. 2. Paris: Ed. l'Harmattan, 1989.

Powell, S.J. 'Drug Therapy of Amoebiasis'. *Bulletin of the World Health Organization* 40, no. 6 (1969): 953.

Prince, Ruth Jane, ed. 'Introduction. Situating Health and the Public in Africa'. In *Making and Unmaking Public Health in Africa: Ethnographic and Historical Perspectives.* Athens: Ohio University Press, 2014.

Pringle, Yolana. 'Neurasthenia at Mengo Hospital, Uganda: A Case Study in Psychiatry and a Diagnosis, 1906–50'. *The Journal of Imperial and Commonwealth History* 44, no. 2 (2016): 241–262.

Prins, Gwyn. 'But What Was the Disease? The Present State of Health and Healing in African Studies'. *Past & Present*, 1989.

Proctor, Robert N. 'Agnotology. A Missing Term to Describe the Cultural Production of Ignorance (and Its Study)'. In *Agnotology: The Making and Unmaking of Ignorance*, edited by Robert N. Proctor and Londa Schiebinger, 1–33. Stanford: Stanford University Press, 2008.

Rafferty, Anne Marie. 'Nurses'. In *Medicine in the Twentieth Century*, edited by Roger Cooter and John Pickstone, 519–29. Amsterdam: Harwood Academic Publishers, 2000.

Ranger, Terence O. 'Godly Medicine: The Ambiguities of Medical Mission in Southeastern Tanzania, 1900–1945'. In *The Social Basis of Health and Healing in Africa*, edited by Steven Feierman and John M. Janzen, 256–82. Berkeley: University of California Press, 1992.

Raponda-Walker, André, and Roger Sillans. *Rites et croyances des peuples du Gabon: essai sur les pratiques religieuses d'autrefois et d'aujourd'hui.* Paris: Présence africaine, 1962.

Raponda-Walker, André, and Roger Sillans. *Les plantes utiles du Gabon: essai d'inventaire et de concordance des noms vernaculaires et scientifiques des plantes spontanées et introduites, description des espèces, propriétés, utilisations économiques, ethnographiques et artistiques.* Fac-Similé (first edition: Paris, 1961). Libreville:

Fondation Raponda-Walker – Sépia – Centre Culturel Saint-Exupéry (Libreville), 1995.

Raponda-Walker, André, and Marcel Soret. *Notes d'histoire du Gabon*. Brazzaville: Institut d'études centrafricaines, 1960.

Ratschiller, Linda. 'Kranke Körper. Mission, Medizin und Fotografie zwischen der Goldküste und Basel 1885–1914'. In *Der schwarze Körper als Missionsgebiet: Medizin, Ethnologie und Theologie in Afrika und Europa 1880–1960*, edited by Siegfried Weichlein and Linda Ratschiller, 41–72. Köln: Böhlau Verlag, 2016.

Ratschiller, Linda, and Siegfried Weichlein. 'Der schwarze Körper als Missionsgebiet 1880–1960. Begriffe, Konzepte, Fragestellungen'. In *Der schwarze Körper als Missionsgebiet: Medizin, Ethnologie und Theologie in Afrika und Europa 1880–1960*, edited by Siegfried Weichlein and Linda Ratschiller, 15–39. Köln: Böhlau Verlag, 2016.

Rehm-Grätzel, Patricia. 'Albert Schweitzers Philosophie der "Ehrfurcht vor dem Leben" und der Friedensgedanke'. In *Albert Schweitzer. Facetten einer Jahrhundertgestalt Referate einer Vorlesungsreihe des Collegium generale der Universität Bern im Frühjahrssemester 2013*, edited by Angela Berlis, Hubert Steinke, Fritz von Gunten, and Andreas Wagner, 87–98. Bern: Haupt Verlag, 2013.

Reiser, Stanley Joel. *Medicine and the Reign of Technology*. Cambridge: University Press, 1978.

Renders, Hans, ed. *Theoretical Discussions of Biography: Approaches from History, Microhistory, and Life Writing*. Lewiston: The Edwin Mellen Press, 2013.

Risse, Guenter B. *Mending Bodies, Saving Souls: A History of Hospitals*. New York: Oxford University Press, 1999.

Rouse, Joseph. 'Two Concepts of Practices'. In *The Practice Turn in Contemporary Theory*, edited by Karin Knorr-Cetina, Theodore R. Schatzki, and Eike Von Savigny, 198–208. London: Taylor and Francis, 2000.

Rutishauser, Armin. 'Wie eine Insel'. In *Wir halfen dem Doktor in Lambarene: Festgabe zum 85. Geburtstag von Albert Schweitzer*, edited by Olga Fausel-Wieber, Ilse Schnabel, and Gertrud Koch, 130–33. Zürich: Schweizer Druck- und Verlagshaus, 1960.

Sadowsky, Jonathan. *Imperial Bedlam: Institutions of Madness in Colonial Southwest Nigeria*. Berkeley: University of California Press, 1999.

Sarraut, Albert. *La mise en valeur des colonies françaises*. Paris: Payot, 1923.

Sautter, Gilles. *De l'Atlantique au fleuve Congo: une géographie du sous-peuplement République du Congo République Gabonaise*. Paris: Imprimerie nationale, 1966.

Scarfone, Marianna. 'Italian Colonial Psychiatry: Outlines of a Discipline, and Practical Achievements in Libya and the Horn of Africa'. *History of Psychiatry* 27, no. 4 (2016): 389–405.

Schatzberg, Michael G. *Political Legitimacy in Middle Africa: Father, Family, Food*. Bloomington: Indiana University Press, 2001.

Schatzki, Theodore R. 'Introduction: Practice Theory'. In *The Practice Turn in Contemporary Theory*, edited by Karin Knorr-Cetina, Theodore R. Schatzki, and Eike Von Savigny, 10–23. London: Taylor and Francis, 2000.

Schiebinger, Londa. 'West Indian Abortifacients and the Making of Ignorance'. In *Agnotology: The Making and Unmaking of Ignorance*, edited by Robert N. Proctor and Londa Schiebinger, 149–62. Stanford: Stanford University Press, 2008.

Schler, Lynn. 'Writing African Women's History with Male Sources: Possibilities and Limitations'. *History in Africa* 31 (2004): 319–333.

Schlich, Thomas. 'Surgery, Science and Modernity: Operating Rooms and Laboratories as Spaces of Control'. *History of Science* 45, no. 3 (2007): 231–256.

Schlich, Thomas. 'The Technological Fix and the Modern Body. Surgery as a Paradigmatic Case'. In *A Cultural History of the Human Body*, edited by Ivan Crozier, 71–92. Oxford: Berg, 2010.

Schlich, Thomas. '"The Days of Brilliancy Are Past": Skill, Styles and the Changing Rules of Surgical Performance, ca. 1820–1920'. *Medical History* 59, no. 03 (2015): 379–403.

Schlich, Thomas, and Christopher Crenner. 'Technological Change in Surgery: An Introductory Essay'. In *Technological Change in Modern Surgery: Historical Perspectives on Innovation*, edited by Thomas Schlich and Christopher Crenner, 1–20. Rochester, NY: University of Rochester Press, 2017.

Schmid, Pascal. 'Mission Medicine in a Decolonising Health Care System: Agogo Hospital, Ghana 1945–1980'. *Ghana Studies* 15/16 (2013 2012): 287–329.

Schnabel, Ilse. 'Medizinisches aus Albert Schweitzers Urwaldspital'. *Sonderabdruck aus der Schweizerischen Medizinischen Wochenschrift.* 66, no. 16 (1936): 1–6.

Schnabel, Ilse. 'Von ärztlichen Verrichtungen'. In *Wir halfen dem Doktor in Lambarene: Festgabe zum 85. Geburtstag von Albert Schweitzer*, edited by Olga Fausel-Wieber, Ilse Schnabel, and Gertrud Koch, 52–60. Zürich: Schweizer Druck- und Verlagshaus, 1960.

Scholl, Johannes. *Albert Schweitzer – von der Ehrfurcht vor dem Leben zur transkulturellen Solidarität: ein alternatives Entwicklungshilfekonzept in der ersten Hälfte des 20. Jahrhunderts.* Weinheim: Beltz Athenäum Verlag, 1994.

Schott, Heinz, and Rainer Tölle. *Geschichte der Psychiatrie: Krankheitslehren, Irrwege, Behandlungsformen.* München: C.H. Beck, 2006.

Schröder, Margrith. 'On fait ce qu'on peut'. In *Wir halfen dem Doktor in Lambarene: Festgabe zum 85. Geburtstag von Albert Schweitzer*, edited by Olga Fausel-Wieber, Ilse Schnabel, and Gertrud Koch, 1969–181. Zürich: Schweizer Druck- und Verlagshaus, 1960.

Schweig, Nicole. *Weltliche Krankenpflege in den deutschen Kolonien Afrikas 1884–1918.* Frankfurt am Main: Mabus-Verlag, 2012.

Schweitzer, Albert. 'Notes et Nouvelles de la part du prof. Albert Schweitzer Lambaréné'. Chambéry, 1913.

Schweitzer, Albert. 'Notes et Nouvelles de la part du prof. Albert Schweitzer. Deuxième rapport'. Chambéry, 1914.

Schweitzer, Albert. *Zwischen Wasser und Urwald: Erlebnisse und Beobachtungen eines Arztes im Urwalde Äquatorialafrikas*. Bern: Paul Haupt, 1921.

Schweitzer, Albert. 'Neues von Albert Schweitzer III. Folge, Oktober 1924'.

Schweitzer, Albert. 'Neues von Albert Schweitzer VII. Folge, Februar 1925'.

Schweitzer, Albert. 'Neues von Albert Schweitzer IV. Folge, März 1925'.

Schweitzer, Albert. 'Neues von Albert Schweitzer VIII. Folge, Advent 1926'.

Schweitzer, Albert. 'Neues von Albert Schweitzer IX. Folge, Pfingsten 1927'.

Schweitzer, Albert. 'Neues von Albert Schweitzer X. Folge, Juli 1927'.

Schweitzer, Albert. *Mitteilungen aus Lambarene. Drittes Heft, Herbst 1925 bis Sommer 1927*. Bern, 1928.

Schweitzer, Albert. 'Mitteilungen aus Lambarene: Erstes Heft, Frühjahr bis Herbst 1924'. In *Mitteilungen aus Lambarene. Erstes und Zweites Heft*. Bern, 1928.

Schweitzer, Albert. 'Mitteilungen aus Lambarene: Zweites Heft, Herbst 1924 bis Herbst 1925'. In *Mitteilungen aus Lambarene. Erstes und Zweites Heft*. Bern, 1928.

Schweitzer, Albert. 'Briefe aus dem Lambarene Spital XI. Folge, März 1930'.

Schweitzer, Albert. 'Briefe aus dem Lambarene Spital XII. Folge, Pfingsten 1931'.

Schweitzer, Albert. 'Briefe aus dem Lambarene Spital XIII. Folge, November 1931'.

Schweitzer, Albert. 'Briefe aus dem Lambarene Spital XIV. Folge, Juli 1933'.

Schweitzer, Albert. 'Briefe aus dem Lambarene Spital XV. Folge, Februar 1934'.

Schweitzer, Albert. 'Briefe aus dem Lambarene Spital XVI. Folge, Januar 1935'.

Schweitzer, Albert. 'Briefe aus dem Lambarene Spital XVII. Folge, Juni 1935'.

Schweitzer, Albert. 'Briefe aus dem Lambarene Spital XVIII. Folge, November 1935'.

Schweitzer, Albert. 'Briefe aus dem Lambarene Spital XIX. Folge, Oktober 1936'.

Schweitzer, Albert. 'Briefe aus dem Lambarene Spital XX. Folge, Mai 1937'.

Schweitzer, Albert. 'Briefe aus dem Lambarene Spital XXI. Folge, März 1938'.

Schweitzer, Albert. *Afrikanische Geschichten*. Bern: Verlag Paul Haupt, 1939.

Schweitzer, Albert. 'Briefe aus dem Lambarene Spital XXII. Folge, Februar 1939'.

Schweitzer, Albert. 'Briefe aus dem Lambarene Spital XXIII. Folge, März 1946'.

Schweitzer, Albert. *Das Spital im Urwald: Aufnahmen von Anna Wildikann*. Bern: Paul Haupt, 1948.

Schweitzer, Albert. 'Briefe aus dem Lambarenespital XXIV. Folge, Oktober 1954'.

Schweitzer, Albert, and William Larimer Mellon. *Brothers in Spirit: The Correspondence of Albert Schweitzer and William Larimer Mellon, Jr*. Edited by Gwen Grant Mellon and Rhena Schweitzer Miller. Syracuse: Syracuse University Press, 1996.

Siefert, Jeanette. *Meine Arbeitsjahre in Lambarene 1933–1935: Erinnerungen an Albert Schweitzer und sein Spital am Ogowe*. Tübingen: Verlag Tübinger Chronik, 1986.

Silla, Eric. *People Are Not the Same: Leprosy and Identity in Twentieth-Century Mali*. Portsmouth, Oxford: Heinemann James Currey, 1998.

Sixt, Barbara. 'Krankenschwester bei Albert Schweitzer – und stellvertretende Mutter für ein verwaistes Gorillakind'. In *Mit dem Herzen einer Gazelle und der Haut eines Nilpferds: Albert Schweitzer in seinen letzten Lebensjahren und die Entwicklung seines Spitals bis zur Gegenwart*, edited by Jo Munz and Walter Munz, 61–64. Frauenfeld: Huber, 2005.

Smithson, Michael J. 'Social Theories of Ignorance'. In *Agnotology: The Making and Unmaking of Ignorance*, edited by Robert N. Proctor and Londa Schiebinger, 209–29. Stanford: Stanford University Press, 2008.

Sorg, Jean-Paul, ed. *Schweitzer, le médecin*. Strasbourg: Editions Oberlin, 1995.

Spangenberg, Izak JJ, and Christina Landman, eds. *The Legacies of Albert Schweitzer Reconsidered*. Cape Town: Aosis Scholarly Books, 2017.

Spivak, Gayatri Chakravorty. 'Can the Subaltern Speak?' In *Marxism and the Interpretation of Culture*, edited by Lawrence Grossberg and Cary Nelson, 271–313. Urbana, Chicago: University of Illinois Press, 1988.

Staewen, Christian. 'Les malades mentaux de l'hôpital de Lambaréné'. In *Schweitzer, le médecin*, edited by Jean-Paul Sorg, 87–91. Strasbourg, 1995.

Staewen, Christian. *Kulturelle und psychologische Bedingungen der Zusammenarbeit mit Afrikanern: Ansatzpunkte für eine komplementäre Partnerschaft*. München: Weltforum Verlag, 1991.

Stanton, Jennifer. 'Introduction'. In *Innovations in Health and Medicine: Diffusion and Resistance in the Twentieth Century*, edited by Jennifer Stanton, 1–18. London: Routledge, 2002.

Stark-Bernhard, Margrit. 'Waschfrauen, Büglerinnen, Schneider und Matratzenmacher, Zimmerdienst, Wildfleisch-Einkauf, Hühner und Trinkwasser'. In *Mit dem Herzen einer Gazelle und der Haut eines Nilpferds: Albert Schweitzer in seinen letzten Lebensjahren und die Entwicklung seines Spitals bis zur Gegenwart*, edited by Jo Munz and Walter Munz, 25–28. Frauenfeld: Huber, 2005.

Stevens, Rosemary. *In Sickness and in Wealth: American Hospitals in the Twentieth Century*. Baltimore: Johns Hopkins University Press, 1999.

Stoler, Ann Laura. *Along the Archival Grain: Epistemic Anxieties and Colonial Common Sense*. Princeton: Princeton University Press, 2009.

Stoler, Ann Laura, and Frederick Cooper. 'Between Metropole and Colony: Rethinking a Research Agenda'. In *Tensions of Empire: Colonial Cultures in a Bourgeois World*, edited by Frederick Cooper and Ann Laura Stoler. Berkeley: University of California Press, 1997.

Studer, Nina Salouâ. *The Hidden Patients: North African Women in French Colonial Psychiatry*. Zürcher Beiträge Zur Geschichtswissenschaft, Band 8. Köln Weimar Wien: Böhlau Verlag, 2016.

Summers, Carol. 'Intimate Colonialism: The Imperial Production of Reproduction in Uganda, 1907–1925'. *Signs* 16, no. 4 (1991): 787–807.

Swiderski, Ŝtanislaw. 'L'Ombwiri société d'initiation et de guérison au Gabon'. *Religioni e Civiltà* 1 (1972): 125–204.

Taap, Erika. *Lambarener Tagebuch*. Berlin: Evangelische Verlagsanstalt, 1970.

Taithe, Bertrand, and Katherine Davis. '"Heroes of Charity?" Between Memory and Hagiography: Colonial Medical Heroes in the Era of Decolonisation'. *The Journal of Imperial and Commonwealth History* 42, no. 5 (2014): 912–935.

Tappan, Jennifer. *The Riddle of Malnutrition : The Long Arc of Biomedical and Public Health Interventions in Uganda*. Athens, Ohio: Ohio University Press, 2017.

Tessmann, Günter. *Die Pangwe: völkerkundliche Monographie eines westafrikanischen Negerstammes Ergebnisse der Lübecker Pangwe-Expedition 1907–1909 und früherer Forschungen 1904–1907*. Vol. 2. Berlin: Ernst Wassmuth, 1913.

Tezi, Rodrigue. 'Une approche socio-historique de l'avènement de la pédiatrie au Gabon par la médecien coloniale au XIXe siècle'. In *Colonisation et colonisés au Gabon*, edited by Fabrice Nguiabama-Makaya, 111–26. Paris: L'Harmattan, 2007.

Thate, Michael J. 'An Anachronism in the African Jungle? Reassessing Albert Schweitzer's African Legacy'. In *Albert Schweitzer in Thought and Action: A Life in Parts*, edited by James Carleton Paget and Michael J. Thate, 295–318. New York: Syracuse University Press, 2016.

Thomas, Lynn M. *Politics of the Womb: Women, Reproduction, and the State in Kenya*. Berkeley: University of California Press, 2003.

Tilley, Helen. *Africa as a Living Laboratory: Empire, Development, and the Problem of Scientific Knowledge, 1870–1950*. Chicago: University of Chicago Press, 2011.

Tonda, Joseph. 'Capital sorcier et travail de Dieu'. *Politique Africaine* 3, no. 79 (2000): 48–65.

Tonda, Joseph. *La guérison divine en Afrique centrale (Congo, Gabon)*. Paris: Éditions Karthala, 2002.

Trensz, Frédéric. 'Le médecin'. In *Rayonnement d'Albert Schweitzer: 34 études et 100 témoignage*, edited by Robert Minder, 208–16. Collection 'Richesses de l'Alsace'. Colmar: Ed. Alsatia, 1975.

Trilles, Henri. 'Les rites de la naissance chez les Fang'. *Bulletin de la Société Neuchateloise de Géographie* 20 (1910 1909): 403–11.

Tröhler, Ulrich. 'Surgery (Modern)'. In *Medicine in the Twentieth Century*, edited by Roger Cooter and John Pickstone, 984–1028. Amsterdam: Harwood Academic Publishers, 2000.

Turrittin, Jane. 'Colonial Midwives and Modernizing Childbirth in French West Africa'. In *Women in African Colonial Histories*, edited by Jean Marie Allman, Susan Geiger, and Nakanyike Musisi, 71–91. Bloomington: Indiana University Press, 2002.

Turshen, Meredeth. 'Reproducing Labor: Colonial Government Regulation of African Women's Reproductive Lives'. In *The Demographics of Empire: The Colonial Order and the Creation of Knowledge*, edited by Karl Ittmann, 217–44. Athens: Ohio University Press, 2010.

Van Der Geest, Sjaak, and Kaja Finkler. 'Hospital Ethnography: Introduction'. *Social Science & Medicine* 59, no. 10 (2004): 1995–2001.

Van Laak, Dirk. 'Kolonien als "Laboratorien der Moderne"?' In *Das Kaiserreich transnational: Deutschland in der Welt 1871–1914*, edited by Sebastian Conrad and Jürgen Osterhammel, 257–79. Göttingen: Vandenhoeck & Ruprecht, 2004.

Van Tol, Deanne. 'Mothers, Babies, and the Colonial State: The Introduction of Maternal and Infant Welfare Services in Nigeria, 1925–1945'. *Spontaneous Generations: A Journal for the History and Philosophy of Science* 1, no. 1 (2007): 110–31.

Vansina, Jan. *Paths in the Rainforests: Toward a History of Political Tradition in Equatorial Africa*. Madison: The University of Wisconsin Press, 1990.

Vaughan, Megan. *Curing Their Ills: Colonial Power and African Illness*. Cambridge: Polity Press, 1991.

Vaughan, Megan. 'Healing and Curing: Issues in the Social History and Anthropology of Medicine in Africa'. *Social History of Medicine* 7, no. 2 (1994): 283–295.

Vaughan, Megan. 'Introduction'. In *Psychiatry and Empire*, edited by Sloan Mahone and Megan Vaughan, 1–16. London: Palgrave Macmillan, 2007.

Vogeler, Karl. *Chirurgie der Hernien*. Berlin: W. de Gruyter, 1951.

Vongsathorn, Kathleen. '"First and Foremost the Evangelist"? Mission and Government Priorities for the Treatment of Leprosy in Uganda, 1927–48'. *Journal of Eastern African Studies* 6, no. 3 (2012): 544–560.

Wall, Barbra Mann. *Into Africa: A Transnational History of Catholic Medical Missions and Social Change*. New Brunswick: Rutgers University Press, 2015.

Warner, John Harley. 'The Uses of Patient Records by Historians: Patterns, Possibilities and Perplexities'. *Health and History*, 1999, 101–111.

Watts, Sheldon J. *Epidemics and History: Disease, Power and Imperialism*. New Haven: Yale University Press, 1999.

Webb Jr, James L.A., and Tamara Giles-Vernick. 'Introduction'. In *Global Health in Africa: Historical Perspectives on Disease Control*, edited by Tamara Giles-Vernick and James L.A. Webb Jr. Athens, Ohio: Ohio University Press, 2013.

Weinstein, Brian G. *Gabon : Nation-Building on the Ogooué*. Cambridge London: M.I.T. Press, 1966.

Wendland, Claire L. *A Heart for the Work : Journeys through an African Medical School*. Chicago: The University of Chicago Press, 2010.

White, Luise. *Speaking with Vampires: Rumor and History in Colonial Africa*. Berkeley: University of California Press, 2000.

Widmer, Alexandra, and Veronika Lipphardt, eds. *Health and Difference: Rendering Human Variation in Colonial Engagements*. New York: Berghahn Books, 2016.

Wilde, Sally. 'The Elephants in the Doctor-Patient Relationship: Patients' Clinical Inter-actions and the Changing Surgical Landscape of the 1890s'. *Health and History*, 2007, 2–27.

Wilde, Sally, and Geoffrey Hirst. 'Learning from Mistakes: Early Twentieth-Century Surgical Practice'. *Journal of the History of Medicine and Allied Sciences* 64, no. 1 (2009): 38–77.

Woodbury, Michael A., Elizabeth S. Palacios, Richard Friedman, and William Thomas. 'Psychiatric Care at the Albert Schweitzer Hospital'. *Psychiatric Services* 16, no. 5 (1965): 145–150.

Worboys, Michael. 'The Colonial World as Mission and Mandate: Leprosy and Empire, 1900–1940'. In *Nature and Empire: Science and the Colonial Enterprise*, edited by Roy MacLeod, 207–18. Chicago: University of Chicago Press, 2000.

Woytt-Secretan, Marie. *Albert Schweitzer baut Lambarene*. Königstein im Taunus: Langewiesche, 1957.

Woytt-Secretan, Marie. 'Souvenirs d'une infirmière'. In *Rayonnement d'Albert Schweitzer: 34 études et 100 témoignage*, edited by Robert Minder, 228–40. Colmar: Ed. Alsatia, 1975.

Wylie, Diana. 'The Ignorance of Mothers and the Health of Children in 20th Century Pondoland'. In *Collected Seminar Papers. Institute of Commonwealth Studies*, 42:104–118, 1992.

Zeller, Christian. *Globalisierungsstrategien – Der Weg von Novartis*. Berlin: Springer, 2001.

Zellweger, Hans. 'Grosskampftag im Spital'. In *Wir halfen dem Doktor in Lambarene: Festgabe zum 85. Geburtstag von Albert Schweitzer*, edited by Olga Fausel-Wieber, Ilse Schnabel, and Gertrud Koch, 84–99. Zürich: Schweizer Druck- und Verlagshaus, 1960.

Zumthurm, Tizian. 'The Colonial Situation in Practice: Food at the Albert Schweitzer Hospital, Lambaréné 1924–65'. *The International Journal of African Historical Studies* 53, no. 1 (2020): 47–69.

Index

Printed in the United States
By Bookmasters